PAIN MANAGEMENT IN SMALL ANIMALS

For Elsevier:

Commissioning Editor: Mary Seager
Development Editor: Rebecca Nelemans
Project Manager: Joannah Duncan
Designer: Andy Chapman
Illustration Manager: Bruce Hogarth
Illustrator: David Graham

PAIN MANAGEMENT IN SMALL ANIMALS

Debbie Grant MA VetMB MRCVS

Veterinary Adviser, Pfizer Animal Health, UK

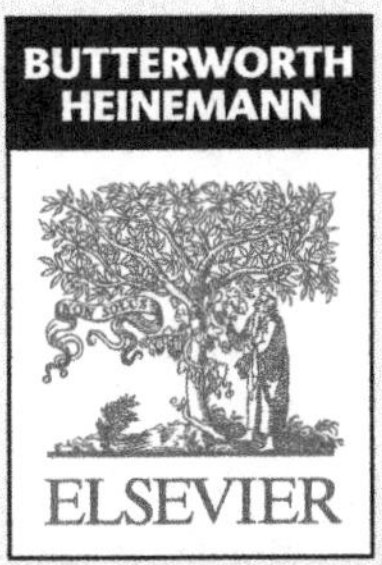

Edinburgh London New York Oxford Philadelphia St Louis Sydney Toronto 2006

BUTTERWORTH
HEINEMANN
ELSEVIER

First published 2006

ISBN 0 7506 8812 2

British Library Cataloging in Publication Data
A catalogue record for this book is available from the British Library

Library of Congress Cataloging in Publication Data
A catalog record for this book is available from the Library of Congress

Knowledge and best practice in this field are constantly changing. As new research and experience broaden our knowledge, changes in practice, treatment and drug therapy may become necessary or appropriate. Readers are advised to check the most current information provided (i) on procedures featured or (ii) by the manufacturer of each product to be administered, to verify the recommended dose or formula, the method and duration of administration, and contraindications. It is the responsibility of the practitioner, relying on their own experience and knowledge of the patient, to make diagnoses, to determine dosages and the best treatment for each individual patient, and to take all appropriate safety precautions. To the fullest extent of the law, neither the publisher nor the author assumes any liability for any injury and/or damage.

The Publisher

The publisher's policy is to use **paper manufactured from sustainable forests**

Printed in China

Contents

Preface

It's taken a good 2000 years or so for humans to readily accept that other animals can experience pain in a similar way to us. This is despite it being a very reasonable premise to make, considering that non-humans possess comparable equipment for the detection and processing of painful stimuli. Even now, in a time when procedures as complex as organ transplantation are on the agenda for veterinary patients, there are still many misconceptions about the presence, recognition and treatment of pain in animals and more than a whiff of reluctance for many clinicians to make pain management a priority. Surely the whole point of the medical profession is to relieve pain and suffering and restore normal body function wherever possible, and in doing so, to maximise a patient's quality of life (maximising life expectancy is often an additional goal particularly in human patients). There can be a tendency for clinicians to focus too much attention on restoring function and unfortunately the management of pain becomes a secondary consideration. Emotive though it seems, putting oneself in the shoes or paws of the patient is not a bad idea to try and realign the goal of treatment to what really matters to the animal: to be free from pain and able to do the things that result in a good quality of life. Making these objectives of paramount importance requires empathy, once defined very well in the following scenario: a man falls down a hole, another person, somebody with sympathy walks past, looks down the hole and says 'oh, how awful for you being stuck in a hole, that's truly terrible' and then walks on. A third person, somebody with empathy, walks up, looks down the hole and says 'oh, how awful for you' then trots off and returns with a pulley, rope and hopefully more than a passing interest in basic load-bearing mechanics.

This book aims to provide veterinary nurses, vets, and vet students with a detailed review of all the available evidence demonstrating that veterinary patients do feel pain and that there are significant detrimental consequences of leaving clinical pain unrelieved. The diagnosis and the assessment of pain are also discussed to enable the reader to recognise and potentially score pain in patients in a practice situation, (analogous to spotting the patients that are down a hole and judging how deep it is). There is a comprehensive explanation of the anatomy and physiology of the pain pathway and all of the available analgesic drugs to provide an understanding of the nature of different types of pain likely to be experienced by patients and how best to alleviate it. This, in turn enables the reader to not only take a rational approach to the provision of analgesia but also to prevent or minimise the development of pain in the first place. The principles of effective pain management are explained to allow practitioners to take an individual approach to each patient in the clinical setting, both for acute or surgical cases and for chronic pain.

In the past few years the treatment and prevention of acute pain associated with surgery has vastly improved in general practice, most cases now routinely receive pre- and postoperative analgesia. Treatment of chronic pain is probably still well below par, mainly due to a lack of recognition of its presence. Unconventional or adjunctive therapies can play an important role in the alleviation of chronic pain and the maximisation of quality of life. Inevitably a lot of information is drawn from the human field where patients can verbalise how the pain makes them feel and the value of therapies. This information can provide valuable insight into the potential usefulness of adjunctive therapies in veterinary patients, the benefit of which may not always be proven, but then again a lack of benefit can't be proven either. Hopefully, the reader will be left with a sense of much greater understanding of their patients' pain and put into practice optimal pain management protocols on an every case basis, i.e. return to the patient in the hole armed with an array of lifting gear, several back-up plans, and an enthusiasm to fill in all the holes they come across in the future.

Debbie Grant, UK 2006

Acknowledgements

Huge thanks to Malcolm McKee for all the photos, references and most of all his kind words of encouragement.

Disclaimer

The views expressed in this book are the views of the author and do not necessarily reflect the views of Pfizer Ltd, who make no representation concerning and do not guarantee or accept responsibility or legal liability for the content, accuracy, completeness, applicability or reliability of the text.

CHAPTER 1 CONCEPTS OF PAIN MANAGEMENT IN ANIMALS

CAN ANIMALS EXPERIENCE PAIN?

There are three components of the overall pain experience. Firstly there is activation of receptors in the body that specifically detect stimuli that could potentially damage tissue. These harmful stimuli are called 'noxious' stimuli such as heat, pressure or chemicals. Once activated the receptors send signals, via nerve fibres, up to the spinal cord and lower parts of the brain. This process is termed 'nociception' and the receptors involved are called 'nociceptors'. The second component is the processing or interpretation of these incoming signals by higher parts of the brain, in the cerebral cortex, which leads to an awareness and appreciation of the unpleasant experience by the animal or human. The third component to the painful experience is changes in behaviour in response to pain.

When comparing the components of a painful experience in animals and humans it has been established that all animals and humans have virtually identical nociceptors and nerve fibres connecting to the spinal cord and brain. The second part, the conscious perception of pain, is an emotional experience that humans are capable of describing verbally but that cannot be directly measured in animals. What can be measured in animals (and humans) are changes in behaviour in response to pain, the third component. These changes can be complex, subtle and very variable between different species and individuals. There are also some characteristic simple reflexes, involuntary responses to the detection of noxious stimuli such as increases in heart rate, blood pressure and stress hormone levels that are measurable and show similar patterns in animals and humans.

It is now widely accepted that animals do experience pain in a similar way to humans and that it can result in suffering. Animals, through domestication, are dependant on humans for their welfare and so we have a moral and ethical obligation to avoid and alleviate pain in animals wherever possible. These current views are based on our knowledge of the anatomy and physiology of the pain pathway, and have been shaped by modern attitudes towards animals and their changing role in our society.

HISTORY AND PHILOSOPHY OF PAIN IN ANIMALS

It is only in recent years that animal pain has become an important topic within the profession and society as a whole. Historically the general attitude towards animals was that they were merely automatons, equivalent to machines, unable to reason, soulless, and therefore incapable of perceiving pain. The most famous advocate of this thinking was the French philosopher René Descartes (1596–1650) who said 'the greatest of all the prejudices we have retained from our infancy is believing that beasts think'. The first significant challenge to Descartes came from an English philosopher Jeremy Bentham (1748–1832) who said 'the question is not can they reason? Can they talk? But can they suffer?' Things started to improve with the passing of the first animal cruelty laws in England in 1821, and the establishment of the forerunner of the RSPCA in 1824. However, none of these moves addressed the majority of animal suffering that is not a result of deliberate cruelty.

With the publication of Charles Darwin's *Origin of the Species* in 1859, and much later the work of scientists and philosophers such as Jane Goodall (*In the Shadow of Man*), Dianne Fossey (*Gorillas in the Mist*), and Dr Bernard E. Rollin, society became much more aware of the common ancestry and similarities between humans and animals. This contributed to a realisation that animals may well experience pain and suffering in a similar way to humans and has helped elevate their moral and legal status.

Over the past few decades there has also been a big change in the role of animals within society.[1,2] Western society has become increasingly concentrated in towns and cities rather than rural areas. A very small percentage of the population is now directly involved with farming. If you ask somebody

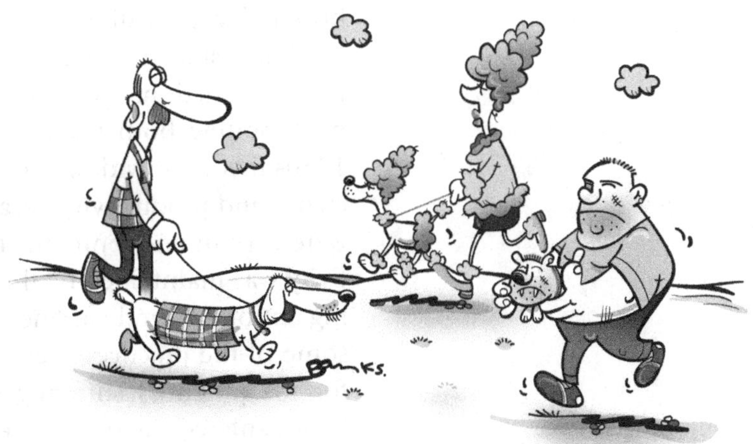

Figure 1.1
Owners and their pets.

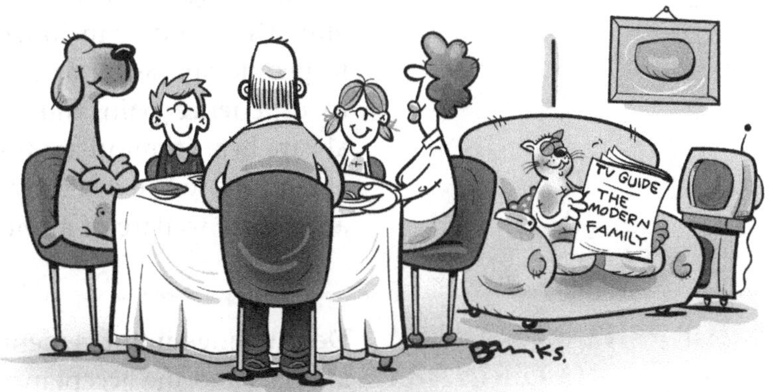

Figure 1.2
The modern family.

today what their experience of animals has been, they will almost inevitably think of a companion animal such as a pet dog or cat that is considered a family member. Before the Second World War the answer would have been a cow or sheep used for food production (and not normally allowed on the sofa!). With increasing prosperity in the West and the decline of extended families, pets have become much more important as a source of companionship. As people have developed strong emotional bonds with their pets they have also become much more concerned for the pets' wellbeing, particularly the prevention and treatment of any pain they may experience.

There have also been big changes in agricultural practices giving rise to a new concern for production animal welfare. Before 1950, successful animal farming was based on good husbandry, providing the optimal environment (e.g. ample food and shelter) for the animals, which in turn optimised their production. This was a rather nicely balanced arrangement suiting both the farmers and their stock. During the 1950s there was widespread industrialisation of farming, efficiency and productivity became paramount, and the animals were kept in environments that were far from ideal. Productivity was maintained by the use of new technologies including antibiotics and vaccines. As public awareness grew about some of the practices, e.g. battery farming, so did a concern for the potential suffering of the animals. Animal welfare issues entered the public arena at a seemingly receptive time when other moral battles were being won, such as equal rights for women and ethnic minorities.

This brings us to today's position on animal ethics, that animals should be included in the moral principles we apply to people and as far as possible we must not allow animals to experience pain and suffering. A useful summary[3,11] to always bear in mind are the so-called five freedoms (see Box 1.1) proposed in 1965 by The Brambell Committee on the acceptable welfare of animals.

CURRENT ATTITUDES IN THE VETERINARY PROFESSION

Despite huge improvements in our general attitude towards animals and the acceptance that they can experience pain in a similar way to humans, the use of analgesics (drugs that relieve pain) by the veterinary profession is still less than ideal. A survey[4,5] in 1996 of 2000 primarily companion animal vets practising in the UK assessed the vets' attitudes towards the provision of perioperative analgesia in cats, dogs and small mammals for a variety of surgical procedures. When asked about surgery in dogs, 97% of vets gave analgesia for major orthopaedic procedures, but only 53% and 32%

Box 1.1 **The five freedoms of acceptable animal welfare**

- Freedom from hunger
- Freedom from physical and thermal discomfort
- Freedom from pain, injury and disease
- Freedom to express normal behaviour
- Freedom from fear and distress

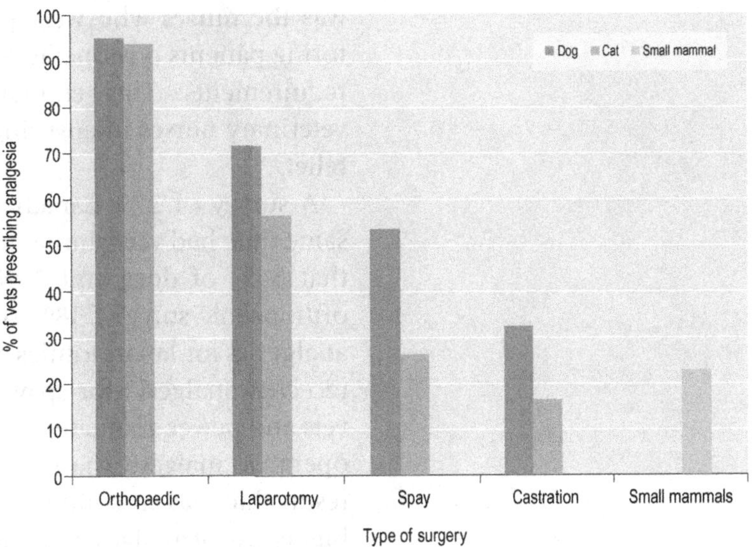

Figure 1.3
Percentage of vets prescribing perioperative analgesia for a variety of surgical procedures in cats and dogs and for any type of surgery in small mammals.[4,5]

gave analgesia for routine ovariohysterectomies (spays) and castrations respectively. The figures for cats were even worse: whilst 94% of vets gave analgesia for orthopaedic surgery, only 26% and 16% gave analgesia for cat spays and castrations (Fig 1.3). The survey also found that 84% of vets gave analgesia for aural surgery in dogs, 72% for ruptured diaphragm repair in cats and 39% for dental surgery in cats. When it came to small mammals such as rabbits, guinea-pigs, ferrets and hamsters, although 93% of respondents performed surgery on them, only 22% routinely administered analgesics.

Interestingly (but maybe not too surprisingly!) the survey also revealed that female vets and newer graduates were more likely to provide analgesics than male vets and older graduates. Respondents were also asked to rank each surgical procedure in terms of the level of pain that they considered would be experienced by the cat or dog undergoing the surgery. A scale of 1 to 10 was used, where 1 represented no pain at all, and 10 represented the worst possible pain. Female vets and newer graduates gave higher scores for each of the procedures. Rather predictably the greatest difference between scores from female and male vets in dogs was for spays (which could reflect a slight lack of empathy on the part of the male vets) and the smallest difference was for castrations (which may reflect a sudden rush of empathy from the male vets). In the majority of practices returning surveys it was the nurses who were principally responsible for monitoring patients postoperatively for signs of pain and analgesic requirements. This emphasises the great importance of veterinary nurses in ensuring the adequate provision of pain relief.

A survey of 275 Canadian vets[6,7] undertaken around the same time had very similar findings to the UK survey. It found that 84% of dogs and 70% of cats received analgesics for orthopaedic surgery, 38% of dogs and 44% of cats received analgesics for laparotomies and 13% of dogs and 17% of cats received analgesia for spays. As with the UK survey, female vets and newer graduates assigned greater importance to perioperative analgesia than their older male colleagues. The only result that was in contrast to the UK survey was the slightly higher use of analgesics in cats than dogs for non-orthopaedic surgery.

Over the past 5 years there has been a significant increase in the awareness of pain management within the profession. Pain management has become a common CPD topic (continuing professional development, i.e. further education for qualified vets who must now participate in at least 35 hours a year). Recently published textbooks, papers and articles all have a greater focus on pain management. It would therefore be reasonable to say that the figures given in the UK and Canadian surveys would be higher today. However there are still some modern misconceptions that contribute to the continuing under-use of analgesics in practice and these are often compounded by several practicalities concerning the recognition of pain and the use of analgesic drugs.

MODERN MISCONCEPTIONS

The following myths remain a barrier to progress in pain management in practice even today.

Myth 1 – Animals don't feel pain or feel less than humans

Animals and humans have almost identical neurological pathways for the detection and processing of painful stimuli. Therefore it is very likely that stimuli causing pain in humans will also cause a similar degree of pain in animals.

Another argument put forward to support this myth is that part of the whole unpleasant experience of pain in people is made up of the fear, anticipation and dread of what may happen. For example, visiting the dentist can be particularly awful for a person who has previously had a very painful extraction or filling. Once they are in the chair there will be the anticipation and dread of a great deal of pain to come. All these emotions may heighten any pain they are then subject to. Similarly for a person who has previously suffered a heart attack, a pain coming from the left arm may be intensified by the fear that it could actually be life threatening.

Part of the myth that animal pain is in some way less then human pain is the false argument that animals just live in the present, their current experiences not influenced by memories or emotions from previous suffering. There is very little evidence to support this argument. The sight of a trembling dog being extricated from under a chair, slid across the waiting room floor and reversed into a vet's consulting room is not uncommon. This behaviour strongly suggests that a previously painful or unpleasant experience at the vet has given rise to fear and anxiety in anticipation of the next visit. It's also likely that this dog will be particularly reactive to any painful stimuli (e.g. an injection) once pinned onto the vet's table, as if in a state of heightened pain perception. Anecdotally, some practices have noticed they have fewer of these reluctant attendees dragged in after the introduction of perioperative analgesia for all routine neutering and surgical procedures. It should also be realised that animals do not have the benefit of the knowledge their pain will be over in a certain time, or that help is on its way, or the final outcome will be better than before the pain started. Part of the human coping mechanism for pain is hope, understanding and a control over their destiny, something that is unavailable to animals.

Myth 2 – Pain can be beneficial for healing/recovery

The recent British survey[4] of vets' attitudes found that 30% of respondents agreed with the statement 'a degree of pain is required to stop the animal being too active post surgery', which is effectively advocating pain as a form of restraint. This myth probably originates from the concept that pain evolved to have a protective function. When an animal is injured the presence of pain prevents the animal using the affected body part and so helps prevent further tissue

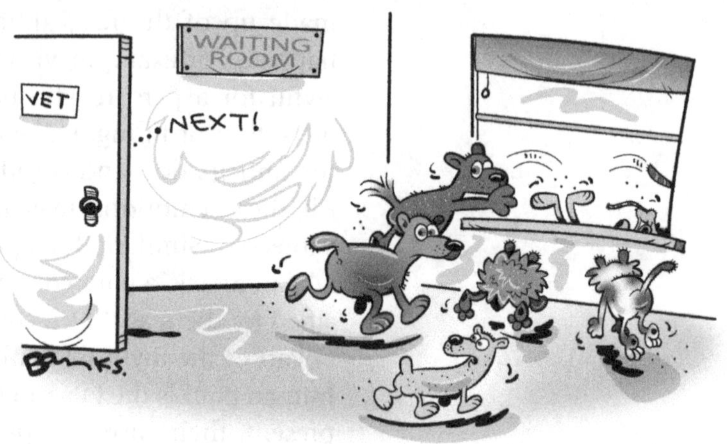

Figure 1.4
'Next please!'

damage. However, it is important to realise that in the clinical situation, where we are taking responsibility for the care of patients and performing surgery on animals, removing the protective role of pain will not have any disadvantages. Contrary to this, it has been demonstrated that there are significant detrimental consequences of leaving animals in clinically unrelieved pain such as a slower recovery time, delayed wound healing and increased risk of sepsis (see Chapter 2). In almost all circumstances the benefits of relieving pain will far outweigh any of pain's apparently protective function. It's also worth noting that analgesic drugs rarely relieve all pain sensations, so excessive use of an injured body part by the animal will still give rise to some pain signals alerting the animal to restrict movement or use of the area. Rather than using pain as a form of restraint postoperatively, additional measures such as bandages, splints and confinement should be used alongside analgesic drugs. Figure 1.5 shows the use of supportive dressings after orthopaedic surgery to help protect the repair whilst the patient is provided with ample analgesia to help recovery.

In some cases, particularly if the patient is anxious or distressed, sedation may be indicated. Adequate analgesia (and support) after orthopaedic surgery will allow a return to normal function and mobility as early as possible, which is after all a primary objective. A specific concern that sometimes crops up is the misconception that animals are more likely to damage sutures or surgical sites if they are 'too comfortable'. Actually, the converse of this is true. Animals in pain

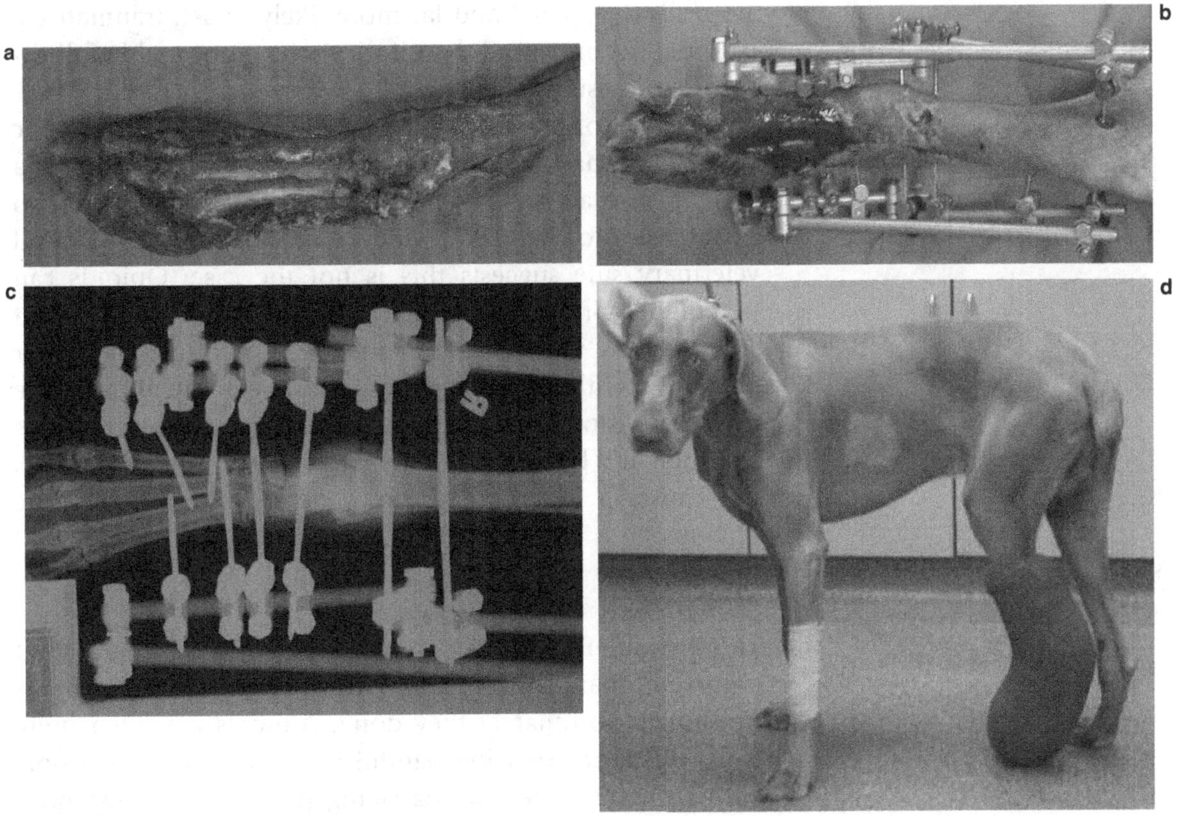

Figure 1.5
(a)–(d) This shear injury was repaired using an external fixator and the repair protected by a dressing.

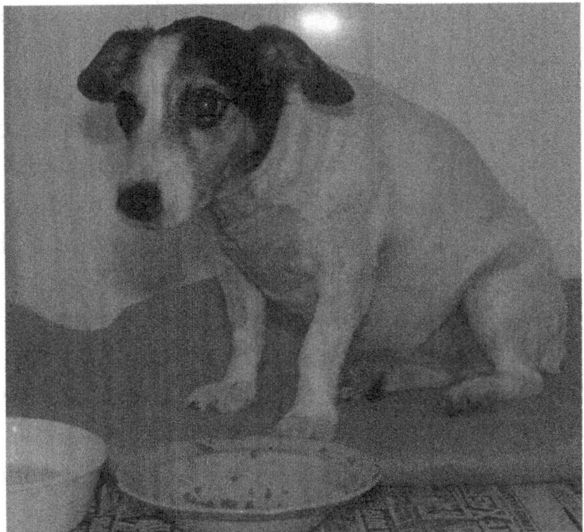

Figure 1.6
Cage rest can be used in spinal cases and analgesia should not be withheld.

are restless, agitated and far more likely to self-traumatise a painful area or wound than if they were comfortable following the provision of analgesia.

Another common concern is that the use of analgesic drugs may mask physiological signs of deterioration in a patient, such as increases in heart and respiratory rate due to hypotension or hypoxia. Evidence on both the human and veterinary side suggests this is not the case. Opioids can potentially produce a bradycardia (slow heart rate), but studies show that when patients are treated adequately for pain, even with large doses of opioids, heart rate in response to hypotension, hypoxia, hypovolaemia or hypercapnia is still high and because the clinician is able to rule out pain as the cause, a deterioration in patient condition is more obvious.

Myth 3 – Animals tolerate pain better than people

This misunderstanding is a result of people's expectation that animals in pain should behave in the same way as humans in pain; unfortunately they don't. Animals are often quite stoic when experiencing painful conditions and so people wrongly assume they are 'managing quite nicely' or just indifferent to the discomfort. This is not a reflection of a tolerance to pain but that animals are designed to hide pain, and may communicate pain in ways that people fail to recognise. The presence of other species, owners, vets, and a strange environment are all factors that can mask an animal's responses to pain (see Chapter 2).

There is also huge variation in pain expression between different species. Prey animals are particularly highly motivated not to show signs of pain as this would alert predators. It's a mistake to wait for a patient to show overt signs of pain like vocalisation before doing anything about it, because by then it's probably already in severe pain. Due to our inability to accurately detect signs of pain in animals we should give them the benefit of the doubt. If an animal is in a situation where a human would be in pain then assume the animal will also be in pain and go ahead with the administration of analgesics. We should not demand 'proof' of pain but instead should demand proof for denying pain relief. Sadly, vets are far more likely to administer antibiotics without evidence of

Box 1.2 Modern *mis*conceptions about pain in animals

- Animals don't feel pain, or feel less than humans
- Pain is beneficial for rest and recovery
- Animals tolerate pain better than humans

infection than they are to administer analgesics without evidence the animal is in pain.[8]

Examples of animals apparently ignoring terrible injuries, and carrying on as if nothing has happened are sometimes used to support the view that they can tolerate pain better than humans or not feel pain. A cat hit by a car may run off immediately afterwards but on later examination be found to be surprisingly squashed and have a fractured pelvis. A dog caught up in a fight with another dog can sustain widespread soft tissue injuries and yet not stop fighting until forcibly separated. This apparent lack of pain in the face of abrupt injury is also well documented in humans. Several studies[9] have been conducted looking at soldiers wounded in combat and people attending accident and emergency departments. A significant proportion of the patients reported that they did not feel any pain at the time of the original injury. This freedom from pain was localised only to the wound, as the patients still complained of any subsequent pain elsewhere such as an intravenous needle being inserted. The studies found that all the victims were eventually in pain within a few hours, certainly by 24 hours. So it seems that both humans and animals may ignore an injury in its early stages. They continue with activities having a higher priority than care of the wound – escaping, defending themselves or finding a safer environment for recovery. The onset of pain maybe delayed but is not absent.

PRACTICAL ISSUES

There are some practicalities regarding pain management that have compounded the under-use of analgesics.

Lack of education

Until literally the past few years there has been a complete lack of emphasis on pain management in veterinary education and textbooks. In the 1996 UK survey of 2000 vets[5] 75% considered that their own knowledge of pain recognition and treatment in animals was inadequate and had been gained mainly through experience in practice rather than as students. Traditionally the primary or sole reason for anaesthetising an animal was just to provide restraint. Even as late as 1973 the first textbook of veterinary anaesthesia published in the USA by Lumb and Jones did not list the control of pain as a reason for using anaesthesia. Vets who qualified in the 1960s would have been taught to carry out surgical procedures using sedatives or paralytic drugs alone, which would not block the pain pathway in any way. There was no dedicated textbook published on pain management in the UK until 2000. This background in education goes some way to explaining why on the whole older graduates have less empathy with animal pain and regard its treatment as a lower priority than most newer graduates.

Limited availability of analgesic drugs

The two classes of analgesics most commonly used for perioperative analgesia are the opioids and non-steroidal anti-inflammatory drugs (NSAIDs). Pethidine, a pure opioid agonist was licensed in 1983, but prior to this there were few if any analgesics available for veterinary use. Currently many of the most potent opioid analgesics such as morphine and fentanyl are still not licensed for veterinary use. Buprenorphine (Vetergesic®), a partial opioid agonist, is now widely used in practices as part of perioperative analgesic protocols but did not have a veterinary license until 1996. In the past 5–7 years the introduction of newer and safer NSAIDs onto the market specifically licensed for preoperative administration has helped transform the management of surgical pain in the UK. Carprofen (Rimadyl®) was licensed pre-op in dogs in 1993 and for cats in 1996. Meloxicam (Metacam®) gained a license claim for pre-op use in dogs in 2000 and then for cats in 2002. Before any of these drugs were on the market, vets were left with a very poor choice of analgesics for use around the time of surgery and for long-term pain control. Even if vets did resort to unlicensed drugs there was very little information available on the effective dosages and durations of analgesics in non-human species. Lack of availability of analgesic drugs is no longer a valid excuse for not providing pain relief. In the 1996 UK survey[4] over 90% of vets had at least one opioid and at least one NSAID available within their practice.

Controlled drugs

Controlled drugs include some of the most potent analgesics, such as morphine. The problem is that controlled drugs require strict record keeping and safe storage, which tends to put busy vets off using them. Controlled drugs (CD) are divided into five schedules by the Misuse of Drugs Act 1971 and the Misuse of Drugs Regulations 1985, according to the degree to which they cause addiction in people or have the potential for abuse (see Chapter 6 Appendix). Practices are understandably reluctant to keep large quantities of controlled drugs on the premises in case it increases the chance of break-ins. Some CDs commonly used for analgesia are:

- Schedule 2 – morphine, pethidine, papaveretum, fentanyl. All purchases and every dose used must be recorded within 24 hours and registers kept for 2 years. The drugs must be stored in a locked secure cabinet. Unused drugs can only be destroyed in the presence of a person authorised by the Secretary of State.
- Schedule 3 – buprenorphine. Invoices from purchases must be kept for 2 years and the drugs must be kept in a secure locked cabinet.

Having the option to use controlled drugs is essential, especially in cases of severe pain. The benefits to the patients far outweigh the extra hassle they create for the practice.

Side effects

All drugs have the potential for side effects. The risk of side effects must be assessed and evaluated against the potential benefits to the patient on an individual case basis. It's fair to say that there is an underlying principle in the profession that above all we must not make matters worse for the patient. This is reinforced by a more recent fear of litigation if we are seen to apparently do the wrong thing for the patient. What may then happen is that vets develop a disproportionate fear of drug side effects and withhold analgesics despite their benefit far outweighing any risk. Traditionally, morphine was not given to cats because it was thought to cause 'morphine mania', a state of excitation. In reality this is only seen at doses approximately 20 times higher than those needed for analgesia. Morphine and other opioids can be given to cats and are very effective analgesics at the right dose.

Opioids are sometimes withheld because of concern over another potential side effect, respiratory depression. However, primates are far more susceptible to this effect than cats and dogs. Reports of significant respiratory depression are very rare and are associated with doses well above those used clinically. Opioid administration after thorocotomy (or laparotomy) may well improve ventilation rather than impair it, due to the pain relief allowing the patient to breathe more easily. There has always been concern over the potential side effects of NSAIDs, particularly an increased risk of renal failure if the animal sustains a drop in blood pressure. The marketing of newer NSAIDs with improved safety profiles has provided the profession with drugs with lower risks of side effects, allowing more widespread use. The risk of side effects can be minimised by the appropriate choice of drugs, supportive therapy (e.g. intravenous fluids), dose adjustment, etc., and more often than not be outweighed by the benefits of alleviating pain.

Cost of analgesics

Practices often try to keep costs to the owner down, whether due to local competition with neighbouring practices or a perceived pressure from the client base. There can be a reluctance to increase the cost of surgical procedures to incorporate preop and postop analgesia, even though the client has never actually been consulted as to whether they mind or not. Everyone in the profession is guilty of 'x-raying clients' pockets' at some time or other, beautifully illustrated by the story of a premier league footballer who took his dog to the local practice, with a suspect ruptured cruciate. The footballer, wearing his carefully ripped designer jeans and limited edition hand crafted t-shirt created by an Italian couture genius, was politely asked by the receptionist (who wasn't a great follower of the celebrity lifestyle weeklies) if he'd like to take advantage of their monthly instalments payment option for the more financially challenged client. The footballer declined, his weekly salary exceeding the entire annual practice turnover by a few noughts.

It's important to make clients aware of what the cost of a procedure includes. Once an owner understands that a price difference is due to the addition of analgesics and the benefits of pain relief are explained, very few people would then quibble about parting with a few more pounds. The vast majority of owners are more than willing to pay for pain relief for their pets, and often won't tolerate anything less than 'doing the very best' for their pet.

Lack of recognition of pain

As touched on earlier, an inability to recognise pain inevitably leads to its under-diagnosis and a failure to treat. Ideally, the presence and degree of pain should always be assessed on an individual case basis along with that animal's requirement for analgesic drugs (such as frequency of repeat dosing) and their response to treatment. However due to the limitations of pain assessment in non-speaking patients, it would be extremely useful to have a standard scheme for pain scoring animals in every day practice. If there were a simple linear pain scale of 1–10, whereby an animal with a score of 6 was in twice as much pain as an animal with a score of 3, it would be easy to have suggested guidelines for the treatment of each level of pain. Unfortunately there is no simple pain scale designed for use in general practice in existence at the moment, although work is ongoing in this area.

Part of an animal's response to pain is a change in behaviour (see Chapter 3); this can obviously vary greatly between species and individuals. The animal may reduce some activities, e.g. grooming, display new behaviours, e.g. restlessness, or deviate from a normal pattern, e.g. lying in sternal recumbency rather than curling up laterally. These changes are much easier to detect if there is good knowledge of the individual animal's normal behaviour, which is where a thorough history from the owner can be very useful. In a practice environment, close observation of patients' behaviour before surgery can provide a normal baseline, which then helps in the assessment of any postoperative pain. This can be an important role for nurses who tend to spend relatively more time with patients in the kennel room and recovery areas

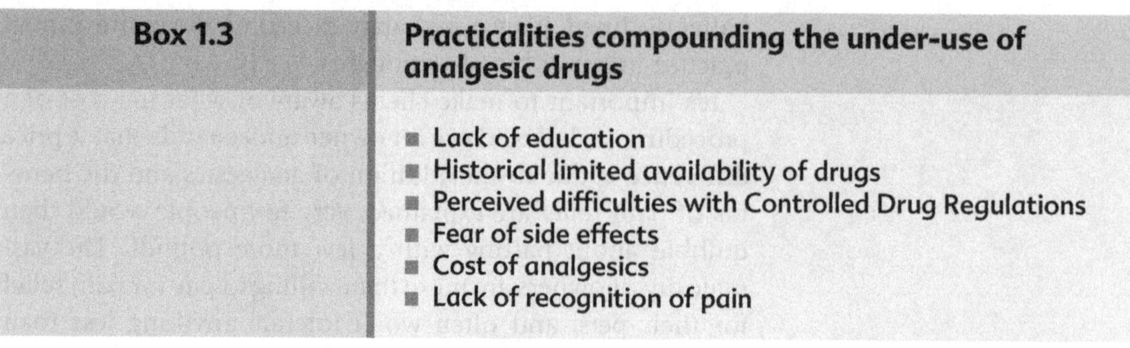

Box 1.3 **Practicalities compounding the under-use of analgesic drugs**

- Lack of education
- Historical limited availability of drugs
- Perceived difficulties with Controlled Drug Regulations
- Fear of side effects
- Cost of analgesics
- Lack of recognition of pain

than vets. If there is any doubt, one of the best ways to diagnose pain is to evaluate the response of the patient when it is given an analgesic and look for the animal's behaviour to return to normal.

PARALLELS IN HUMAN MEDICINE

It is not only veterinary medicine that has until recently managed to ignore pain – there have been similar attitudes and developments on the human side as well, particularly in the field of neonatal medicine.

In the late 19th century it was believed that newborn babies were not sufficiently developed to experience pain. At this time even Charles Darwin refused to accept that the cries, convulsive movements, facial expressions, vascular and breathing changes seen in children were anything more than simple reflex actions, involving no conscious perception of an unpleasant experience.[10] He was quoted as saying that these changes in 'animals, children, savages and the insane' should not simply imply the awareness of pain. In 1968 a report[10] on paediatric pain relief from the USA stated that 'paediatric patients seldom need medication for relief of pain.[10] They tolerate discomfort well. The child will say he does not feel well or that he is uncomfortable or that he wants his parents, but often he will not relate this unhappiness to pain'. Maybe the authors came across some of the most incredibly well behaved, abnormally quiet children, ever in existence. Again, like animals, it was mistakenly believed that babies had no memory of pain so it was thought that pain would have no lasting effects on behaviour and development. It was common practice even as recently as the 1980s for babies to have major surgery such as open-heart surgery without full anaesthesia or analgesia, but just using muscle paralysing drugs. In the seventies a study looking at the provision of analgesia on a paediatric surgical ward in Iowa, USA, found that only 48% of 4–8-year-olds received any analgesics during their stay in hospital.

A series of studies[10] and a new public awareness in the late 1980s finally changed the concept of pain and its management in neonates and children. Babies undergoing heart surgery were found to mount a massive physiological stress response when operated on under minimal or no anaesthesia. When full anaesthesia was provided the stress response was reduced and the clinical outcome was possibly improved. This work started a great deal of debate in the medical world, and caused a public outcry when it was featured in the tabloid newspapers of the time, under headlines such as 'Pain-killer shock in babies' operations' and 'Inhumane baby operations slammed'. It was at this time that the medical world accepted that the anatomical and physiological pathways involved in pain are intact and functional in neonates and they have the capacity to perceive pain from birth. In the 1990s work was done that clearly demonstrated that children do retain a memory of a previously painful experience and that it can affect their response to a subsequent painful stimuli.[10] A group of baby boys, previously circumcised, and another group of intact baby boys were studied during administration of vaccines 4–6 months later. It was found that circumcised boys displayed more pain behaviours than uncircumcised boys at vaccination, and had the higher pain scores.

Some of the reasons for the under-treatment of pain in humans are the same as for animals including misconceptions about pain, lack of recognition of pain in children and neonates, lack of education and a fear of side effects of analgesics. There was no information on pain assessment or management to be found in the 10 leading paediatric textbooks in the late 1980s; fortunately since then dedicated chapters have appeared. Over the past 15 years, human pain management has also become a hot topic for conferences and policy makers and pain-scoring scales have come into common use in hospitals and clinics, leading to significant improvements in the treatment of human pain.

Key concepts in pain management for animals

The following key principles should be applied in every day veterinary practice to ensure that pain management is made a priority and that animal pain is diagnosed and treated appropriately:

1. The veterinary profession has a moral and ethical obligation to avoid (or minimise) pain and treat pain in our patients wherever possible.
2. Clinically unrelieved pain is never beneficial, and should not be used as a form of restraint.
3. If a surgical procedure, medical condition or injury is expected to cause pain in a human, then assume it will cause pain in an animal and provide appropriate analgesia. This is sometimes referred to as 'The Principle of Analogy'.
4. Don't wait for proof that an animal is in pain, but give the patient the benefit of the doubt and provide analgesia.
5. To determine if an animal is in pain, give an analgesic and look for the animal's behaviour to return to normal.

REFERENCES

1. Edenburgh N. Changing roles of animals in society. In: Hellebrekers LJ, ed. Animal pain. The Netherlands: Van Der Wees; 2000: 39–51
2. Rollin BE. The ethics of pain control in companion animals. In: Hellebrekers LJ, ed. Animal pain. The Netherlands: Van Der Wees; 2000:17–39
3. Lascelles BDX, Main DCJ. Surgical trauma and chronically painful conditions – within our comfort levels but beyond theirs? J Am Vet Med Assoc 2002; 221(2): 215–222
4. Capner CA, Lascelles BDX, Waterman-Pearson AE. Current British attitudes to perioperative analgesia for dogs. Veterinary Record 1999; 145:95–99
5. Capner CA, Lascelles BDX, Waterman-Pearson AE. Current British veterinary attitudes to perioperative analgesia for cats and small mammals. Veterinary Record 1999; 145: 601–604
6. Dahoo SE, Dahoo IR. Postoperative use of analgesics in dogs and cats by Canadian veterinarians. Canadian Veterinary Journal 1996(37):546–551
7. Dahoo SE, Dahoo IR. Factors influencing the postoperative use of analgesics in dogs and cats by Canadian veterinarians. Canadian Veterinary Journal 1996(37):552–556
8. Read R, Pearson M, Holmes R, et al. Proceedings of a canine pain management round table conference, Pfizer Animal Health. Sydney: Aug 2000
9. Wall P. Pain the science of suffering. London: Phoenix; 2000:4–21
10. Howard Lee B. Managing pain in human neonates – applications for animals. J Am Vet Med Assoc 2002; 221(2):233–237
11. Brambell FWR. Report of technical committee to enquire into the welfare of animals kept under intensive husbandry systems. London: HMSO; 1965

FURTHER READING

Flecknell P, Waterman-Pearson A, eds. Pain management in animals. London: Saunders; 2000

Robertson SA. What is pain? J Am Vet Med Assoc 2002; 221(2):202–205

CHAPTER 2 EVIDENCE THAT ANIMALS FEEL PAIN AND ITS CONSEQUENCES

EVIDENCE THAT ANIMALS FEEL PAIN

One of the reasons for the reluctance to accept that animals feel pain and a tendency to give its treatment a low priority is that scientists like to be able to measure things that are easily quantifiable or have an absolute amount (i.e. an objective measure such as volume or weight). The problem with pain is that it can't be measured directly, so it is unknown how much is present in the first place. It therefore follows that trying to measure any reduction in pain as a result of treatment all becomes a bit foggy, there is a rapid loss of interest by everyone involved and the assumption is made that it can't be all that important to start with. Objective measures such as heart rate and levels of stress hormones can be used to assess pain but are not entirely reliable by themselves. Pain assessment has to include more subjective elements (i.e. indirect measures) by looking at associated behaviour changes that rely more on the observer's judgement than concrete numbers. However, several very clever studies have been conducted that provide excellent scientific evidence, not just assumptions based on anthropomorphism (attributing human traits to animals), to show animals do feel pain.

Animals learn to avoid noxious stimuli

Examples of avoidance of noxious stimuli by animals can be seen everyday, e.g. dogs that have been hit by an owner will show a very swift ducking action if they see a hand raised over them and horses very quickly learn not to go near an electric fence after receiving a shock on their first entanglement with it. Laboratory studies have demonstrated that animals exhibit the same avoidance behaviours as humans in response to a

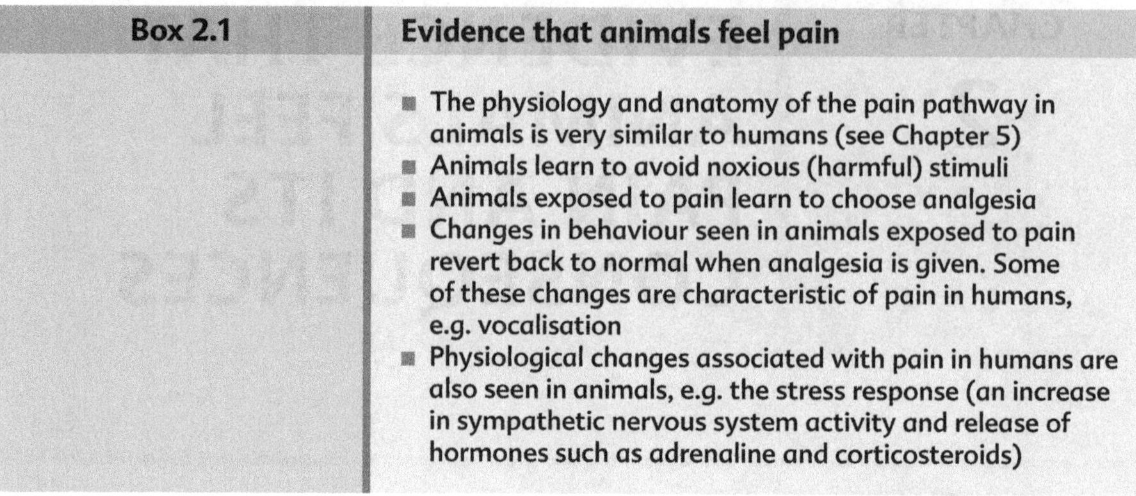

Box 2.1 **Evidence that animals feel pain**

- The physiology and anatomy of the pain pathway in animals is very similar to humans (see Chapter 5)
- Animals learn to avoid noxious (harmful) stimuli
- Animals exposed to pain learn to choose analgesia
- Changes in behaviour seen in animals exposed to pain revert back to normal when analgesia is given. Some of these changes are characteristic of pain in humans, e.g. vocalisation
- Physiological changes associated with pain in humans are also seen in animals, e.g. the stress response (an increase in sympathetic nervous system activity and release of hormones such as adrenaline and corticosteroids)

painful stimulus including simple withdrawal reflexes and unlearned behaviours such as vocalisation or escape. More complex learned behaviours have also been demonstrated, e.g. rats will learn to jump barriers to avoid noxious stimuli such as small electric shocks.

Similar studies have shown that animals will work out a system that involves pressing levers to control a noxious stimulus and will reduce the stimulus down to a level below the pain threshold. From personal experience of Labrador ownership, the learning process may well be interrupted by the presence of food (especially if it's rotting), so it can take many years of head compression before a Labrador realises a swing-top bin lid can be a source of pain! What's really happening here is that a certain level of mild discomfort is acceptable to the dog when it's suitably rewarded. Once the stimulus exceeds a noxious threshold, such as cutting its nose on an opened tin can, the animal will show avoidance behaviour.

Animals learn to choose analgesia

Rat studies have demonstrated not only that animals will choose analgesia when in pain but that the amount of self-medication with analgesic drugs depends on the severity of pain experienced. A model for the study of chronic pain in rats has been established by looking at arthritis in rats induced by inoculating an adjuvant (a substance that stimulates the immune system), causing inflammation in multiple joints.

These studies are primarily used for research into human rheumatoid arthritis. By 3 weeks after inoculation of the adjuvant, the hind paws and joints of the rats have swollen and this is thought to be the period of most severe pain, which persists up to about 5 weeks after inoculation. The swelling then slowly subsides and the paws and joints gradually decrease in diameter over the following 6–8 weeks. During this time the rats are probably experiencing less severe chronic pain interspersed with bouts of more acute severe pain as a result of using affected joints during movement and activity.

In the first study[1] the fluid intakes of two groups of rats (arthritic rats and normal rats) were monitored for an 11-week period after inoculation of the arthritic rats. All the rats were offered both sweetened water and water containing an analgesic, suprofen (a NSAID – non-steroidal anti-inflammatory drug). The daily consumption of sweetened water and suprofen water by all the rats was measured along with the size of swelling of the hind paws and joints of arthritic rats. Total fluid intake by both groups was the same. The normal rats showed a strong preference for the sweetened water; their average consumption of the suprofen water was only 1–2 % of their total intake over the study period. This contrasted with the arthritic rats, whose consumption of suprofen water markedly increased during weeks 3–5 to reach 16% of their total intake. Their suprofen intake then started to drop off and returned to levels slightly above the normal rats by week 9. This difference in suprofen intake between the two groups closely followed changes in paw and joint swellings (measured by diameters in mm) of the arthritic rats. Diameters increased from baseline to sizes greatly exceeding normal rats over the first 4 weeks. The swelling then gradually decreased, but joints remained larger than normal to the end of the study. Figure 2.1 shows the difference in suprofen consumption between the two groups of rats, and how it reflects the progression of pain associated with joint and paw swelling.

One possible flaw in the suprofen study was that the rats may have been choosing suprofen for its anti-inflammatory effect, enabling better joint mobility rather than for purely an analgesic effect. The study was repeated using fentanyl,[2] an opioid analgesic, with no anti-inflammatory properties. The results were very similar; both groups of rats had the same total fluid intake, but the consumption of fentanyl water

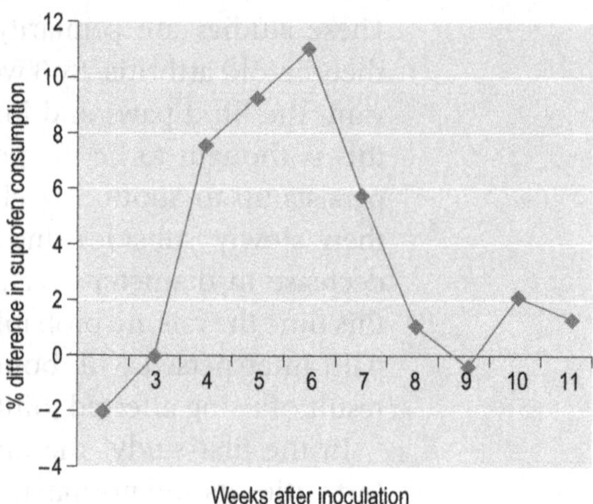

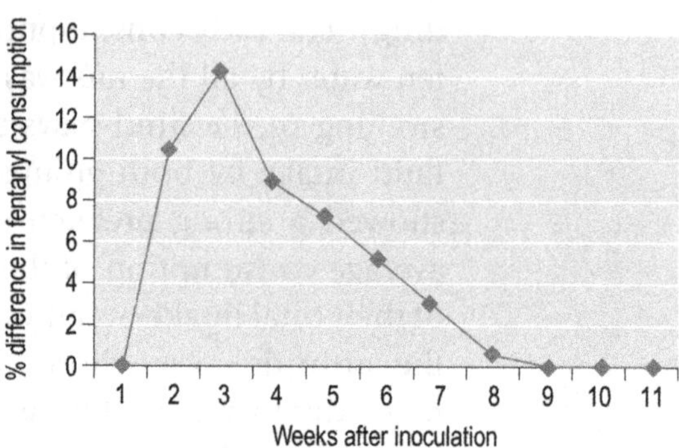

Figure 2.1
Percentage differences in analgesic consumption by arthritic and normal rats over an 11-week period after induction of arthritis. (Upper graph from Colpaert F, De Witte P, Maroli A, et al. Self administration of the analgesic suprofen in arthritic rats: evidence of Mycobacterium butyricin-induced arthritis as an experimental model of chronic pain. Life Sciences 1980; 27:921–928, reproduced with permission.) (Lower graph from Colpaert F, Meert T, De Witte P, Schmitt P. Further evidence validating adjuvant arthritis as an experimental model of chronic pain in the rat. Life Sciences 1982; 31:67–75, reproduced with permission.)

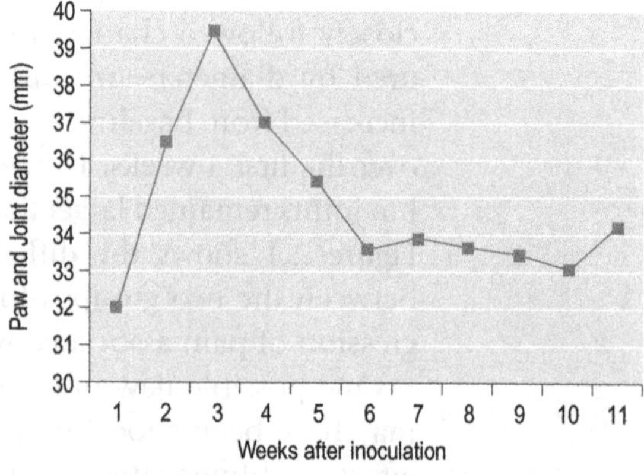

Figure 2.2
Changes in paw and joint swelling, measured as diameters, of arthritic rats over the same 11-week period. (From Colpaert F, De Witte P, Maroli A, et al. Self administration of the analgesic suprofen in arthritic rats: evidence of Mycobacterium butyricin-induced arthritis as an experimental model of chronic pain. Life Sciences 1980; 27:921–928, reproduced with permission.)

by arthritic rats was significantly greater than normal rats in weeks 3–5. The difference in fentanyl consumption between normal and arthritic rats also closely followed the progression of joint and paw swelling (both peaked at week 3) (Fig 2.2). These studies clearly demonstrated that rats with arthritis will choose to self-medicate with analgesics when they are available, strongly suggesting they are experiencing pain associated with joint inflammation[3] (as seen in humans with similar conditions). The degree of self-medication corresponds remarkably well with the severity of pain expected from the arthritis over time.

There have been some very elegant studies looking at the humble broiler chicken beautifully demonstrating that even these birds, not exactly renowned for their great intellect, will learn to choose analgesia. Broiler chickens are bred for meat and have the misfortune of being the Sumo wrestlers of the avian world, with the legs of sparrows. They are designed for rapid growth and often suffer from lameness, basically because the chickens become too heavy for their legs and their abnormal body shapes put excessive stresses on the leg joints. This leads to gait abnormalities, impairs the birds' ability to walk and results in chronic pain.

In the first of these studies[4] it was established that lameness was painful and that carprofen (Rimadyl®) was an effective analgesic in the chickens. Two groups of chickens, a lame group and a normal group, were sent off round an obstacle course and timed as to how long it took them to complete it.

Figure 2.3
'I could murder a gin and tonic!'

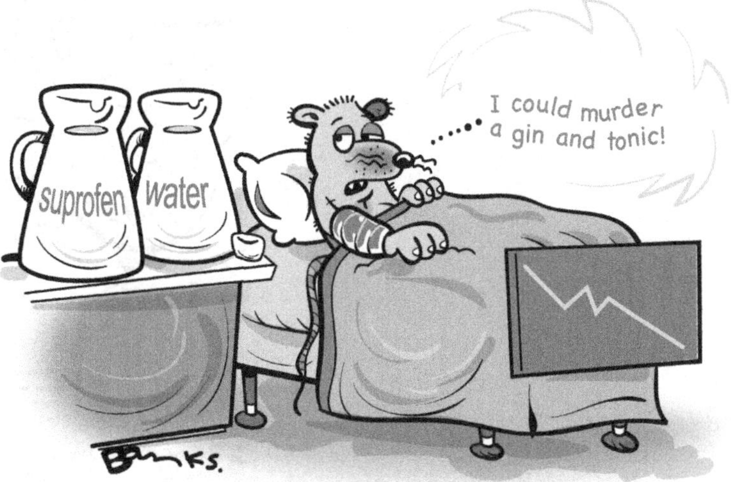

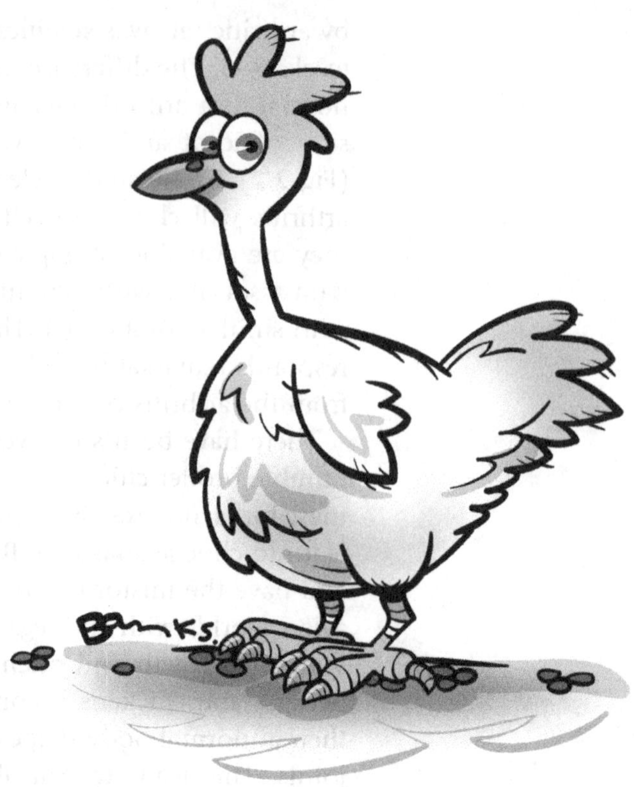

Figure 2.4
The humble broiler chicken.

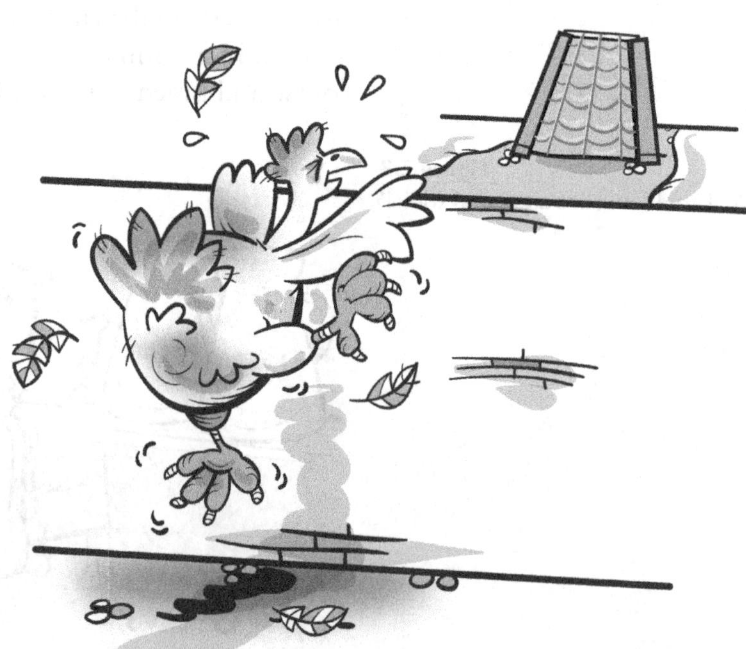

Figure 2.5
Difficulties with the obstacle course.

All the chickens were then treated with carprofen, sent back round the obstacle course and re-timed. The normal chickens completed the course in an average of 11 seconds both before and after treatment. The lame chickens took an average of 34 seconds to complete the course before treatment, but after treatment were significantly speedier, completing the course in just 18 seconds. The study results suggested that carprofen reduced the pain associated with lameness in chickens and as a result significantly improved locomotion.

In the next study[5] normal and lame chickens were offered both ad libitum plain food and ad libitum medicated food containing carprofen. Although total food consumption was the same for both groups of chickens, the lame chickens showed a significant preference for the medicated food, whilst the normal chickens showed a significant preference for the plain food. On average, lame birds ate 42% more medicated food than sound ones. Within the group of lame birds, it was also found that as the severity of lameness increased, the greater was the consumption of medicated food by the chicken. This study provides very good evidence that chickens will choose to self-medicate with an analgesic

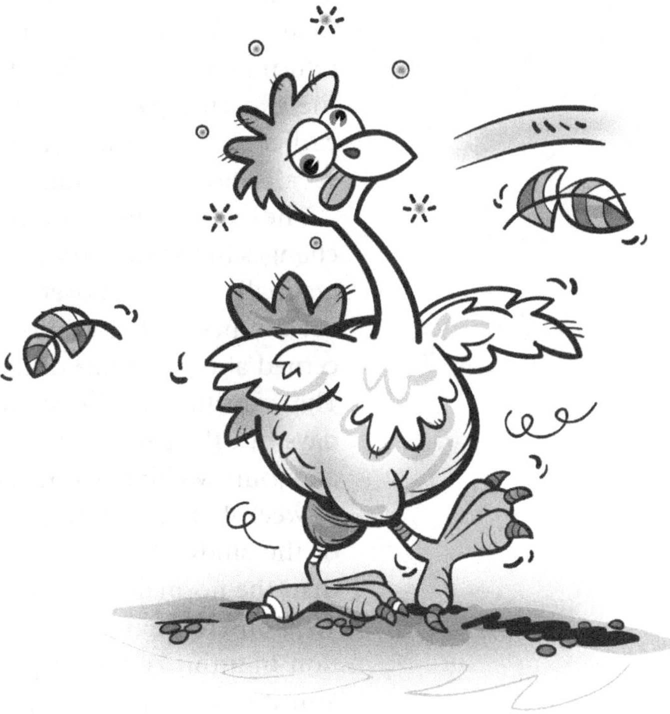

Figure 2.6
In one experiment the broilers simply could not resist the offer of opioids.

drug, and are able to balance their intake to match their level of pain. Just as an aside, apparently they tried running the study using an opioid, but all the chickens self-medicated to the point of coma and fell over, so they could not assess any lameness anyway.

Changes seen in behaviour

There are several behavioural changes characteristic of human chronic pain that have been studied in animals – irritability, disturbances in food intake and loss of body weight. The arthritic rat studies have used the frequency of vocalisations (squeaks) of rats housed in small groups as a possible indicator of irritability associated with pain. In one study,[2] normal and arthritic rats were housed in groups of 5, and provided with ad lib food and plain water (no analgesic drugs were administered). The number of vocalisations made by the rats was measured over 20 minutes, on a daily basis, for 11 weeks after arthritis was induced. The number of vocalisations by normal rats remained low throughout the study. Vocalisations by arthritic rats increased sharply at the same time that the paws and joints started to swell, from day 10, up to nine times more frequently than the normal rats. The arthritic rats continued to squeak significantly more often than normal rats through to week 7, and frequency didn't return to normal levels until week 11, again closely following the expected pain levels from paw and joint swellings. An earlier study[3] found that analgesic drugs reduced the hypervocalisation in such rats.

The vocalisation study also monitored body weight changes in the two groups of rats. Body weight of normal rats gradually increased over the 11 weeks as they basically could eat as much as they wanted (and probably weren't overly concerned about the size of their bum in a study environment). The arthritic rats also started to gain weight in the first few days but then suffered weight loss from day 10 (when paw and joint swelling developed). They continued to lose weight to week 4, and despite 'piling on the grams' in the last weeks of the study, they always remained at a lower body weight than the normal rats. Results from a previous study[3] found a 15% difference in bodyweight even at 11 weeks after induction of arthritis. One explanation for the weight changes in arthritic rats is that the arthritis impaired their ability to reach the food and actually consume it. However in this study the food was so accessible the rats did not have to move significantly to have a feed. A different explanation is that chronic pain directly depresses hunger in the rats, clinically reducing food intake in a parallel way that chronic pain can lead to mental depression in humans. Unfortunately, weight changes were not monitored in a group of arthritic rats that were provided with analgesia, so it was unknown whether administration of analgesics would return feeding behaviour to near normal levels.

A more recent study in rats[6] has looked very closely at more subtle changes in behaviour that could be indicative of post-operative pain, by assessing the frequency of several activities using video recordings. The study compared groups of rats that underwent exploratory laparotomy with or without analgesia (in the form of a NSAID) with groups of rats that did not undergo surgery. Surgery was found to greatly increase the frequency of four activities – twitching, staggering, back arching and writhing. Administration of an analgesic significantly reduced the frequency of all these behaviours. The results provide further evidence that rats experienced pain associated with surgery because the procedure led to changes in behaviour that were reverted back to a more normal pattern by the provision of analgesia.

Physiological changes associated with pain

When there is tissue injury and stimulation of pain receptors, the pain signals that are generated go to the spinal cord and

Figure 2.7
Pain and the stress response.

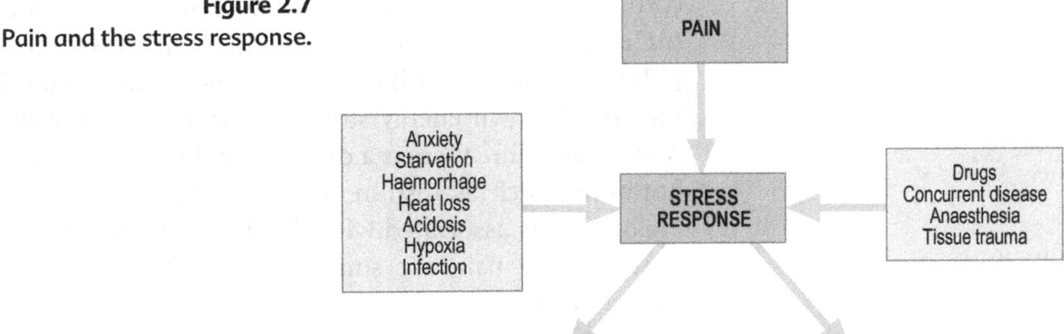

Box 2.2

Clinically unrelieved pain, such as postoperative pain, can result in increased morbidity and mortality in patients.

higher centres of the brain where they lead to activation of the 'stress response' in patients.

The stress response is characterised by cardiovascular, endocrine and metabolic changes resulting from stimulation of the sympathetic nervous system and the release of certain hormones (mainly from the adrenal glands). The stress response results in profound physiological changes that in the wild would prepare an animal for surviving the short-term situation by 'flight' or 'fight', but in a clinical setting have no purpose. In fact these changes have adverse consequences that ultimately result in increased patient morbidity, prolonged hospitalisation and even mortality.

The stress response involves over-stimulation of the sympathetic nervous system that is part of the involuntary, or autonomic nervous system, responsible for maintaining normal body functions such as heart rate, breathing and body temperature. Sympathetic activity produces a flight or fight response, increasing heart rate and blood pressure, and is normally offset or balanced by the parasympathetic nervous system that predominates during more restful situations. Parasympathetic activity lowers heart rate and blood pressure (the put-your-feet-up with pizza response). The stress response also involves the release of hormones, in particular cortisol (a glucocorticoid), adrenocorticotrophic hormone (ACTH), catecholamines (e.g. adrenaline), growth hormone (GH) and glucagon. All of these hormones are catabolic, i.e. they break down energy stores and increase metabolic rate. At the same time there is a decrease in the release of anabolic hormones such as insulin. The overall detrimental physiological effects associated with unrelieved acute pain, such as postoperative pain are summarised in Table 2.1 and discussed below.

The stress response occurs as a result of painful stimuli, but there are other factors that contribute to the overall

Table 2.1
The detrimental effects of unrelieved pain

Body system	Pain-associated change	Consequences
Cardiovascular	Increased heart rate Increased blood pressure Increased cardiac output Increased risk of arrhythmias	Impaired cardiovascular function
Respiratory	Increased respiratory rate Reduced ventilation	Hypoxaemia Hypercapnia Acidosis Increased risk of atelectasis Increased risk of pneumonia
Gastrointestinal	Increased intestinal secretions Paralytic ileus	Vomiting Anorexia Increased risk of gastric ulceration Intestinal pain
Urinary	Urine retention Water and sodium retention	Electrolyte changes
Metabolism	Increased metabolism and O_2 consumption Breakdown of muscle, fat and glucose stores	Delayed wound healing Increased tissue breakdown Weight loss
Immune system	Impaired immune function	Increased risk of infection and sepsis Enhanced metastatic tumour spread Increased risk of tumour recurrence
Nervous system	Sensitisation of pain pathway	Hyperalgesia and allodynia, heightened pain perception and chronic pain

endocrine, metabolic and neuronal changes (see Fig 2.7). Infection, haemorrhage, heat loss, starvation, anxiety, hypoxia and acid–base changes and degree of tissue damage are all involved in the mechanisms of the stress response. Anaesthetic agents, concurrent disease and other drugs can all affect the physiological changes seen in the patient. This makes it very difficult to use these parameters as a direct measure of pain, although some are more useful than others, e.g. cortisol levels, blood pressure and heart rate, respiratory rate can be helpful in assessing pain (see Chapter 3). However, it has been shown in both animals and humans that the provision of adequate analgesia will help abolish or minimise the detrimental consequences of pain.

Cardiovascular system

Pain results in sympathetic over-activity leading to increased heart rate, increased blood pressure and increased cardiac output (the volume of blood pumped by the heart per minute), and peripheral vasoconstriction (narrowing of peripheral blood vessels which diverts blood away from the extremities, skin and intestines to vital organs). This results in the myocardium (heart muscle) having to work harder and therefore require more oxygen. There is evidence that intense sympathetic activity can result in vasoconstriction of the coronary artery, reducing the main blood supply to the heart muscle itself. If this is combined with an increase in oxygen demand the end result could potentially be myocardial ischaemia. Studies in humans[7] have shown that postoperative analgesia using epidurals, NSAID infusions or opioid infusions improved oxygen supply to the myocardium and reduced myocardial ischaemia. High levels of circulating catecholamines, such as adrenaline, also increase heart rate and blood pressure and can induce cardiac arrhythmias. All of these effects will impair cardiovascular function in the patient.

Respiratory system

Chest and abdominal pain commonly result in respiratory dysfunction, seen clinically as rapid shallow breathing. This arises because the patient may consciously reduce muscle movement and because pain signals from the injured area result in reflex muscle spasm in and around the region of tissue damage. This leads to 'muscle splinting' where there is muscle contraction either side of the injury creating a natural splint to prevent movement and minimise further pain. The splinting can be associated with partial closure of the glottis producing a grunting sound during breathing. The end result is a small tidal volume, high inspiratory and expiratory pressures, impairment of pulmonary gas exchange, a ventilation perfusion mismatch (V/Q inequality) and therefore hypoxaemia (deficiency of oxygen in the blood) and hypercapnia (high blood CO_2 levels) can develop. If enough CO_2 is retained through poor ventilation the patient can develop acidosis. These changes in respiration can make the patients more prone to atelectasis (areas of lung collapse). Muscle splinting also prevents coughing and secretion clearing which increases the risk of infection and pneumonia. Effective pain relief will abolish these respiratory abnormalities.

Gastrointestinal tract

Sympathetic activity increases intestinal secretions and smooth muscle sphincter tone, and decreases intestinal motility. This can result in a greater risk of gastric ulceration, gastric stasis and paralytic ileus (loss of peristalsis), nausea and vomiting and intestinal pain. Anorexia is one of the commonest signs of pain in animals and may be a result of these changes in the GI tract but there may also be a central depressant effect on appetite as a direct result of pain.

Renal system and urinary tract

The stress response also leads to the increased release of vasopressin (also known as antidiuretic hormone, ADH) and aldosterone, resulting in water and sodium retention. Increased sympathetic activity due to pain may be expected to reduce renal blood flow via vasoconstriction of the afferent arteriole, reducing glomerular filtration rate (GFR) and impairing renal clearance. However, there appears to be few studies reporting the occurrence of this effect in either animals or humans. Sympathetic activity will increase urinary sphincter activity, which may result in urine retention.

Metabolism

There is an increase in metabolic rate and oxygen consumption and a general shift from anabolism to catabolism as the release of stress hormones results in the breakdown of glycogen stores, fat and muscle. This can create a 'double whammy' situation, where the animal's energy demands go up as metabolic rate increases and energy stores are being depleted, but the energy or calorie intake goes down as the first thing an animal does when it's in pain is to stop eating. On top of all this there is often a rather large surgical incision that needs a bit of healing. The net result in the longer term is weight loss and cachexia, but in the short term this energy deficit will lead to delayed wound healing and increased tissue breakdown. In cats, inappetence secondary to pain can result in hepatic lipidosis.

Blood clotting

There is some speculation that platelet function may be reduced, resulting in clotting disorders and an increased risk of haemorrhage although the mechanism for this effect is not clear.

Immune system

Suppression of the immune system (from the release of glucocorticoids and ACTH) is a feature of the stress response and can result in increased rates of postoperative infection and sepsis. Studies in humans have shown that adequate perioperative analgesia reduces surgery-induced immunosuppression and results in decreased incidence of infections.[9]

Effects of pain in cancer patients

Recent studies have found that postoperative pain associated with surgery in cancer patients can promote metastatic spread (and recurrence) of the tumour. This enhancement of tumour metastases can be greatly reduced by the provision of adequate analgesia at the time of surgery. Several studies[8,9] have been carried out looking at a certain type of mammary adenocarcinoma in rats that very predictably metastasises to the lungs. In the first study[8] it was established that an exploratory laparotomy (without analgesia) in rats inoculated with tumour cells resulted in a doubling of the number of lung metastases found in the lungs 3 weeks later, compared with a group that did not undergo surgery. In the next part of the study two groups of rats underwent exploratory laparotomy. One group of rats was given morphine preoperatively and for at least 10 hours postoperatively whilst the other group was not given any analgesia. Three weeks after surgery the rats given morphine had a 36% reduction in the number of lung metastases compared with the rats not receiving analgesia.

In a later study in rats with mammary adenocarcinoma, even more dramatic results were obtained using fentanyl, another potent opioid analgesic. Surgery in a group of rats not receiving analgesia resulted in a 3–4-fold increase in tumour cells retained in the lungs, compared with rats not

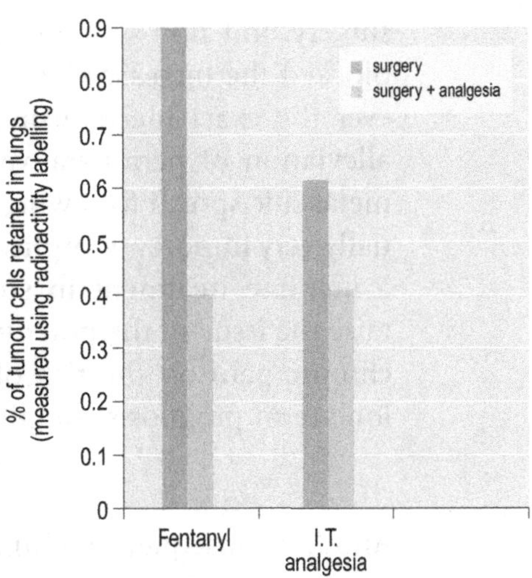

Figure 2.8 The effect of fentanyl administration and intrathecal bupivacaine and morphine on lung retention of tumour cells in rats. (From Page GG, Blakely WP, Ben-Eliyahu S. Evidence that postoperative pain is a mediator of the tumour promoting effects of surgery in rats. Pain 2001; 90:191–199, reproduced with permission.)

undergoing surgery. Fentanyl administration resulted in a 65% reduction in lung tumour cell retention, compared with the rats not receiving any analgesia at the time of surgery. This study also looked at a group of rats given intrathecal analgesia (bupivacaine and morphine injected directly around the spinal cord). This was to see if the reduction in metastases still occurred even though the analgesic was not systemic. The reduction in tumour cells in the lungs was still significant – 45% fewer than the group without analgesia (Fig 2.8).

These studies demonstrate that the provision of pain relief can greatly attenuate the surgery-induced increase in metastatic spread of tumours. The exact mechanism of how pain leads to the enhancement of tumour spread and how analgesia blocks this is not fully known. It is known that surgery suppresses the immune system, and in particular the activity of NK (natural killer) cells, which seem to be closely involved in resistance against metastatic spread of tumours. It's been shown that a drop in NK cell activity occurs post-op in the rat model and seems to allow the enhanced spread of the mammary adenocarcinoma. Human studies have found low NK activity post-op to be associated with higher rates of cancer recurrence in colorectal, breast, head & neck and lung cancers. It's unlikely that the analgesic drugs have a direct effect on the tumour or immune cells, as provision of analgesia had no effect on tumour spread in rats not undergoing surgery and non-systemic administration of analgesics still blocked the increase in metastases caused by surgery. Whatever the exact mechanisms, all the work suggests that the alleviation of perioperative pain may be protective against metastatic spread following cancer surgery, which has potentially very important implications considering surgery is often a first-line treatment in such patients. These findings also raise the issue of the potential effects of unrelieved acute and chronic pain on the risk of recurrence of tumours and the long-term prognosis overall.

Chronic pain

Another consequence of unrelieved pain can be the development of ongoing chronic pain. If the pain pathway (primarily at the level of neurons in the dorsal horn of the spinal cord) is subject to a bombardment of afferent signals from nociceptors, morphological changes can occur in the pathway that result in the amplification of subsequent painful stimuli. This is sensitisation (see Chapter 5) and can lead to heightened pain perception. The changes can fail to return to normal and persist even after the original injury or stimulus has resolved. This scenario can leave an animal with chronic pain. It's thought that the degree of sensitisation probably depends on the size and duration of the initial painful experience. The degree of sensitisation and the potential for chronic pain can be minimised by the administration of analgesics as soon as the noxious stimulus is experienced or ideally before it even occurs (preoperatively).

PSYCHOLOGICAL EFFECTS OF PAIN

It is impossible to prove that animals suffer any of the psychological effects of severe unrelieved pain known to occur in humans, however it is also impossible to prove that they don't occur. Changes seen in people include[7] increased fear and anxiety, self-absorption, withdrawal from inter-personal contact, increased sensitivity to external stimuli such as light and sound. If severe pain is prolonged, patients may feel anger and resentment, and become demoralised and depressed at the lack of control over their environment. In a few rare cases, reported in intensive care units, acute pain has been a factor contributing to a state of delirium and psychosis in patients. Factors that can exacerbate acute pain in the

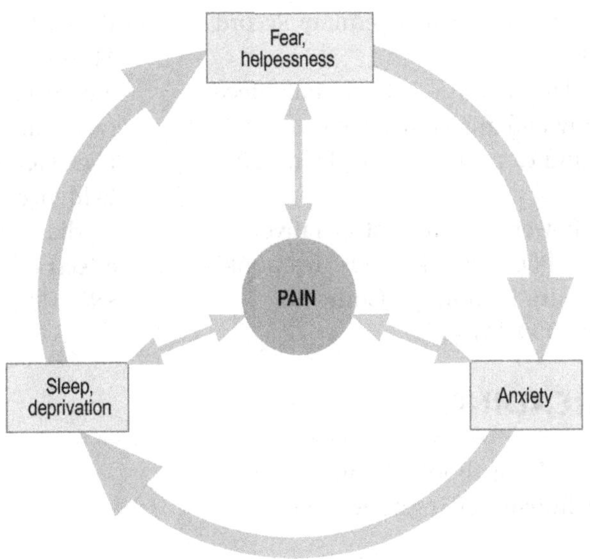

Figure 2.9
Vicious circle of pain, anxiety and sleep deprivation in humans. (From Cousins M, Power I. Acute postoperative pain. In: Wall PD, Melzack R, eds. Textbook of pain, 4th edn. Edinburgh: Churchill Livingstone; 1999:447–491, reproduced with permission.)

hospital situation in people and could be realistically applied to veterinary patients include: sleep deprivation and sleep pattern disturbances, excessive noise, disturbing sounds, lack of communication, lack of windows, deprivation of normal day–night cycles, and general boredom. In people a vicious circle of pain, anxiety and sleep deprivation can become established when pain is persistent and unrelieved (Fig 2.9).

It is worth considering the possible psychological effects of pain on animals, making every effort to provide optimal surroundings for inpatients as well as administering analgesic drugs to try to minimise the effects of pain.

REFERENCES

1. Colpaert F, De Witte P, Maroli A, et al. Self administration of the analgesic suprofen in arthritic rats: evidence of Mycobacterium butyricum-induced arthritis as an experimental model of chronic pain. Life Sciences 1980; 27:921–928
2. Colpaert F, Meert T, De Witte P, Schmitt P. Further evidence validating adjuvant arthritis as an experimental model of chronic pain in the rat. Life Sciences 1982; 31:67–75
3. Colpaert F. Evidence that adjuvant arthritis in the rat is associated with chronic pain. Pain 1987; 28:201–222
4. McGeown D, Danbury TC, Waterman-Pearson AE, Kestin SC. Effect of carprofen on lameness in broiler chickens. The Veterinary Record 1999; 144:668–671
5. Danbury TC, Weeks CA, Chambers JP, Waterman-Pearson AE, Kestin SC. Self-selection of the analgesic drug carprofen by

lame broiler chickens. The Veterinary Record 2000; 146:307–311

6. Roughan JV, Flecknell PA. Behavioural effects of laparotomy and analgesic effects of ketoprofen and carprofen in rats. Pain 2001; 90:65–74
7. Cousins M, Power I. Acute postoperative pain. In: Wall PD, Melzack R, eds. Textbook of pain, 4th edn. Edinburgh: Churchill Livingstone; 1999:447–491
8. Page GG, Ben-Eliyahu S, Yirmiya R, et al. Morphine attenuates surgery induced enhancement of metastatic colonization in rats. Pain 1993; 54:21–28
9. Page GG, Blakely WP, Ben-Eliyahu S. Evidence that postoperative pain is a mediator of the tumour promoting effects of surgery in rats. Pain 2001; 90: 191–199

FURTHER READING

Wall PD, Melzack R. Textbook of pain, 4th edn. Edinburgh:Churchill Livingstone; 1999

CHAPTER 3 ASSESSING PAIN IN ANIMALS

PROBLEMS WITH PAIN ASSESSMENT IN ANIMALS

One of the main reasons for the under-treatment of pain in veterinary practice is the inability to recognise and diagnose pain in our patients. The International Association for the Study of Pain (IASP) has defined pain as an unpleasant sensory and emotional experience associated with actual or potential tissue damage. They also added that the inability to communicate in no way negates the possibility that an individual is experiencing pain or is in need of appropriate pain-relieving treatment. It's clearly established that the sensory experience of pain, nociception (the detection and perception of damaging or potentially damaging stimuli) occurs in animals in a very similar way to humans, so they do experience pain, but the emotional component cannot be expressed because emotions are described using language. However, the lack of ability to communicate emotions, with words such as unbearable, awful, or distressing etc. does not imply a lack of emotions. For example it's readily accepted that neonatal humans and non-verbal humans can experience pain and the associated emotions that go with it.

Interestingly, the ability to verbalise doesn't necessarily result in the provision of optimum pain management by carers. Even on the human side there is a tendency for medics to underestimate patients' pain, inevitably leading to its under-treatment. A study[1] conducted in an emergency department in France compared the pain scores of 200 patients rated by themselves with the scores given by the attending physicians. Physicians gave significantly lower pain scores than the patients, both on arrival at the department and at discharge. The extent of the mismatch between doctor and patient scores was greatest with more expert physicians than inexperienced ones and depended upon physician

Box 3.1

Pain is an unpleasant sensory and emotional experience associated with potential or actual tissue damage. The inability to communicate in no way negates the possibility that an individual is experiencing pain.

Box 3.2

Assessment of pain in animals is largely based on recognising changes in behaviour for each individual patient in response to pain. A good knowledge of a patient's normal behaviour is therefore essential.

gender, patient gender and the obviousness of the cause of pain. These results are consistent with previous findings that 50–80% of patients may have inadequate control of pain at some point during a hospital stay.[2] Another human study[3] compared patient-controlled administration (PCA) of i.v. morphine versus nurse administered i.m. morphine for 48 hours following abdominal surgery in 20 adults. The patients were divided into two groups and received one of the treatments for the first 24 hours, then changed to the other route for the next 24 hours. Patients reported significantly less discomfort whilst on the PCA morphine and the majority stated a preference for PCA for any future procedures.

When it comes to veterinary patients there is a reliance on the recognition of behavioural and physiological changes associated with pain to diagnose its presence, severity and whether there is an adequate response to analgesic therapy. The fact that there is no simple pain scale established yet for widespread use by general practitioners is a reflection of the difficulties involved in interpreting behavioural observations, and the physiological parameters associated with pain as there are so many other factors influencing both of them. A thorough knowledge of an individual's 'normal' behaviour is essential to establish whether a change has occurred. It is therefore very important to get a good history from the owner or take time to observe a hospital patient before surgery.

Some responses to pain may not even be detectable, or not known about, and there are also differences between the people doing the observing, which can affect patient assessment. One major mistake to avoid when assessing animal pain is to assume an animal isn't in pain if we can't see any obvious anthropomorphic signs that actually require an extremely painful experience to occur in most animals, e.g. vocalisation. Similarly, it may be observed that one patient reacts very obviously to a painful stimulus, whilst another patient may seemingly react very little to the same stimulus. This frequently results in the incorrect assumption that the less reactive animal has felt 'less pain'. However, the anatomy and physiology of the nociceptive pathway is very similar across species and individuals, so it's reasonable to accept that the threshold for experiencing pain is very similar for all animals. Therefore it's likely that the two patients will be feeling the same 'amount of pain'.

The variation comes about because individuals may have different tolerances of a given amount of pain and different behavioural patterns in response to it. As the intensity or duration of a noxious stimulus increases, an animal's behaviour becomes dominated by attempts to avoid or escape it when their tolerance of the pain is exceeded. This may not necessarily occur at the same point in different individuals. One animal may tolerate pain a lot longer before showing overt behavioural changes, but this does not mean it is experiencing less pain. An animal tolerating a lot of pain is not the same as an animal being free of pain. There are also many factors influencing the resulting behaviour changes associated with pain, both between species and within the same species, which are discussed below.

Box 3.3

The threshold for experiencing pain is very similar between animals. Different observable responses to the same painful stimulus are due to variation in tolerances to pain and the resulting behaviour changes.

VARIATION IN REACTIONS TO PAIN

Behaviour associated with the presence of pain and the degree of its severity can be influenced by the following factors.

Species

Interpretation of behaviour changes depends upon a good knowledge of normal behaviour for a given species, and behavioural signs of pain can rarely be extrapolated between different species. A prey species such as a rabbit has evolved over many thousands of years not to show overt signs of pain, as this would merely attract the attention of predators and result in the rabbit getting eaten quicker. Thus rabbits are extremely difficult to assess for pain as they are beautifully designed to disguise signs of pain and injury. Animals that live in herds may actually benefit from informing other members of the group that they are in pain, depending on the social organisation. This may be the case with horses, which are fairly uninhibited when it comes to signs of pain and don't think twice about a bit of thrashing around during colic. Generally, species more interactive with humans, e.g. dogs, tend to be more outwardly expressive of pain to a human observer than species that have a more distant relationship, like cats.

Environment

When animals are brought into a strange environment, typically the veterinary practice, the animal's normal territory is disrupted, there are novel smells, noises, bright lights, changes in temperature and the presence of people and other species (some of which will be natural predators). This makes patients anxious, apprehensive or excited, which will modify their behaviour and potentially mask signs of pain. It seems that the animal's focus of attention is temporarily distracted away from behaviours related to pain when an environmental factor takes priority in motivating the animal's outward responses. Cats will dramatically change their behaviour, becoming very stressed, in the company of barking dogs; dogs will often alter behaviour to please or protect an owner in a strange environment, and small mammals such as rabbits and guinea-pigs will usually become immobile when being observed by humans.

The motivation to eat has been shown to reduce pain-associated behaviours shown by chickens[4] and would no doubt be true of many canine patients presented with a nice plump pet rabbit sat on an adjacent chair innocently waiting for a nail trim. Ill animals are often brought in on their own, even if they are normally kept in groups, again leading to changes in their observable responses. A common example of the impact of the practice environment on a patient's behaviour is the classic case of the hopping lame dog, rushed in at night by an owner convinced of the diagnosis of multiple fractures, only to see the dog sprint athletically across the waiting room in the opposite direction to the vet on arrival.

Location of pain

Behavioural patterns may be altered by the site of pain. It's easier to assess a painful joint, due to overt lameness than it is to detect and assess a comparable level of back pain, which would result in more subtle posture changes. The severity and even the presence of bilateral limb pain or lameness can be underestimated, compared with a unilateral lameness, because the animal will appear to have a more normal gait as it is unable to avoid weight-bearing on both affected limbs. Visceral pain may well be more difficult to diagnose and quantify than some somatic pain because there is a reliance on more general signs of demeanour, reduced appetite, etc. rather than any characteristic behaviour changes associated with guarding or not using an area of tissue injury. The danger is to underestimate the severity of pain, as its diagnosis becomes more difficult.

INDIVIDUAL DIFFERENCES IN REACTIONS TO PAIN

Even within a species there can be great variation in responses to the same painful stimulus by two individuals. Some of the factors involved in this individual variation in reaction to pain are as follows.

Age

Generally speaking younger animals, particularly neonates, are more reactive to pain than adults. The vocal protests of a 9-week-old West Highland White terrier having its first vaccination far exceed the moderate flinch shown by most adult 'Westies' (albeit a nice one), coming in for a booster vaccination, even though the stimulus is the same.

Genetics

Genetics, or breed, can play a large part in determining a patient's behavioural responses. The motivation of a stoic working Labrador to obey an owner can often exceed or override that of showing signs of pain. They will often just sit quietly despite experiencing quite severe pain. This can be in stark contrast to toy breeds like a Mini Yorkshire terrier that may require the assistance of the entire practice lay-staff team, several towels and possibly a whiff of chemical restraint just to perform a nail clip.

Gender

Human studies have shown differences in tolerances between men and women for different painful stimuli, but the direction of the effect can vary according to stimulus type. Differences in reactivity to pain could be due to an actual variability in pain thresholds between the sexes (see below under 'factors influencing the expected degree of pain').

Previous conditioning

Previous painful experiences of an animal will inevitably affect its behaviour in the future, as it may anticipate an unpleasant situation with the resulting anxiety and apprehension leading to a reaction not in proportion to the actual degree of pain. A dog with a long history of otitis externa may be extremely reactive to an otoscopic ear examination, even if there is no current ear disease as it is expecting a very painful experience and responds accordingly.

Temperament

The character and temperament of an animal will also determine its reaction to pain. A normally dominant dog will often become more aggressive when in pain, whilst a quiet dog will often become dull and anxious. Bear in mind that aggression can also be a reaction to a psychological stimulus when there is a perceived threat or attack rather than just pain. A common example would be some dogs' reaction to

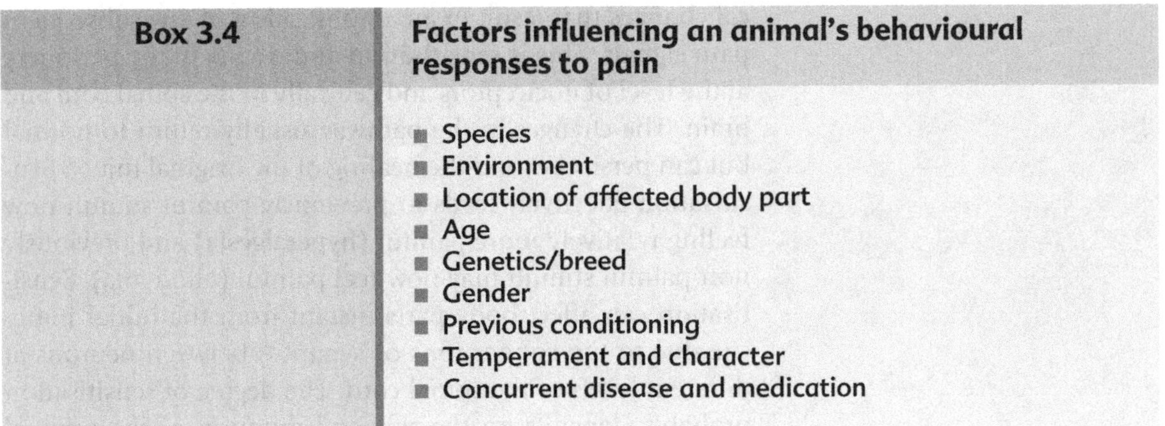

Box 3.4 **Factors influencing an animal's behavioural responses to pain**

- Species
- Environment
- Location of affected body part
- Age
- Genetics/breed
- Gender
- Previous conditioning
- Temperament and character
- Concurrent disease and medication

an intranasal vaccine, which doesn't involve any tissue damage on behalf of the patient but could result in severe trauma for the vet in such cases.

Other factors

Anything influencing an animal's normal behaviour can also change pain-associated behaviour, e.g. anaesthetic and sedative agents, other medications, concurrent disease.

FACTORS INFLUENCING THE EXPECTED DEGREE OF PAIN

Having said that the threshold for experiencing pain is fairly consistent between different species and individuals, there are some factors that may genuinely alter the nature or degree of pain experienced by one patient compared with another. This variability is primarily due to differences between individuals in the anatomy and physiology of their pain pathway as a result of morphological changes in the nociceptive pathway from previous painful stimuli, i.e. sensitisation (see Chapter 5), gender (as recent evidence suggests) or concurrent disease. The degree of pain expected from a particular surgical procedure can also vary due to differences in technical skills between surgeons, and sometimes the degree of expected pain cannot be easily estimated in veterinary patients because there is no human equivalent.

Sensitisation

If the pain pathway is subject to a bombardment of incoming signals from a painful stimulus, it can show morphological changes that result in an amplification of any subsequent pain signals. This is sensitisation and occurs in the periphery at the level of nociceptors and centrally in the spinal cord and brain. The changes in the pathway usually return to normal but can persist beyond the healing of the original injury. Sensitisation effectively leads to previously painful stimuli now feeling relatively more painful (hyperalgesia) and previously non-painful stimuli may now feel painful (allodynia). Sensitisation can affect body parts distant from the initial injury site due to the connections or synapses between neurons at different levels of the spinal cord. The degree of sensitisation probably depends on the size and duration of the original painful stimulus.

The presence of sensitisation in an individual patient is very likely to enhance a painful experience beyond that of a patient with no sensitisation. This effect was demonstrated in a study[5] looking at bitch spays, comparing groups of dogs given preoperative analgesia in the form of carprofen (Rimadyl®) with a group not given analgesia. Administering analgesics before the pain pathway is stimulated in the first place, i.e. preoperatively, has been shown to reduce subsequent sensitisation (see Chapter 5). The pain threshold of all the dogs was measured pre- and postoperatively by mechanical threshold testing, applying a probe to the ventral abdomen (wound site) and to the distal tibia (amongst other places). The probe applied an increasing force to the skin and the reading at which the dog reacted (such as withdrawing) was used to determine the pain threshold.

Dogs not given any analgesia (control group) had a significantly greater degree of sensitisation and hyperalgesia at 12 and 20 hours postoperatively at these two test sites than the dogs given carprofen. At 12 hours there was on average a 74% drop in the pain thresholds of the control dogs (compared with preop values) at the wound site, whilst the dogs given analgesia had a 55% drop in their thresholds. At the tibia, the control dogs experienced a 29% drop in threshold, whilst it was only 5% in the dogs receiving analgesia. Patients with a greater degree of sensitisation will require more analgesia to control their postoperative pain than animals that have been premedicated with an analgesic and subsequently have pain thresholds nearer to normal preop values.

Gender

Human and animal studies[6] have shown that there can be sex differences in pain due to a multitude of underlying differences in genetics, anatomy, physiology, neural and hormonal mechanisms between the sexes (in addition, lifestyle and cultural factors also play a role on the human side). Women generally report greater and more varied pain than men, but seem to have more ways of dealing with it and derive more benefit from analgesic strategies. This difference is not just a consequence of women being more willing to report pain and seek help. Studies looking at somatic painful stimuli, e.g. pressure and electrical stimuli, consistently show women have lower thresholds than men. However, the direction of sex differences in pain can depend on the site and type of painful stimulus experienced. Men show greater sensitivity to painful stimuli applied in the lower abdominal region nearer the genitalia rather than to limbs, whilst women are more sensitive to thermal stimuli, but not when they are delivered repeatedly. Experimental evidence in both animals and humans show pain sensitivity to change at puberty, during the menstrual cycle, pregnancy and lactation.

The mechanisms underlying these findings are not yet established but recent work has focused on anatomical structures, sex-linked genetic differences and the influence of sex hormones on nociception. Obviously the main area of anatomical difference is the reproductive tract. Afferent nociceptive neurones (C fibres) running from the pelvic organs into the spinal cord diverge widely as they enter the spinal cord and synapse with dorsal horn neurons at many different levels of the cord, including upper cervical. A greater proportion of the female reproductive tract is internal and trauma and disease (e.g. pregnancy, parturition, pyometra) are more common than in males. Therefore sensitisation of the C fibres, and the resulting widespread hyperalgesia and allodynia of other tissues, may well occur more often in female patients. This helps explain the higher incidence of multiple referred pain reported in women, particularly in muscles of the head and neck. Studies in rodents have discovered there are sex-linked genetic differences coding for metabolising enzymes, receptors (e.g. opioid receptors) and some of the chemicals involved in sensitisation and transmission of pain.

The sex hormones can play a role in the organisation of the CNS during development, which could contribute to sex differences in nociception, but they also exert an influence on the cells of the CNS throughout life. Evidence from animal studies reveals the following sex differences in CNS neuroactive agents (chemicals involved in the transmission of nerve impulses): the levels of the agents and the numbers of their receptors in different parts of the CNS, variation in function with reproductive status, and changes in their expression by hormones. Some of these neuroactive agents are involved in sensitisation, so it may be that hormonal status at the time of injury has importance for the subsequent development of hyperalgesia and allodynia. Sex hormones can also modify the stress response (sympathetic over-activity and hypothalamic-pituitary hormone response) responsible for many of the physiological changes associated with pain. Oestrogen, progesterone and testosterone are all associated with both increased pain and conversely an apparent analgesic effect in humans at various stages of life. This suggests it may be relative changes in levels of sex hormones rather than their absolute concentrations at any one time that affect pain. It's also been found that the nociceptive threshold increases during oestrus, in late pregnancy and immediately after birth. However it is worth noting that many veterinary patients in practice are neutered and therefore are subject to much less hormonal fluctuations than humans.

Other significant factors contributing to sex differences revealed in human pain studies that would not be applicable to veterinary patients include the experimental setting (clinic versus science lab), personal beliefs about efficacy and self-control and the sex and attractiveness of the experimenter!

Surgical technique

Some idea of the extent of tissue injury and invasiveness of a surgical procedure can provide a basis for the expected level of pain and appropriate treatment, but even this will vary with the experience and technique of the surgeon. A new graduate can cause a lot of tissue trauma and postoperative pain in a patient, handling nearly every major abdominal and pelvic organ trying to locate those elusive uterine horns in a cat spay. Prior to surgery, consideration should be given

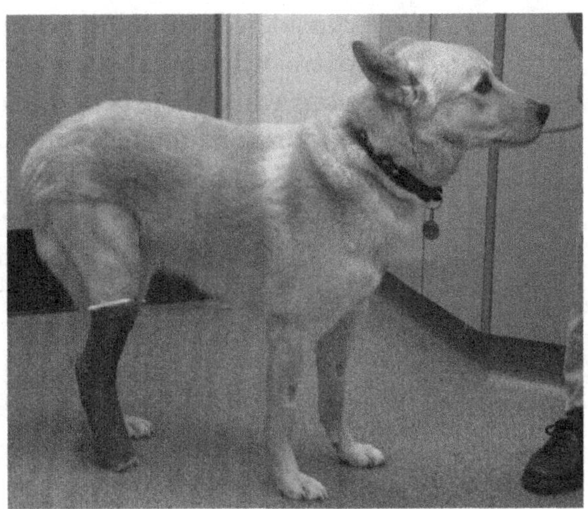

Figure 3.1 Supportive dressings help immobilise orthopaedic repairs, but care must be taken to ensure they are not too tight as this will cause more pain.

where possible to using the surgical approach that causes the least trauma and tissue disruption, e.g. going between muscle bellies rather than sectioning them. It makes sense that the smaller the incision and tissue exposure the less surgical stimulus of the pain pathway, but if an incision is too small the surgeon can cause even greater trauma in the end as a result of forceful retraction.

Exposed tissues should be kept viable and covered in saline soaked swabs. Tourniquets are known to cause intense pain in conscious animals after about 20 minutes, so this should be borne in mind under anaesthesia, when the nociceptive pathway will still be firing (just without the conscious 'ouch' response), and appropriate analgesia provided. Suture knots will cause intense irritation and pain if pulled too tightly, but still need to secure the repair. Unstable orthopaedic repairs will cause a lot of pain in patients if free ends of a fracture are still able to move, supportive dressings can be used to ensure immobilisation of the site, but care must be taken to ensure they aren't too tight. Over-tight bandages will cause ischaemia and trauma of underlying tissue which itself is very painful.

Lack of human equivalence

Another starting point for judging the degree of pain is to use the Principle of Analogy (See Chapter 1) and assume any procedure or injury reported to be painful by a verbal human is considered painful in an animal, even if they aren't showing overt behavioural signs of pain. However, there are limitations when there is no direct human equivalent, such as tail docking or aural haematomas. It therefore seems appropriate in these situations to look at the extent of injury, the tissues involved, and known innervations of the affected area to establish a guideline. Tail docking involves bone and large nerve trunk trauma, both of which can be associated with severe pain.

VARIATION BETWEEN OBSERVERS SCORING PAIN IN ANIMALS

The amount of pain ascribed to a patient will also be affected by differences between the people doing the assessing. Observer knowledge of the species and normal behaviour for the individual patient, mood, attitude, previous experience, personal opinions, value-judgements, empathy and observational skills will all influence pain assessment, as may the duration of the observation period. Ideally the same trained, experienced observer should be used whenever possible for establishing drug protocols and looking at responses to treatment to ensure adequate analgesia has been administered to a patient.

MANIPULATION AND FUNCTION IN ASSESSING PAIN

Another important basic approach to assessing pain in animals is not only to observe the patient when they are undisturbed, but also to look at responses to human approach, manipulation and palpation of the injured area and function compared to normal. Where appropriate it's also useful to assess patients when they are walking around. This 'manipulation pain' is particularly useful in animals suffering from milder pains where behaviour at rest appears normal, and is also particularly useful in cats, who tend to be less demonstrative of pain than dogs. Handling the patient may exacerbate a chronic low-grade pain and elicit an acute transient severe pain comparable to that experienced by the animal when it attempts normal activities. A painful joint may not become apparent until the animal is weight-bearing and it is flexed or extended. The range of movement is reduced because of pain but any mechanical restrictions (such as changes in joint anatomy) must also be taken into account.

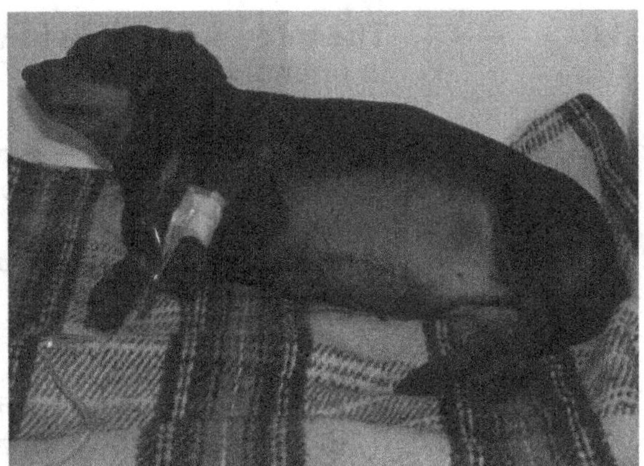

Figure 3.2
Patients should be carefully handled around the painful area to help assess pain.

Box 3.5	Basic starting points for pain assessment in animals
	■ Have a good knowledge of the species-specific behaviour of the patient. ■ Have a good knowledge of the patient's normal behaviour. ■ Be aware that behaviour changes in response to pain can be influenced by many external factors. ■ Assess the patient over an adequate period of time, undisturbed, on approach and on manipulation and palpation. Evaluate the level of function of an injured area where appropriate. ■ Use the 'Principle of Analogy' as a guideline for the presence and severity of expected pain. ■ Where there is no human equivalent, look at site, extent and type of tissue damage to gauge the potential pain level expected. ■ Take into account surgical technique and experience. ■ Take into account individual patient factors affecting pain such as sensitisation and concurrent disease.

GENERAL SIGNS OF PAIN IN ANIMALS

Animals usually display three types of behaviour changes in response to pain. In the face of acute pain, when tissue is being damaged, animals will predominantly show avoidance and escape behaviours. Experimental animal models of pain[7] show that animals try to escape a noxious stimulus of about the same intensity that causes human subjects to first report pain. Increasing the intensity of the acute noxious stimulus

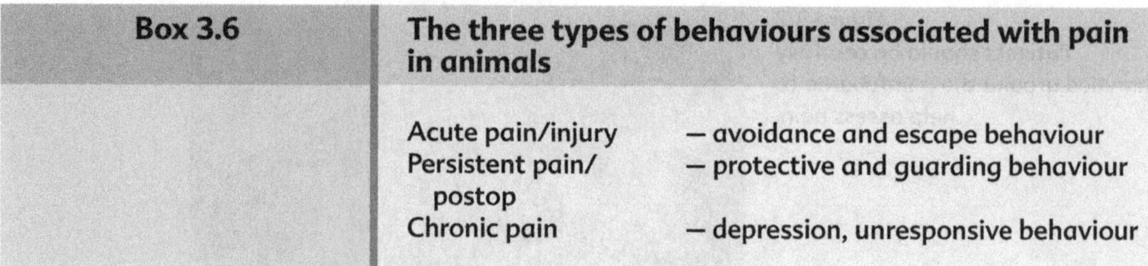

Box 3.6 **The three types of behaviours associated with pain in animals**

Acute pain/injury	– avoidance and escape behaviour
Persistent pain/ postop	– protective and guarding behaviour
Chronic pain	– depression, unresponsive behaviour

increases the escape force, and in some species vocalisation by the animal. As the pain becomes more persistent (e.g. the immediate postoperative period) or tissue continues to be damaged, animals start to show more protective or guarding behaviours to try and minimise any stimulation of the affected body part, and often change body position to one that causes the least discomfort. When chronic pain becomes established, behaviour is suggestive of depression, and animals tend to become inactive and unresponsive. Chronic pain is even harder to evaluate than acute pain as often the signs are insidious in onset and often go unnoticed even by the owner until a very advanced stage. Chronic dental, cancer or osteoarthritic pain may just manifest as weight loss, lethargy, or loss of body condition. Two of the commonest indicators of pain in animals are reduced appetite and reduced activity levels.

For all species it's apparent that it requires an extremely painful experience for the most obvious behaviours to occur, e.g. vocalisation, aggression on palpation of painful area, rolling. If analgesia is withheld until this time, then the patients will already have experienced a great deal of pain and their welfare has been severely compromised. It's vital to be able to detect the earlier more common signs of moderate pain, e.g. changes in body position and posture, changes in eating, sleeping, grooming patterns and locomotion. Table 3.1 lists the common behaviour changes indicative of pain in animals,[2,8] and species-specific behaviours are discussed below.

SIGNS OF PAIN IN DOGS

Acute pain

Acute pain in dogs invariably produces an avoidance or escape reaction, which can vary from a mild flinch when

Table 3.1
Common behaviours indicative of pain in animals

Aspect of behaviour	Pain-associated change
Vocalisation	Spontaneous, or in response to movement or palpation of affected area
Facial expression	Dullness of eyes, 'staring into space', drooping of head and ears. Excessive tear formation Fearful expression, or grimace, dilated pupils and pinned back ears on approach or handling by human
Self-awareness	Lick, bite, kick, scratch, chew painful area; self-mutilation if pain is severe
Activity level	Restlessness, frequent changes in position, or unwilling to move at all Overall decrease in activity Disturbed sleep patterns, often insomnia
Attitude	More aggressive or more withdrawn and anxious Aggression in response to manipulation of painful area
Appetite	Reduced Weight loss, or reduced growth rate
Grooming	Reduced, loss of coat condition, hair standing on end Reluctance to move can result in soiling from faeces and urine
Posture and locomotion	Guarding and reluctance to use painful area resulting in abnormal postures, e.g. Severe abdominal pain: hunching, falling, and or rolling Limb pain: lameness or stilted gait, stiffness

injected subcutaneously in the scruff, to hiding behind an owner's legs or making a break for freedom through a closed door. As discussed earlier there are huge individual differences in reactions for a variety of reasons. Generally, as the severity of the painful stimulus increases, the stronger the avoidance reaction. Vocalisation and aggression (out of character for a dog) are often associated with more severe pain, particularly if the dog was taken by surprise by the painful incident, such as after a road traffic accident.

Table 3.2
Common behaviours indicative of pain in dogs[2,7–10]

Aspect of behaviour	Pain-associated change
Vocalisation	Howling, barking, groaning, whimpering, whining, growling. Often stops when dog is comforted. (May be none at all)
Facial expression	Fixed stare, dilated pupils, glazed appearance, furrowing of brows (analogous to human wincing), panting May just move eyes rather than head
Self-awareness	Protects, licks, chews, rubs or looks at painful area (self-trauma)
Locomotion	Unusual gait or unable to walk Limping, non-weight-bearing on a painful limb
Activity	Trembling, shivering, restlessness, or reluctance to move, play or perform normal tasks. Lying quietly not moving for hours, in a stupor, slow to rise
Attitude	Escaping, increased aggression or fearfulness. May attack human or other animals when painful area touched Weak tail wag, poor response to owner
Appetite	Decreased, picky or absent
Urination and bowel movements	Urine retention and constipation if pain reduces mobility or failure in housetraining and increased urination
Grooming	Reduced, loss of coat sheen (especially with chronic pain)
Response to palpation	Withdrawing, protecting, vocalisation, aggression
Posture	Tail between legs Drooped head Lying on side in flat extended position Prolonged sitting Twisted body to protect painful site Hunched, arched back, tucked abdomen Abdominal pain can produce: Prolonged standing, or sternal recumbency with little movement Praying mantis, elbows on ground with hind limbs straight and weight bearing

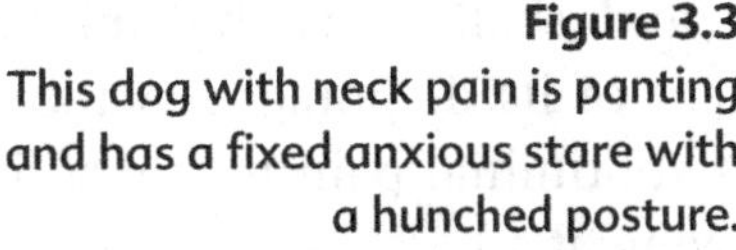

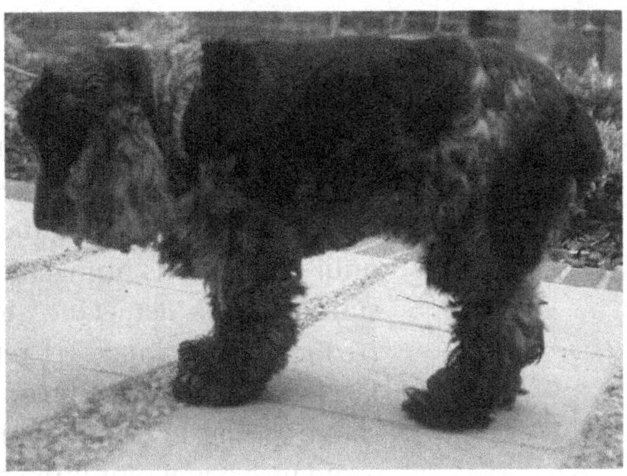

Figure 3.3
This dog with neck pain is panting and has a fixed anxious stare with a hunched posture.

Postoperative or immediate postinjury persisting pain

Dogs that are in pain will recover consciousness from anaesthesia more rapidly as the pain prevents sleep. Whimpering is a common form of vocalisation due to pain on recovery, posture is adjusted to minimise pressure or weight on the painful body part, and movement restricted. For example, a dog that is uncomfortable after a laparotomy will stand as soon as possible and refuse to sit or lie down. If the sutures at an op site are under tension and causing pain the dog will position itself to minimise skin tension in that area once it's coordinated enough. Changes in facial expression are commonly obvious in dogs experiencing moderate to severe pain. Pawing at painful areas may occur and specific reactions to localised pain include head shaking with ear pain, blepharospasm (sustained tight closure of eyes) with eye pain and drooling with mouth pain.

After orthopaedic surgery a dog left in pain from an unstable repair or overly tight dressing that is causing ischaemia may vocalise, chew at the dressing and be very restless. The dog may lie in lateral recumbency with the unaffected limbs held rigidly out from the body, trembling. If the pain persists the dog will become depressed, withdrawn, comfort seeking or aggressive depending on its temperament. Severe abdominal pain can lead to what's known as the 'praying mantis position' where the dog's front end is on the ground with elbows flexed, and the hindquarters are up in the air, with straight weight bearing hind limbs. The abdominal wall is tense and breathing is rapid and shallow as the animal attempts to minimise movement of its diaphragm. A more sedated patient with persistent abdominal pain may just lie in sternal recumbency, not moving at all.

When dogs are discharged from the practice after surgery, the excitement of seeing the owner often masks signs of pain until the dog gets home and settles down again into familiar surroundings. Reluctance to move and a reduced appetite (reduced food intake is reflected in a reduced amount of faeces which may also be noticed by owners) commonly indicate ongoing low-grade pain postop, with vocalisation and avoidance behaviour if the painful area is manipulated. Dogs will persistently try to chew and remove dressings where there is localised pain.

A study[11] looking at behaviour of dogs in the first 24 hours after ovariohysterectomy using videotaping and handler interaction found several interesting differences between dogs operated on with or without analgesia in the form of oxymorphone (a potent opioid agonist). A total of 42 pet dogs and well socialised laboratory dogs were enrolled into one of four groups: anaesthesia only, anaesthesia with oxymorphone only, anaesthesia and ovariohysterectomy with no analgesia, anaesthesia and ovariohysterectomy with oxymorphone analgesia. All the dogs that had surgery spent more time sleeping, less time standing, less time grooming and more time licking the abdominal wound than dogs that just had an anaesthetic without surgery. This suggested that surgery was a tiring, painful experience that reduced movement and focussed the animals' attention on the incision site.

Interactive greeting behaviours with handlers such as movement, tail wagging, orienting, lip licking, vocalisation, pawing and attempts to get out of the kennel were reduced by surgery. Greeting behaviour was also decreased during abdominal palpation by handlers. Lip lifting (an obvious sign of aggression) was only seen in the group of dogs that had surgery without analgesia. When comparing dogs that had surgery with or without analgesia, the dogs receiving oxymorphone still had reductions in their spontaneous and interactive behaviours, but this was probably due to the sedative effects of this analgesic. However, it was demonstrated that when oxymorphone was given to dogs undergoing surgery, the pain relief resulted in a faster return to more normal greeting behaviours, standing and movement.

Chronic pain

Chronic pain scenarios are discussed in more detail in Chapter 11. The severity of chronic pain is easily underestimated because it is not necessarily correlated to the apparent degree of tissue injury or disease progression because of changes that may have occurred in the pain pathway over time (i.e. sensitisation). Chronic pain often has an insidious onset so even the owner doesn't see the changes in behaviour that are occurring. Osteoarthritis is the commonest cause of chronic pain in dogs, and owners often mistake the dog's lack of activity and stiffness as signs of 'old age' rather than chronic pain. Muscle wasting and uneven nail wear are good indicators of chronic limb pain; arching of the spine to transfer body weight onto forelimbs may reflect bilateral hind limb pain or lower spinal pain. Chronic dental pain in both cats and dogs is often left untreated and may present as uneven accumulation of tartar, with a greater build-up on the painful side of the mouth.

SIGNS OF PAIN IN CATS

Cats are far less demonstrative of pain than dogs, so assessment can be even more difficult in this species. It's very important to get a good history from the owner to ascertain the patient's normal behaviour and therefore be able to recognise any pain-related changes.

Acute pain

Cats respond to acute painful stimuli like an injection by flinching, a short growl, cowering or marked aggression (depending on the individual), and attempts to escape. If the pain is ongoing they again show a lot of aggression, hissing, spitting and more vigorous attempts to escape.

Postoperative or immediate postinjury persisting pain

Cats often appear depressed, inappetent, immobile, silent, tense and distanced from their environment when in postop pain or after acute trauma. They do not respond to petting or attention and often try to hide at the back of a cage or in an

Table 3.3 Common behaviours indicative of pain in cats[2,7–10]

Aspect of behaviour	Pain-associated change
Vocalisation	Groan, growl, hissing, moaning, purring, spitting, (crying, screaming)
Facial expression	Furrowed brow, squinting eyes, dilated pupils May just move eyes rather than head
Self-awareness	Protects, licks, chews, rubs painful area (self-trauma) Tends to hide painful body part
Locomotion	Unusual gait or unable to walk Limping, non-weight-bearing on a painful limb
Activity	Restricted movement, may show repeated meaningless movements Often immobile, positioned far away from observer (at back of cage, under blanket) No interest in play or normal tasks
Attitude	Hiding, aggression, comfort seeking Dissociation from environment with severe pain
Appetite	Reduced
Urination and bowel movements	Failure to use litter tray
Grooming	Failure to groom (especially chronic pain)
Response to palpation	Protecting, escaping, attacking, hissing, biting, scratching, vocalising
Posture	Generally in sternal recumbency, limbs and abdomen tucked Arched or hunched head and neck or back. Does not curl up in lateral recumbency. May be lying flat, slumped body or have a drooped head

enclosed space. Postoperatively cats in pain often sit hunched in sternal rather than in curled lateral recumbency, and show aggression and resentment of handling. Most people will have had the experience of spending several frantic hours dismantling part of the practice premises to retrieve an escapee feline patient from a corner nobody knew existed. This withdrawal behaviour can be seen after major trauma such as a road traffic accident where the cat doesn't return home but finds a secluded location and remains there for several days. After severe trauma some cats hyperventilate (which responds to analgesic therapy) or show manic aggression, rolling around and tearing at bandages or dressings. Vocalisation is much more rare than in dogs, apart from the occasional growl.

Cats recovering from abdominal surgery adopt a sternal position, their elbows well back and stifles well forward with tense abdominal muscles and anxious facial expression. Nasal, ocular and anal pain leads to rubbing or scratching of the affected area. Cats with head pain (including aural, ocular and nasal pain) often appear depressed, very quiet and still with their head hanging down, and again try to hide away from any observers. Self-mutilation of any painful area can occur as seen in dogs.

Chronic pain

There are few specific signs of chronic pain in cats, and because they are less interactive with owners (for example they self-regulate their exercise and aren't walked) long-term behaviour changes are often missed. As with dogs the most notable signs of chronic pain are reduced appetite and activity levels. This usually presents as weight loss, more time spent sleeping, venturing outside less often and reduced jumping, playing and climbing, and a poor coat (with a 'paint-brush' matted appearance) from lack of grooming. Drinking is rarely altered unless the pain is very severe. Limb pain can result in lameness and disuse muscle atrophy, multiple limb pain causes overall reduction in activity levels, stiffness and a doddery gait (as seen in dogs). Inappropriate urination and failure to use a litter tray can be a manifestation of pain, and should be considered as well as the usual causes.

OTHER CAUSES OF BEHAVIOUR CHANGES

Any abnormal behaviour can be associated with pain. However, it is worth bearing in mind that many diseases can alter behaviour without having a painful component. For example, hyperthyroidism in cats often produces weight loss and increased aggression, neither of which are directly due to pain. Lymphoma often causes anorexia, but again isn't normally associated with pain. Lameness can be due to an underlying mechanical problem (although more often than not a painful element will contribute). Apprehension and anxiety alone can be associated with trembling, agitation, panting, changes in temperament (poor response to owner, aggression, depression) low tail carriage, restlessness, hiding (cats) and vocalisation, and even poor grooming.

Poor general health can produce reduced activity levels, decreased appetite, changes in urination and defecation, recumbency and depression. Dogs generally chew at dressings when the body part beneath them is painful or the bandage is too tight. However, cats will often try to remove all bandaging even if it's not painful or too tight. Bandages around the chest or abdomen of a cat can produce a manic response or great agitation, suggestive of pain, but very often the cat is simply reacting to the pressure of bandage material around its torso. Conversely, cats in pain with a torso bandage often sit in a sternal position, immobile, with their heads down.

OTHER SMALL ANIMALS

All animals tend to display the three types of behaviour associated with pain as described earlier: avoidance and escape at the time of acute pain or injury, protective and guarding behaviours as the pain persists in the immediate postinjury or postop period, and then depression and general unresponsiveness with chronic pain. Animals in pain invariably reduce their food intake, and exotic species are no exception. Pain assessment in exotics is very tricky – not only are we less familiar with the normal behaviour but changes due to pain are very subtle. Referral to veterinarians who are very familiar with these species is strongly recommended as few general practitioners (without a special interest) can honestly differentiate between a depressed gecko sat on a log with a throbbing headache and a perfectly happy gecko going about its everyday business of sitting on a log. Frankly, not every vet could identify a gecko in the first place. Assessing the behaviour of small mammals is made even more difficult by the fact they often become completely immobile in the presence of an observer and are sometimes nocturnal.

Table 3.4
Signs of pain in other small mammals and exotic species[2,10,12]

	Rabbit	Guinea-pig	Small rodents	Birds	Reptiles
Posture	Anxious, facing back of cage, hiding Hunched with abdominal pain	Anxious, hiding, recumbent	Persistently recumbent, hiding or hunched Stretching and back arching with abdominal pain (rats)	Prolonged sitting on feet Drooping of wings,head and neck. Head turned under wing, hiding	Abnormal
Temperament	Aggressive, docile, kicking, scratching	Quiet, terrified, agitated	Aggressive or docile	Docile, appears asleep or increased aggression. Less social interaction (people and other birds)	Increased aggression
Vocalisation	Piercing squealing	Repetitive squealing	Squealing (rare)	Excessive noise or quiet (less 'talking' or singing)	
Locomotion	Accelerated or depressed movement	Drags back legs	Accelerated or depressed movement. Sudden short movements when resting	Reluctance to move, not using wings. Collapse	Immobility
Appetite	Reduced	Reduced	Reduced	Reduced	Reduced
Other	Grind teeth Increased respiratory rate	Increased respiratory rate	Abnormal writhing, self-trauma, eating bedding Piloerection, soiled coat from lack of grooming Salivation, regurgitation Seizures Increased respiratory rate	Ruffled feathers, picking or plucking over painful area, reduced preening Increased respiratory rate, or mouth breathing	Dull colouration

Most small mammals reduce their overall levels of spontaneous activity (e.g. rearing, grooming) when in pain and become completely immobile, hiding in a corner or small space, separating themselves from any other members of the group if present. Rabbits and small rodents may squeal when experiencing severe pain. Rabbits with abdominal pain have a tensed hunched up appearance and may grind their teeth. Rats show a characteristic stretching and back arching, maybe pressing the abdomen onto the floor with abdominal pain and making sudden short movements when resting. Reduced grooming in rats due to pain can lead to the build up of a reddish brown secretion from the harderian glands (porphyrin) around the eyes and nose. This is a non-specific sign of stress but may well be associated with pain.

A reduced food intake is hard to detect in small mammals but may be reflected in a reduced amount of faeces or smaller faecal pellets in the cage along with loss of body weight and condition. Changes in food intake can have dire consequences in rabbits and guinea-pigs as it can trigger fatal gastrointestinal disturbances, so it's very important to provide adequate postop analgesia to ensure they start eating normally again as soon as possible. There is a bit of a myth around about the 'immobility response' of rabbits when they are manually held in dorsal recumbency and scruffed. It's been suggested this is a form of anaesthesia and analgesia. However, studies have shown that although it may seemingly reduce a withdrawal response to a painful stimulus, physiological changes in heart rate and respiratory rate indicate distress, and it should not be used as a substitute for analgesia, sedation or general anaesthesia.

There is considerable variation between different species of birds in pain reactions. Usually they will vocalise, flap their wings and try to escape an acute painful stimulus. Parrot species will react with a lot of vocalisation and strong avoidance reactions, whilst raptors and wild birds may be more likely to become quiet and unresponsive when experiencing similar pain. Birds will show an increased respiratory rate and even 'mouth breathe' when in pain; feathers may be ruffled and wings become drooped after initial flapping. There is a reduction in the time spent preening, so the feathers continue to look ruffled. Localised pain can lead to birds excessively preening and plucking over the affected area, and they may also show guarding behaviour of that body part. Prolonged pain will lead to reduced activity overall, a reduced appetite with weight loss, and less interaction of tame birds with people or less socialising with other birds. Birds with leg pain spend a lot of time lying down with the painful leg extended.

Little is known about pain-associated behaviour in amphibians, reptiles, even fish and invertebrates. However, they all have apparatus for appreciating pain and so it must not be ignored despite our ignorance about its outward signs. Careful observation is required to detect changes in behaviour, posture, locomotion and overall activity. At the moment current knowledge indicates that these species have a more 'on-off' nature to pain responses, with less gradation than is seen in mammals.[10]

PHYSIOLOGICAL MEASUREMENTS

As described in Chapter 2, pain can result in many physiological changes. Unfortunately they are non-specific and are inconsistent and unreliable as a sole measure of pain. The majority of physiological changes are a result of the stress response which is also affected by psychological factors, disease states, surgery and tissue trauma, heat loss, haemorrhage, anaesthetic agents and other drugs, all of which are common in surgical and trauma patients alongside pain per se. The other drawback of physiological measures is that there can be a ceiling effect, whereby the parameter reaches a maximum level even though the pain may continue to increase (after all, there is only so much cortisol or adrenaline an animal can produce). It may therefore be worth measuring the duration of change of the parameter, rather than just its magnitude as an indicator of the severity of pain.

However, physiological parameters can be useful when used in conjunction with behavioural observations to assess pain. Probably the most useful physiological measures indicative of pain are increased heart and respiratory rates, increased blood pressure and raised serum levels of cortisol and adrenaline. The release of endogenous opioids (β-endorphins) from the pituitary gland in response to stress are also being studied as markers of pain. Acute stress has been shown to markedly increase plasma β-endorphin levels in cats (up to an 8-fold increase), rats and horses.[13] Other

Table 3.5
Physiological signs of pain in animals

Body system	Signs associated with pain
Neurological	Twitching, tremors, convulsions, paralysis, dilated pupils, hyperaesthesia, sluggish reflexes, absent or exaggerated areas of numbness
Cardiovascular	Tachycardia, hypertension, arrhythmias (increased stroke volume and cardiac output, vasoconstriction, decreased CRT) NB very severe pain can lead to shock
Respiratory	Increased respiratory rate, panting, reduced blood oxygen saturation (hypoxia, hypercapnia, acidosis)
Musculoskeletal	Lameness, stiffness, doddery gait, muscle atrophy, reluctance to move, muscle flaccidity or twitching, tetanus, rigidity
Digestive	Loss of body weight, poor growth, reduced amount of faeces (and changes in faecal consistency, colour), vomiting
Urinary	Urine retention, decreased volume (reduced fluid intake), changes in specific gravity.
Endocrine and metabolic	Raised cortisol and adrenaline, ACTH, catecholamines and endogenous opioid levels (β-endorphins). Increased blood glucose and lactic acid levels
Miscellaneous	Increased body temperature (or decreased), swellings and changed skin colour at affected area, depression, insomnia, sluggishness, or hyperactivity, crepitus. Reduced pain thresholds, measured by mechanical threshold testing

(From Short C. Pain in animals. In: Wall PD, Melzack R, eds. Textbook of pain, 4th edn. Edinburgh: Churchill Livingstone; 1999:1013, reproduced with permission.)

measurements can be selected depending on the site and duration of tissue injury and disease. Table 3.5 lists some of the physiological changes that can be detected on physical examination and blood sampling. Another useful tool (but not terribly realistic in practice) is mechanical threshold testing (described earlier under 'Sensitisation'). Hyperalgesia and allodynia can be measured quite accurately and changes in wound sensitivity may be a good measure of localised pain, although in theory it may not reflect pain emanating from other affected tissues.

EXAMPLES OF STUDIES LOOKING AT PHYSIOLOGICAL MEASURES OF PAIN

Although there are studies[13,14] showing rather a clear lack of correlation between physiological measures and surgical pain in practice, there are some examples where a relationship has been nicely demonstrated. A study[15] looking at cat spays compared a group of cats receiving a general anaesthetic, with no subsequent surgery, with groups of cats undergoing anaesthesia, followed by ovariohysterectomy, without analgesia (placebo group) or with postoperative analgesia in the form of butorphanol (a partial opioid). Immediately postop, before butorphanol administration, cats that had undergone surgery had greater cortisol levels than cats not undergoing surgery. At 1 and 2 hours postop the placebo group still had significantly higher cortisol levels than cats that had received analgesia, or hadn't undergone surgery (Fig 3.4).

Cats undergoing surgery without analgesia also showed on average a 16–17% increase in their systolic blood pressure from baseline values, whereas blood pressure in cats that received analgesia returned to baseline after butorphanol was administered. Blood pressure values in the placebo group were significantly higher than the other groups at most time points postop (Fig 3.5). In this study another group of cats just received butorphanol and nothing else; they had no significant changes from baseline in any of the parameters, which supported the assumption that butorphanol had its effects on the physiological parameters measured by its pain relieving action, not because of any direct effect of the drug itself. Unfortunately this paper found no clear correlation between heart rate, respiratory rate, adrenaline levels or blood glucose levels and pain.

Another study[16] looked at cortisol levels, heart rate, respiratory rate, and blood pressure of dogs undergoing ovariohysterectomy, with or without pre- and postop analgesia in the form of oxymorphone (the same study that measured behaviour patterns[11] mentioned earlier). Again, this study found cortisol levels to be the most useful physiological indicator of pain. Dogs undergoing surgery had significantly higher cortisol levels than control dogs that did not have any

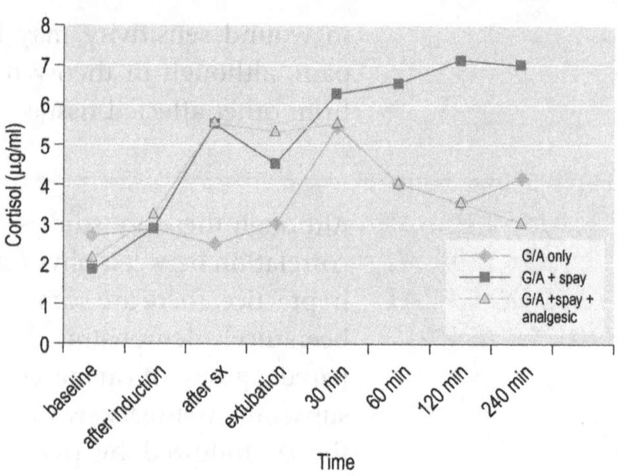

Figure 3.4 Plasma concentrations of cortisol in cats undergoing anaesthesia only or anaesthesia and spay with or without postoperative butorphanol given at 30 mins after extubation. (From Smith JD, Allen SW, Quandt JE, et al. Indicators of postoperative pain in cats and correlation with clinical criteria. American Journal of Veterinary Research 1996; 57(11):1674–1678, reproduced with permission.)

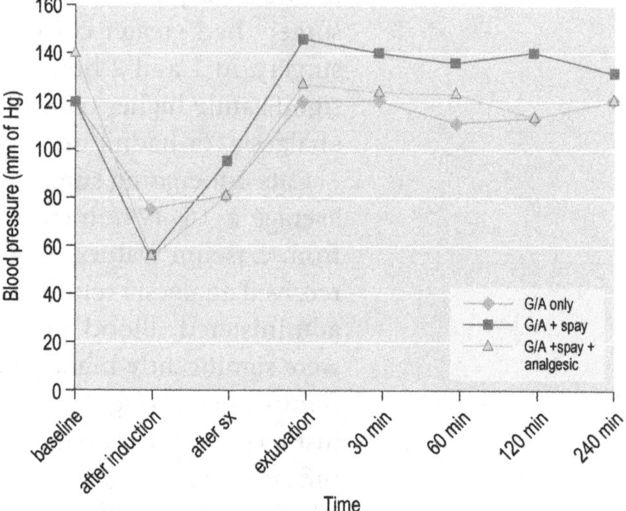

Figure 3.5 Systolic blood pressure in cats undergoing anaesthesia only or anaesthesia and spay with or without postoperative butorphanol given at 30 mins after extubation. (From Smith JD, Allen SW, Quandt JE, et al. Indicators of postoperative pain in cats and correlation with clinical criteria. American Journal of Veterinary Research 1996; 57(11):1674–1678, reproduced with permission.)

surgery, 3–12 hours postop. The surgery group, not receiving oxymorphone (placebo group) developed the highest cortisol levels of all dogs and they were higher than the surgery with analgesia group postop (Fig 3.6). Dogs given just oxymorphone (with no surgery) did not show any drop in cortisol levels, so the effect seen in the surgery with analgesia group was likely to be due to pain relief, not a direct effect of oxymorphone on cortisol levels.

The same study also found that the placebo group maintained higher heart rates postop than the surgery with analgesia group, suggesting that pain was causing a measurable

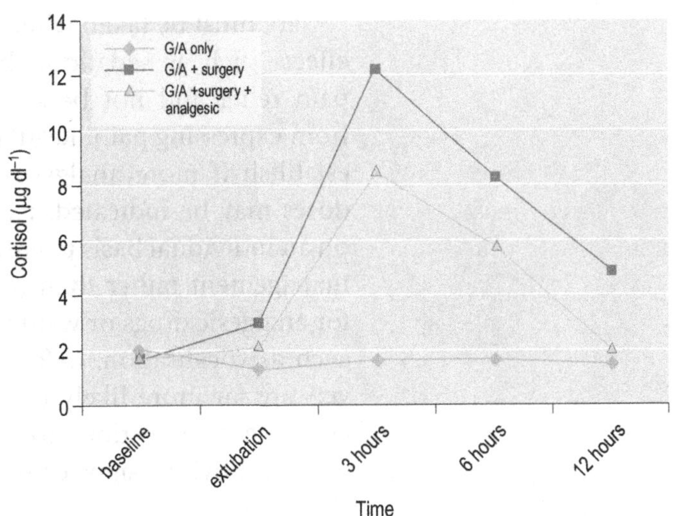

Figure 3.6
Mean plasma cortisol level of dogs undergoing anaesthesia only or anaesthesia and ovariohysterectomy with or without perioperative oxymorphone. (Data from Hansen BD, Hardie EM, Carroll GS. Physiological measurements after ovariohysterectomy in dogs: what's normal? Applied Behaviour Science 1997; 51:101–109.)

tachycardia. However, the group of dogs that just received oxymorphone without any surgery also showed lower heart rates, so it's difficult to attribute this effect to pain relief rather than a direct effect of oxymorphone on heart rate. There was no clear or consistent correlation established in this study between respiratory rate, blood pressure or body temperature and surgical pain.

DIAGNOSIS OF PAIN USING ANALGESICS

One of the most effective and straightforward ways to assess pain in animals is to give an analgesic drug and evaluate the response. This is a particularly useful technique of learning about assessing pain in patients, especially where outward behavioural signs are equivocal or subtle. This approach is also useful with outpatients when assessing chronic pain in patients presenting with non-specific signs such as reduced exercise tolerance, changes in temperament and general lack of enthusiasm for life. Owners may notice a huge improvement in a pet's overall demeanour during or after a course of analgesics. This is often the case in osteoarthritis where owners commonly return at a 7-day recheck saying their old dog is now like a puppy again. Basically, if in doubt, provide analgesia and monitor the animals' response both in spontaneous undisturbed activities and their behaviour when interacting with a handler (usually the attending nurse).

Care must be taken when using analgesic drugs with other effects such as sedation, that the response seen is due to pain relief and not because the drug prevents the patient from expressing pain. Regular re-examination of patients will establish if more analgesia is required and when repeated doses may be indicated. Patients should always be assessed on an individual basis to ensure effective pain assessment and management rather than relying on set durations of action for analgesic drugs or waiting for a prerequisite of behaviour, such as vocalisation, before administering analgesics. Sadly, vets are far more likely to administer an antibiotic without evidence of infection, than they are to give an analgesic without obvious signs of pain.

Key principles of pain assessment in animals

1. The threshold for experiencing pain is very similar between different species and individuals.
2. Variations in observable reactions to the same painful stimulus are due to differences in individual tolerances to pain and the associated behavioural responses, rather than the 'amount of pain experienced'.
3. The tolerance for a noxious stimulus is exceeded when an animal's behaviour becomes dominated by responses to the pain being experienced.
4. An animal tolerating pain is not the same as an animal being free of pain, even if there are no obvious behavioural changes.
5. An animal may already be experiencing moderate to severe pain before showing outwardly obvious signs of pain (so don't wait for one before providing analgesia).
6. If accurate assessment of the presence or severity of pain is not possible then give animals the benefit of the doubt and provide analgesia.
7. One of the best ways to diagnose pain is to give an analgesic and evaluate the response.

REFERENCES

1. Marquie L, Raufaste E, Lauque D, et al. Pain rating by patients and physicians: evidence of systematic pain miscalibration. Pain 2003; 102(3):289–296
2. Short C. Pain in animals. In: Wall PD, Melzack R, eds. Textbook of pain, 4th edn. Edinburgh: Churchill Livingstone; 1999: 1007–1015
3. Bollish SJ, Collins CL, Kirking DM, et al. Efficacy of patient controlled versus conventional analgesia for postoperative pain. Clin Pharm 1985; 4(1):48–52
4. Rutherford KMD. Assessing animal pain. Animal Welfare 2002; 11:31–53
5. Lascelles BD, Jones A, Waterman-Pearson AE. Efficacy and kinetics of carprofen,

administered preoperatively or postoperatively, for the prevention of pain in dogs undergoing ovariohysterectomy. Veterinary Surgery 1998; 27:568–582

6. Berkley KJ, Holdcroft A. Sex and gender differences in pain. In: Wall PD, Melzack R, eds. Textbook of pain, 4th edn. Edinburgh: Churchill Livingstone; 1999:951–965
7. Mathews KA. Pain assessment and general approach to management. Vet Clinics of North America: Small Animal Practice 2000; 30(4):729–755
8. Hardie EM. Recognition of pain behaviour in animals. In: Hellebrekers LJ, ed. Animal pain. The Netherlands: Van Der Wees; 2000: 51–69
9. Lascelles BDX, Gaynor JS. Recognition of pain in dogs and cats. Recognition and management of acute and chronic pain: a clinical perspective. Proceedings of WSAVA 26th Congress, August 2001, Vancouver, British Columbia
10. Dobromylskyj P, Flecknell PA, Lascelles BDX, et al. Pain assessment. In: Flecknell P, Waterman-Pearson A, eds. Pain management in animals. London: Saunders 2000
11. Hardie EM, Hansen BD, Carroll GS. Behaviour after ovariohysterectomy in dogs: what's normal? Applied Behaviour Science 1997; 51:111–128
12. Redrobe S. Practical analgesic treatment in exotic animal species. In: Hellebrekers LJ, ed. Animal pain. The Netherlands: Van Der Wees; 2000:145–160
13. Cambridge AJ, Tobias K, Newberry RC, et al. Subjective and objective measurements of postoperative pain in cats. JAVMA 2000; 217(5):685–690
14. Conzemius MG, Hill CM, Sammarco JL, et al. Correlation between subjective and objective measures used to determine severity of postoperative pain in dogs. JAVMA 1997; 210(11):1619–1621
15. Smith JD, Allen SW, Quandt JE, et al. Indicators of postoperative pain in cats and correlation with clinical criteria. American Journal of Veterinary Research 1996; 57(11): 1674–1678
16. Hansen BD, Hardie EM, Carroll GS. Physiological measurements after ovariohysterectomy in dogs: what's normal? Applied Behaviour Science 1997; 51: 101–109
17. Sukumarannair SA, Anil L, Deen J. Challenges of pain assessment in domestic animals. JAVMA 2002; 220(3):313–319

CHAPTER 4 METHODS OF PAIN SCORING IN ANIMALS

PAIN SCORING IN GENERAL PRACTICE

Currently there is no established simple pain scoring system available for use in general practice that enables patients to be assigned a score depending on the presence of pain, its severity and the response to analgesic therapy. The widespread use of a standard pain scale would help ensure the optimal management of pain in practice by increasing its recognition and form the basis of recommended guidelines for analgesic protocols at each level of pain on the scale. The goal is for the score to be reduced to as near normal as possible in response to analgesic therapy. In theory it would be very helpful to be able to say a dog with a pain score of 4 was in twice as much pain as one with a score of 2, and this would indicate the administration of say both an opioid and a non-steroidal anti-inflammatory drug (NSAID). After analgesia is given, reassessment would ideally show the score had dropped to 1 or less; if not, then more analgesia is required. The pain scales that are available are not quite this simple and require training and experience in their use. However, there is no reason why vets and nurses can't become an in-house expert and put a chosen system into practice.

A pain scale needs to be proven to be reliable, sensitive and valid to be a useful tool. Reliability means that the same score is given when the scale is used in lots of individuals with similar levels of pain, i.e. the scoring is reproducible. Reliability also entails a good degree of agreement between the scores of different observers assessing the same patients. A sensitive scale is one that's able to detect and measure small differences in levels of pain. Validation is extremely difficult (and not without controversy), as this means demonstrating that the scoring system is actually measuring what it's supposed to, not anything else, such as inadvertently assessing

Box 4.1	The measurement of pain is important to:
	■ Aid in its diagnosis ■ Determine pain intensity, quality and duration ■ Help decide on the choice of therapy ■ Evaluate the relative effectiveness of therapies

depth of sedation or degree of socialisation. In humans, pain scales used by physicians can be validated by patients' verbal self-reporting. The problem in animal pain is that there are no established objective measures of levels of pain against which a pain score can be compared and checked. At the moment, validation for new animal pain scales relies on demonstrating a correlation with several different independent measures, e.g. expected levels of pain with particular surgical procedures, physiological parameters, and currently available pain scales.

Pain scales that are used in veterinary medicine are adaptations of those used for pain measurement in humans and are primarily designed for acute pain assessment. They are mainly based on observer assessment of a patient's spontaneous behaviours, and may also incorporate behaviours on handling, interaction and manipulation by the observer, plus some physiological measures. Chapter 9 discusses suggested analgesic protocols for use once the presence of acute pain and its severity has been established. Pain scores should be reassessed regularly as pain can wax and wane; the intensity may not always be constant. Repeated assessments should continue after analgesics have been given, to ensure there has been an adequate response to treatment and to find out when repeat dosing or additional analgesia is required. Ideally the same experienced clinician should pain score a patient to minimise observer variation.

Simple descriptive scales (SDS)

These are the most basic pain scales that have 3–5 grades for the observer to choose from. Each grade of pain is defined by a short description; the observer watches and handles the patient then allocates the appropriate number from the scale to the patient, as seen in the examples below.

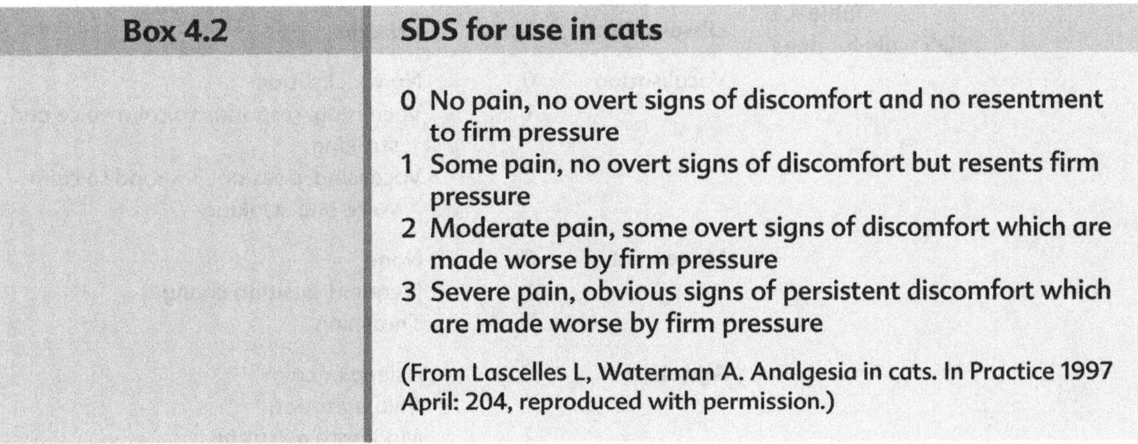

Box 4.2 **SDS for use in cats**

0 No pain, no overt signs of discomfort and no resentment to firm pressure
1 Some pain, no overt signs of discomfort but resents firm pressure
2 Moderate pain, some overt signs of discomfort which are made worse by firm pressure
3 Severe pain, obvious signs of persistent discomfort which are made worse by firm pressure

(From Lascelles L, Waterman A. Analgesia in cats. In Practice 1997 April: 204, reproduced with permission.)

Box 4.3 **Recognition of pain**

0 No pain
1 Happy cat, purr and friendly. Flinch with wound pressure, but not with stroke over area
2 Happy cat, flinch on wound stroke
3 Looks uncomfortable but can touch wound
4 Worst possible pain. Looks uncomfortable and cannot touch wound. Growl and hiss.

(After Hardie EM. Recognition of pain behaviour in animals. In: Hellebrekers LJ, ed. Animal pain. The Netherlands: Van Der Wees; 2000:51–71, reproduced with permission.)

SDS scales can be applied to several particular behaviours (or observations) associated with pain, then added together to give an overall pain score. These are sometimes called multifactorial pain scales (MFPS).[3] An example of such a pain scale is given in Table 4.1 for use in dogs and cats.

The SDS is easy to use in practice but is very subjective and there is the potential for big variation in scoring between different observers. The other limitation is lack of sensitivity; the scale isn't very good at detecting small changes or differences in pain. The SDS doesn't distinguish patients that are 'just a 2' from those that are 'nearly a 3'. It also implies that there are equal steps in pain intensity between each score; there is the assumption that the increase in pain from a '3' to a '4' is

Table 4.1
SDS scale for dogs

Observation	Score	Criteria
Vocalisation	0	No vocalisation
	1	Vocalising, responds to calm voice and stroking
	2	Vocalising, does not respond to calm voice and stroking
Movement	0	None
	1	Frequent position changes
	2	Thrashing
Agitation	0	Asleep or calm
	1	Mild agitation
	2	Moderate agitation
	3	Severe agitation

(From Conzemius MG, Hill CM, Sammarco JL, et al. Correlation between subjective and objective measures used to determine severity of postoperative pain in dogs. J Am Vet Med Assoc 1997; 210(11):1619–1621, reproduced with permission.)

the same magnitude as a '2' to a '3', which may not be the case at all. Unfortunately, when attempting to make something user-friendly, over simplification can occur, and this is probably true of these pain scales, where there are such a small number of pain levels and non-specific definitions. A human study looking at chronic pain reported that a 10–20-point scale provided sufficient levels of discrimination to describe pain intensity.[5] Another paper looking at bitch spays identified 166 possible pain associated behaviours,[6] which could not be easily incorporated into a standard SDS!

Visual analogue scale (VAS)

This pain scale consists of a line 100 mm in length, where one end represents 'no pain at all' and the other end represents 'the worst possible pain'. The observer marks a point on the line that corresponds to the pain intensity for the patient. The distance between the 'no pain' end of the line and the mark is the pain score, so the range is from 0 to 100 (Fig 4.1). Sometimes the distance to the mark is divided by the total length of the line, giving a range of 0–10. The use of a blank line prevents the scorer being influenced by numerical cues.

It's a good idea to apply a more specific definition to the end of the VAS for the different situations it's used in, e.g.

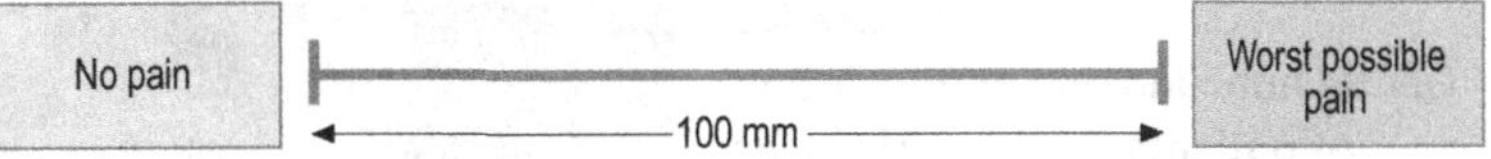

Figure 4.1 Example of a VAS.

100mm corresponds to the worst possible pain for a particular surgical procedure, as the worst pain for a castration will probably differ from the worst pain after a thoracotomy. The VAS has been widely used in human medicine and veterinary studies. It does appear to be quite sensitive and allows for much better gradation of pain intensity than the SDS, but is still very subjective, relying on the observer's overall judgement of the patient. There is some criticism[7] from the veterinary and human side that VAS are influenced by the visual and motor coordination of the observer, reducing the ability of users to accurately place the mark on the line, resulting in errors of up to 7mm being reported. This is not a clinical tool to be used with a hangover. The VAS may also allow for over-interpretation – can human observers realistically differentiate up to 100 distinct levels of pain? VASs require observers that are experienced and well trained to give a reliable score as there is little 'in-built' guidance on what exactly to look for in different patients.

Dynamic and interactive visual analogue scale (DIVAS)

This is a modified VAS that incorporates an interactive and dynamic assessment.[8] Not only is the patient observed whilst it's undisturbed but their responses to approach, handling, palpation of the painful area, and walking around are also assessed. A mark on a 100mm line is then made, and the distance from the start (no pain at all) is taken as the pain score. The DIVAS overcomes some of the deficiencies of a purely observational score. A dog lying still because of a very painful wound would get a low score on just observation (see Table 4.1) and the pain would remain undetected unless the dog was also handled. The VAS and DIVAS are generally considered inherently more sensitive than the SDS.[3,8]

Figure 4.3a illustrates the results of a DIVAS used to assess pain in bitches for 20 hours after ovariohysterectomy.[8] The graph compares scores between the group of dogs not

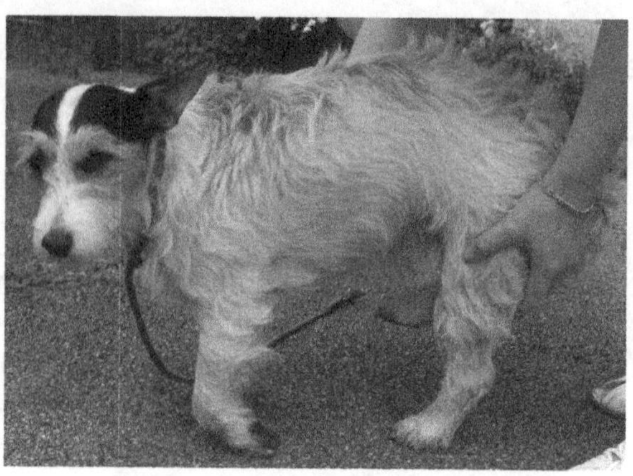

Figure 4.2
Gentle handling and manipulation of patients significantly helps evaluate pain. This dog with spinal pain may just lie very still in a kennel but the level of discomfort is more obvious when standing.

given analgesia, to a group given preoperative carprofen (Rimadyl®) a NSAID, which seemed to provide a significant degree of analgesia.

Figure 4.3b illustrates the results of a DIVAS used to assess postoperative pain in cats that underwent ovariohysterectomy with or without preoperative analgesia (carprofen or pethidine – an opioid).[9] The DIVAS scores differentiated between groups given pain relief and those that were not, and also differentiated between treatment groups that had low or high doses of the analgesics.

Numerical rating scale (NRS)

This is very similar to the VAS, but the observer assesses the patient and then chooses a rating on a scale of 0–10 (or 0–100) rather than placing a mark on a line. On a NRS 0 represents no pain at all and 10 (or 100) represents the worst possible pain (see Fig 4.4).

Again the NRS seems to be more sensitive than the SDS.[3] It has been suggested that the NRS is a good compromise between the lack of sensitivity of SDS and the unreliability of VAS, for pain scoring dogs in practice.[7] The same authors however still found a lot of variability between four very experienced observers using all three types of scale (SDS, VAS and NRS) to pain score dogs after a variety of surgical procedures.

Variable rating scale (VRS)

The VRS incorporates objective physiological data (HR, RR, pupil size, rectal temp) as well as spontaneous behaviours, posture, interactive behavioural responses to palpation,

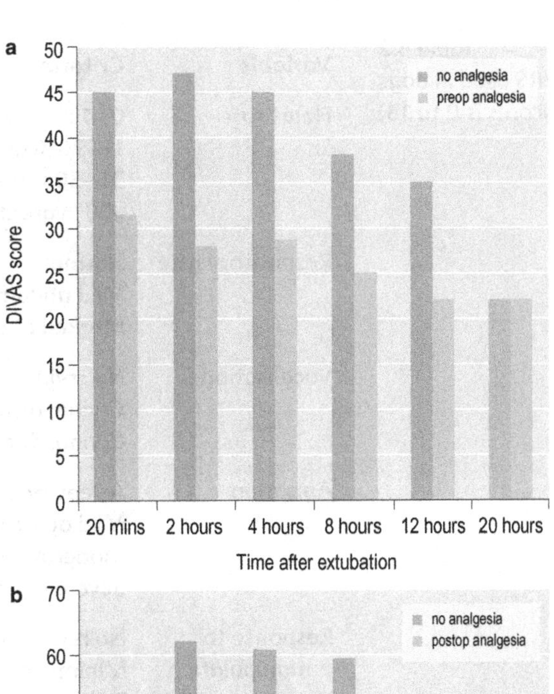

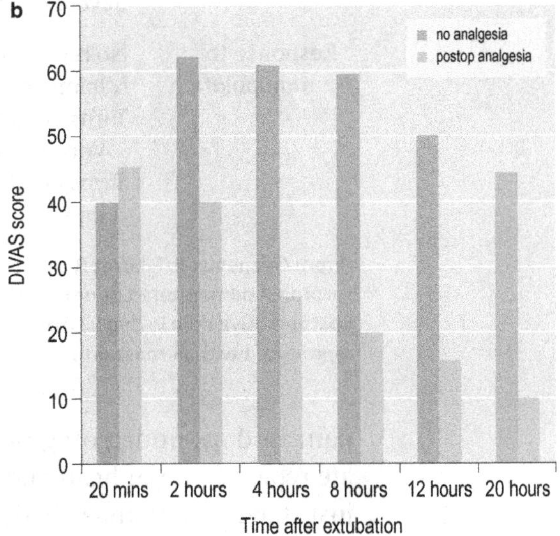

Figure 4.3 (a) Mean DIVAS pain scores of dogs for the first 20 hours after undergoing ovariohysterectomy, with or without analgesia (preop carpofen at 4mg/kg s.c.). (After Lascelles BDX, Cripps PJ, Jones A, et al. Efficacy and kinetics of carprofen, administered preoperatively or postoperatively for the prevention of pain in dogs undergoing ovariohysterectomy. Veterinary Surgery 1998; 27:568–582, reproduced with permission.) (b) Mean DIVAS scores for cats (10 per group) undergoing ovariohysterectomy, with or without carprofen analgesia (at 4mg/kg s.c.) given at extubation. (After Lascelles BDX, Cripps P, Mirchandani S, et al. Carprofen as an analgesic for postoperative pain in cats: dose titration and assessment of efficacy in comparison to pethidine hydrochloride. Journal of Small Animal Practice 1995; 36:535–541, reproduced with permission.)

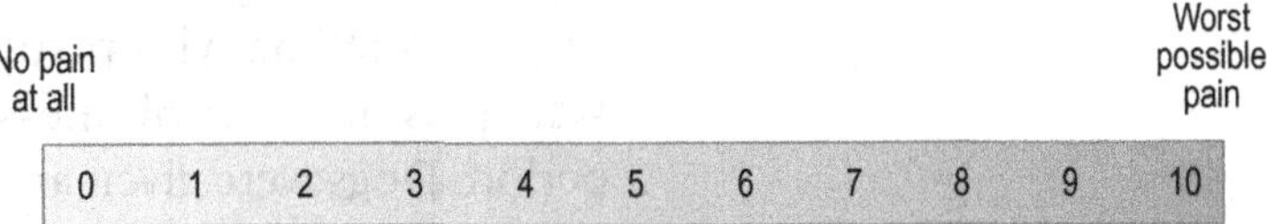

Figure 4.4 Example of a NRS.

mental status and vocalisation. The observer assigns a number from the scale to each patient variable according to the definitions (or descriptors) provided. The numbers are then added up to give the total score. These scales seem to be quite sensitive and reliable between different assessors. Table 4.2 gives an example of a VRS that was used to assess postop

Table 4.2
Example of a VRS used in dogs (range of scores is 0 to 13)

Variable	Criteria	Score
Heart rate	0–10% greater than preop value	0
	11–30% greater than preop value	1
	31–50% greater than preop value	2
	>50% greater than preop value	3
Respiratory rate	Normal	0
	Mild abdominal assistance	1
	Marked abdominal assistance	2
Vocalisation	No crying	0
	Crying, responsive to calm voice	1
	Crying, does not respond to calm voice	2
Agitation	Asleep or calm	0
	Mild agitation	1
	Moderate agitation	2
	Severe agitation	3
Response to manipulation	No response	0
	Minimal response, tries to move away	1
	Turns head towards site, slight vocalisation	2
	Turns head with intention to bite, howls	3

(From Grisneaux E, Pibarot P, Dupuis J, et al. Comparison of ketoprofen and carprofen administered prior to orthopaedic surgery for control of postoperative pain in dogs. J Am Vet Med Assoc 1999;215(8):1105–1110, reproduced with permission.)

pain in dogs undergoing orthopaedic surgery (cranial cruciate repair, femoral head and neck excision) and control dogs just having an anaesthetic for radiography without any surgery.[10] Results of pain scores for control dogs and groups of surgery dogs given no preop analgesia, and a group given carprofen (Rimadyl®) preop are illustrated in Fig 4.5, alongside plasma cortisol measurements taken over the same period. Dogs were given an opioid analgesic (oxymorphone), termed intervention treatment, if their pain score reached 7 on the scale during the study.

Both pain scores and cortisol levels for control dogs were significantly lower than the surgery dogs at most time points. The surgery dogs receiving analgesia also had significantly lower pain scores than the group not receiving analgesia at most time points. The study rather nicely supported the reliability and validity of this VRS.

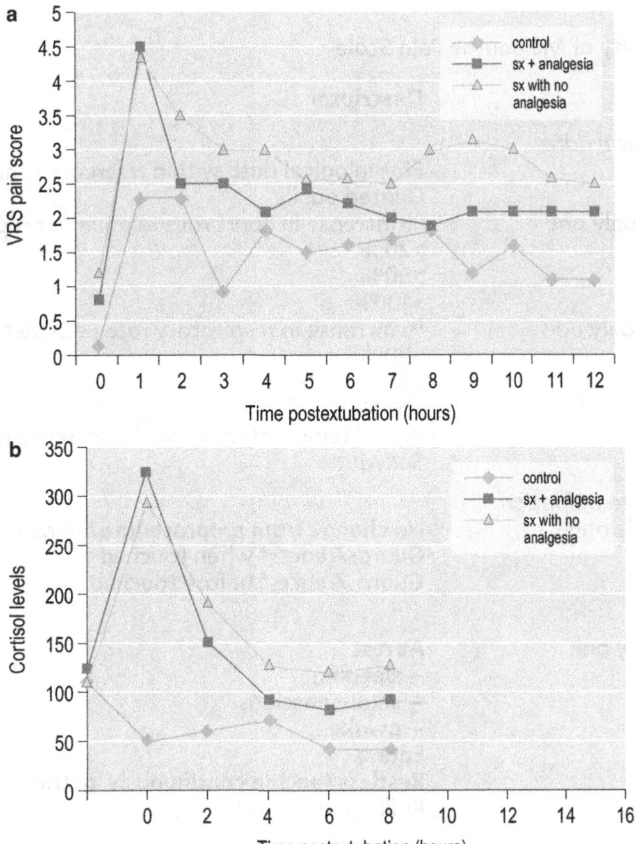

Figure 4.5 (a) Mean VRS postop pain scores in dogs undergoing an anaesthetic only (controls) and dogs undergoing ovariohysterectomy with or without carprofen. (b) Mean plasma cortisol levels postop of dogs undergoing anaesthesia only, and dogs undergoing surgery with or without carprofen analgesia. ((a) and (b) after Grisneaux E, Pibarot P, Dupuis J, et al. Comparison of ketoprofen and carprofen administered prior to orthopaedic surgery for control of postoperative pain in dogs. J Am Vet Med Assoc 1999; 215(8): 1105–1110, reproduced with permission.)

The University of Melbourne pain scale[11]

This is a VRS that incorporates even more physiological parameters and behaviour variables. It has 6 categories (physiological data, response to palpation, activity, mental status, posture and vocalisation) and 12 variables, giving a score range of 0–27. When used on dogs following ovariohysterectomy it showed good agreement between different assessors and the scale also differentiated between dogs that were anaesthetised but not subject to surgery, and those that did have surgery with or without analgesia. The scale also discriminated between different surgery treatment groups, showing that changes in scores followed the expected duration of action of the analgesic drugs, providing good evidence of validation. It looks very promising for use in clinical practice. (See Table 4.3.)

Table 4.3
The University of Melbourne Pain Scale

Category	Descriptor	Score
Physiological data		
a.	Physiological data within reference range	0
b.	Dilated pupils	2
c. choose only one	% increase in heart rate relative to preprocedure rate	
	>20%	1
	>50%	2
	>100%	3
d. choose only one	% increase in respiratory rate relative to preprocedure rate	
	>20%	1
	>50%	2
	>100%	3
e.	Rectal temperature exceeds reference range	1
f.	Salivation	2
Response to palpation		
choose only one	No change from preprocedure behaviour	0
	Guards/reacts* when touched	2
	Guards/reacts* before touched	3
Activity		
choose only one	At rest	
	– sleeping	0
	– semi-conscious	0
	– awake	1
	Eating	0
	Restless (pacing continuously, getting up & down)	2
	Rolling/thrashing	3
Mental status†		
choose only one	Submissive	0
	Overtly friendly	1
	Wary	2
	Aggressive	3
Posture		
a.	Guarding or protecting affected area (includes foetal position)	2
b. choose only one	Lateral recumbency	0
	Sternal recumbency	1
	Sitting or standing, head up	1
	Standing, head hanging down	2
	Moving	1
	Abnormal posture (e.g. prayer position, hunched back)	2
Vocalisation‡		
choose only one	Not vocalising	0
	Vocalising when touched	2
	Intermittent vocalisation	2
	Continuous vocalisation	3

Some descriptors are grouped under 'choose only one' as they are mutually exclusive, i.e. the dog cannot be standing at the same time as sitting
*Includes turning head toward affected area; or tense muscles and a protective (guarding) posture
†For mental status the assessor must have obtained a baseline score of the dog's normal aggressive/dominant behaviour, before the painful procedure. The mental status score is taken as the absolute difference between the pre-procedure and the post procedure scores
‡Does not include alert barking
(From Firth AM, Haldane SL. Development of a scale to evaluate postoperative pain in dogs. J Am Vet Med Assoc 1999; 214:651–659, reproduced with permission.)

Descriptive pain assessment scale[5]

This is a suggested guide to pain assessment that could be used in practice, ideally in conjunction with an idea of the anticipated level of pain for each surgical procedure (see Chapter 9), physiological measures of heart rate and respiratory rate, and with a good knowledge of pain-associated behaviours detailed in the previous chapter. This scale is used as a teaching tool at the Ontario Veterinary College. The weakness in this scale is that not all possible combinations or permutations of behaviour associated with each level of pain on the scale are documented, so essentially the scale is incomplete, and as yet there hasn't been a controlled study to fully validate it. The scale follows (from Mathews KA. Pain assessment and general approach to management. Vet Clinics of North America: Small Animal Practice 2000; 30(4): 729–755, reproduced with permission):

0 No pain

- Patient is running, playing, eating, jumping, bouncy
- Sitting or walking normally
- Sleeping comfortably with dreaming
- Normal, affectionate response to caregiver
- Heart rate should be normal, if elevated it is due to excitement
- Cats rub their face on the caregiver's hand or cage, may roll over and purr
- Cats and dogs groom themselves when free of pain
- Appetite is normal
- Behaviour different from this not associated with pain may be associated with apprehension or anxiety. Apprehension or anxiety can be a feature of hospitalised patients.

1 Probably no pain

- Patient appears to be normal, but condition is not as clear-cut as first category
- Heart rate should be normal or slightly increased because of excitement.

2 Mild discomfort

- Patient still eats or sleeps but may not dream
- May limp slightly or resist palpation of the surgical wound, but otherwise shows no signs of discomfort
- Not depressed
- There may be a slight increase in respiratory rate; heart rate may or may not be increased

- Dogs may continue to wag their tails and cats may still purr during interaction with the caregiver
- Reassess within the hour, and then give an analgesic if condition seems worse

3 Mild pain or discomfort

- Patient limps or guards incision, or the abdomen is slightly tucked up if abdominal surgery was performed
- Looks a little depressed
- Cannot get comfortable
- May tremble or shake
- Seems to be interested in food and may still eat a little but somewhat picky
- This could be a transition from category 2, so you notice a change from being comfortable to becoming restless as though analgesia is wearing off
- Respiratory rate may be increased and a little shallow
- Heart rate may be increased or normal, depending on whether an opioid was given previously
- Cats may continue to purr and dogs may wag their tail even when they are in pain so disregard these behavioural patterns as indicators of comfort.

4 Mild to moderate pain

- Patient resists touching of the operative site, injured area, painful abdomen, or neck, for example
- Guarding or splinting of the abdomen, or stretching of all four legs
- May look at, lick or chew the painful area
- Patient may lie or sit in an abnormal position and is not curled up or relaxed
- May tremble or shake
- May or may not seem interested in food; may start to eat and then stop after 1 or 2 bites
- Respiratory rate may be increased or shallow
- Heart rate may be increased or normal
- Pupils may be dilated
- May whimper (dogs) or give a plaintive meow (cats) occasionally; slow to rise and hang the tail down
- There may be no weight bearing or only a toe touch on the injured limb
- Somewhat depressed in response to the caregiver
- Cats may lie quietly and not move for prolonged periods.

5 Moderate pain

- Similar to previous category but condition progressing
- Patient may be reluctant to move, depressed or inappetent and may bite or attempt to bite when the caregiver approaches the painful area
- Trembling or shaking with head down may be a feature, depressed
- The patient may vocalise when caregiver attempts to move it or when it is approached
- Definite splinting of abdomen if affected here (e.g. pancreatitis, peritonitis, hepatitis, abdominal incision), or the patient is unable to bear weight on the operated or injured limb
- Ears may be pulled back
- Heart and respiratory rates may be increased
- Pupils may be dilated
- The patient lies down but does not really sleep or may stand in the praying position if there is abdominal pain.

6 Increased moderate pain

- Similar to previous category but patient may vocalise or whine frequently without provocation and when attempting to move
- Heart rate may be increased or within normal limits if an opioid has been given previously; respiratory rate may be increased with an abdominal lift (where the patient attempts to cry but there is no associated vocalisation)
- Pupils may be dilated.

7 Moderate to severe pain

- Includes signs from categories 5 and 6
- Patient is quite depressed and not concerned with its surroundings but usually responds to direct voice (this may be seen as a stop to whining, turning of the head or eyes)
- Patient urinates and defecates (if diarrhoea) without attempting to move, cries out when moved or spontaneously or continually whimpers
- Occasionally an animal does not vocalise
- Heart and respiratory rates may be increased
- Hypertension may be present
- Pupils may be dilated.

8 Severe pain

- Signs same as previous category
- Vocalising may be more of a feature, or animal is so consumed with pain it does not notice caregiver's presence and just lies there
- With severe trauma, the patient may not be able to move or cry because of the increased pain with this activity and therefore remains motionless and extremely depressed
- May thrash around cage intermittently
- With some traumatic or neurological pain the patient may scream, especially cats, when being approached
- Increased heart rate (tachycardia), with or without increased respiratory rate (tachypnea), with increased abdominal effort and hypertension is usually present even if an opioid has been given previously – although these can be unreliable parameters if not present.

9 Severe to excruciating pain

- Signs same as previous category, but patient is hyperaesthetic (increased or exaggerated response to any stimuli, especially touch)
- Patient trembles involuntarily when any part of the body in close proximity to the wound or injury is touched because of the neuropathic or severe inflammatory pain
- This degree of pain can cause death.

10 Worst possible pain?

- Same as category 9, but worse
- Patient emitting piercing screams or almost comatose
- Patient is hyperaesthetic or hyperalgesic
- The whole body is trembling, and pain is elicited wherever you touch the patient
- This degree of pain can cause death.

N.B. Dogs may continue to wag their tail in response to touch or commands even though they may be experiencing moderate to severe pain. Therefore a tail wag should not be used to assume a dog is pain free. Cats may continue to purr when in any degree of pain, in fact up until death. Depressed in the context of this scale means a slow or hangdog response in situations where normally the dog or cat would act as described at level 0 (no pain). The level of depression can vary from the patient appearing tired, with partially closed eyes and low head carriage through to a poor or no response at all to the caregiver.

Glasgow composite pain scale[12]

This pain scale is currently in development at Glasgow Vet School for the assessment of acute pain in practice. It is based on the McGill Pain Questionnaire used in humans (see below). The scale consists of a questionnaire for clinicians with 6 behavioural categories (vocalisation, attention to painful area, mobility, response to touch, demeanour and comfort/posture). Each category has 4–6 descriptors for levels of pain, and the score from each category is added up to give an overall (or composite) pain score (similar to the VRS examples described above). Initially the descriptors of each pain level within the behaviour categories were established by asking vets for terms they would use to describe pain in their patients (300 words were collected in the end). The assessor observes the patient undisturbed, then approaches the kennel, interacts and encourages the patient to lead walk. The scale is still being worked on to try and take into account patient variables not related to pain such as differences in breed that can greatly affect temperament.

Box 4.4 **Pain scales and physiological measures**

Pain scales available for assessing acute pain in animals

- Simple Descriptive Scale (SDS) – behavioural only
- Visual Analogue Scale (VAS) – behavioural only
- Dynamic and Interactive Visual Analogue Scale (DIVAS) – behavioural only
- Variable Rating Scales (VRS) – behavioural + physiological measures (e.g. University of Melbourne Pain Scale)
- Descriptive Pain Assessment Scale – behavioural + physiological measures
- Glasgow Composite Pain Scale – behavioural only

Useful physiological measures (see Chapter 3) to use with pain scales

- Heart rate, respiratory rate, blood pressure, (blood cortisol levels, β-endorphin levels, pupil size)
- Mechanical threshold testing of pain thresholds

CHRONIC PAIN SCORING

Chronic pain is even harder to assess than acute pain, where sudden changes in behaviour are more obvious to an observer, because the signs of chronic pain are often subtle and insidious in onset, and only usually recognisable by owners. Even so, owners often fail to detect gradual changes in their pets' behaviour over long periods of time as they often forget what the animal used to be like. Common causes of chronic pain include osteoarthritis, cancer, dental disease, cystitis and otitis externa, and the signs are often mistaken for ageing, just 'getting old', and owners just don't realise that analgesic treatment can make a huge difference. When the pets are medicated, owners often comment on how the dog is acting like a puppy again and only then realise that it wasn't normal for a 6-year-old Labrador to only manage to walk 20 feet before collapsing in a heap or stopping for a nap.

As discussed in Chapter 3, chronic pain usually presents as signs of depression, loss of appetite, reduced activity, a general lack of interest in life and a reduced pain threshold. There are very few formal studies looking at chronic pain scoring in animals – the model most commonly studied is chronic lameness, typically due to osteoarthritis. The degree of lameness is taken as a measure of limb pain, and can be scored subjectively using types of the SDS (see below) or VAS (Fig 4.6), and objectively by using kinesiology (studies on movement) such as force plate gait analysis and kinematic gait analysis. The diagnosis and scoring of chronic pain is generally very reliant on a thorough owner history, and pain questionnaires may be very useful for capturing relevant information. N.B. The most effective diagnostic technique for the presence of chronic pain is response to analgesic therapy.

Force plate gait analysis

Force plate (or kinetic) gait analysis is currently used experimentally to evaluate lameness and response to treatments for osteoarthritis. Force plate analysis involves measuring the forces applied by the patient to each limb, whilst it is running in a controlled manner on a treadmill. Dogs need to be trained to use the treadmill before measurements can be taken, and are required to run within a set speed range. Gait

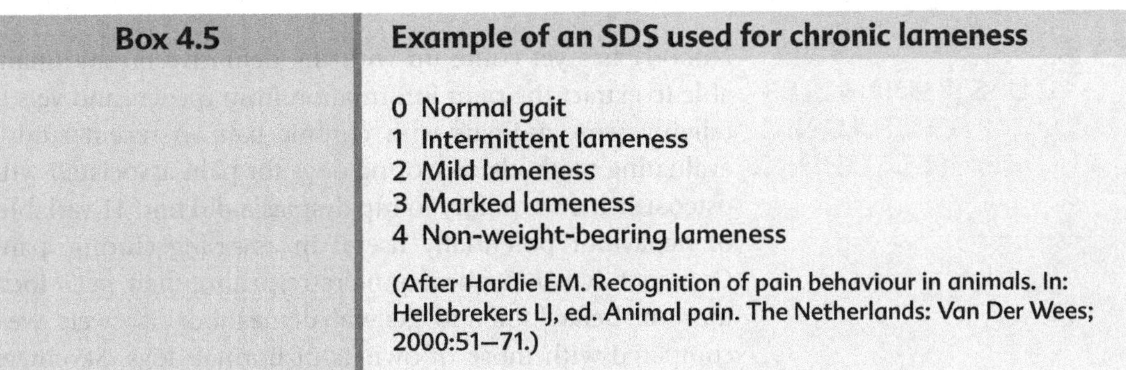

Box 4.5 Example of an SDS used for chronic lameness

0 Normal gait
1 Intermittent lameness
2 Mild lameness
3 Marked lameness
4 Non-weight-bearing lameness

(After Hardie EM. Recognition of pain behaviour in animals. In: Hellebrekers LJ, ed. Animal pain. The Netherlands: Van Der Wees; 2000:51–71.)

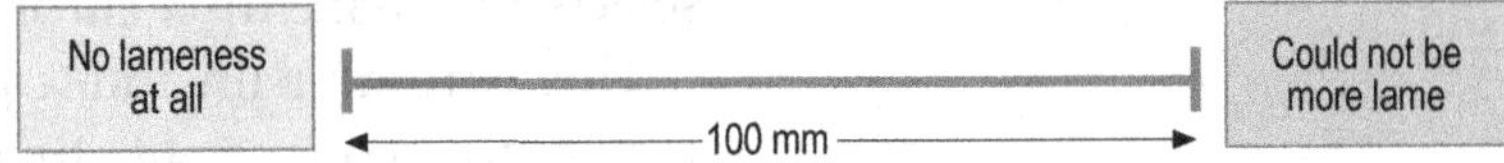

Figure 4.6
Example of a VAS used for chronic lameness. (After Hardie EM. Recognition of pain behaviour in animals. In: Hellebrekers LJ, ed. Animal pain. The Netherlands: Van Der Wees; 2000:51–71.)

is divided into two phases, the swing phase is the time the foot is in the air, and the stance phase is the time when the foot is in contact with the ground. The swing and stance phase add together to give one stride. The force plate measures ground reaction forces in three planes: vertical, mediolateral (side to side) and craniocaudal (front to back). Lots of data can be generated using this technique – peak vertical force and vertical impulse and amplitude of craniocaudal forces seem to be the most useful, all being reduced by lameness.[13]

Kinematic gait analysis

This technique of measuring lameness looks at joint movements, rather than the forces applied. This technique involves analysing joint movement data, obtained by putting fluorescent spots on joints and filming the patient running on a treadmill. The latest developments involve combining force plate and kinematic data to give information on the forces and movements for limbs and joints. Normal values for all these measurements need to be clearly established before any scaling can be done for scoring the degree of joint dysfunction and pain.

OWNER QUESTIONNAIRES FOR CHRONIC PAIN SCORING

Nobody has yet come up with the definitive questionnaire able to extract the right information from owners and vets to reliably score animals with chronic pain. A recent study[14] evaluating methods of scoring dogs for pain associated with osteoarthritis secondary to hip dysplasia did find 11 variables of behaviour potentially useful in assessing chronic pain. Owners filled in a questionnaire regarding their pet's locomotion, behaviour and general demeanour. Answers were compared with those of owners of normal dogs. Seventeen questions were found to give significantly different scores between the two groups of owners, and 11 were finally selected to make up a chronic pain index (Table 4.4).

This chronic pain index gives a lowest score of 0, and a maximum score of 44. In the study, normal dogs had an index or score of 0–5, whilst dogs with osteoarthritis had scores of 7–35. The authors suggest that a score <6 indicates a normal dog, and scores >6 indicates the presence of chronic pain (a score of 6–11 is a grey area for whether dogs presently have chronic pain). Other categories that weren't included in the final index but did show significant increases in dogs with chronic pain compared to normal dogs were excessive panting, and vocalisation when stretching legs caudally. Painful dogs were significantly less willing to jump and pace, and had significantly greater scores for problems climbing and descending stairs. Interestingly, the study found many owners had not considered that their dogs might be in pain because there had been no vocalisation. Vocalisation with chronic pain (if it's present at all) is probably only limited to grunting on expiration, whining or whimpering and yet humans still seem to innately consider it an essential necessity for acknowledging the presence of pain in animals. It's analogous to thinking that people are only truly feeling sad if they are observed in floods of uncontrollable tears, accompanied by some wailing and gnashing of teeth, and that if they're not they must be perfectly happy. This study concluded that chronic pain assessment using a multifactorial questionnaire, is most accurate when both the owner and vet are involved. The owner can give valuable information on changes in demeanour and behaviour, whilst the vet may be better placed to assess functional changes such as lameness

Table 4.4

Chronic pain index (scale) for dogs with hip osteoarthritis, forming an owner questionnaire[14]

Category	Descriptor	Score
Positive behaviour		
Mood	Very alert	0
	Alert	1
	Neither alert nor indifferent	2
	Indifferent	3
	Very indifferent	4
Willingness to participate in play and games	Very willing	0
	Willingly	1
	Reluctantly	2
	Very reluctantly	3
	Does not participate at all	4
Negative behaviour		
Vocalisation (audible complaining)	Never	0
	Hardly ever	1
	Sometimes	2
	Often	3
	Very often	4
Locomotion, willingness to		
Walk	Very willingly	0
	Willingly	1
	Reluctantly	2
	Very reluctantly	3
	Does not participate in action at all	4
Trot	Very willingly	0
	Willingly	1
	Reluctantly	2
	Very reluctantly	3
	Does not participate in action at all	4
Gallop	Very willingly	0
	Willingly	1
	Reluctantly	2
	Very reluctantly	3
	Does not participate in action at all	4
Locomotion, ease with which the dog		
Lies down	With great ease	0
	Easily	1
	Neither easily nor with difficulty	2
	With difficulty	3
	With great difficulty	4
Gets up from prone position	With great ease	0
	Easily	1
	Neither easily nor with difficulty	2
	With difficulty	3
	With great difficulty	4
Locomotion, frequency dog has		
Problems in moving after rest	Never	0
	Hardly ever	1
	Sometimes	2
	Often	3
	Very often	4
Problems in moving after major activity	Never	0
	Hardly ever	1
	Sometimes	2
	Often	3
	Very often	4

Table 4.5
Behaviour disturbances likely to be associated with chronic pain in dogs, and the percentage of owners of 13 dogs who reported them

Behaviour			
Decreases or disappears		***Appears or increases***	
Mobility	85%	Dependence	15%
Activity	62%	Aggression	23%
Appetite	23%	Anxiety	38%
Curiosity	31%	Compulsive behaviour	23%
Sociability	46%	Daytime sleeping	38%
Playfulness	38%	Drinking	8%
Marking	8%	Fearfulness	15%
Positive demeanour	*	Vocalising	38%
		Restlessness	15%
		Negative demeanour	*

*No value given
(After Wiseman ML, Nolan AM, Reid J, Scott EM. Preliminary study on owner-reported behaviour changes associated with chronic pain in dogs. Vet Record 2001; 149:423–424, reproduced with permission.)

and gait abnormalities and help direct owners' awareness to the potential signs of pain in their pets.

Another recent paper,[15] from Glasgow University, has also used owner-reported changes in their dogs' behaviour to help establish signs likely to be associated with chronic pain and therefore useful in the development of a chronic pain scale. Owners of 13 pet dogs diagnosed with chronic osteoarthritis were interviewed about any changes they had noticed since the dog developed the painful condition or since its treatment. Table 4.5 lists the behaviours identified by owners that are likely to be associated with chronic pain plus the direction of change and the percentage of owners who reported the disturbance (which gives an indication of how common each of these signs of chronic pain may be).

PHYSIOLOGICAL AND OBJECTIVE MEASURES OF CHRONIC PAIN

The role of stress hormones and changes in their concentrations in chronic pain in animals is unknown. In the study looking at a chronic pain index for dogs with hip osteoarthritis,[14] blood levels of the stress hormones, cortisol, adrenaline, noradrenaline and also β-endorphin were measured. The results suggested that chronic pain may decrease plasma β-endorphin concentration, but increase adrenaline, cortisol and vasopressin (antidiuretic hormone) levels. However, there was no correlation between the pain scores given by the assessors and hormone concentrations and much more work needs to be done before these parameters can be established as a useful tool in chronic pain scoring. Other potentially useful measures that could be incorporated into chronic pain scoring systems and/or owner questionnaires include mechanical threshold testing, changes in body weight, changes in growth rate, total food consumption, time taken to consume food or start locomotion, kinesiology studies (for lameness, described earlier), total time spent sleeping, and total activity time.

HUMAN PAIN SCALES

The animal pain scales in use now have been derived from human pain scales, hence the information and experience gained from pain scoring in humans, particularly the non-verbal kind such as young children, can be very useful in the veterinary setting. There are three approaches to the measurement of pain in people; self-reporting either verbally or using self-rating scales, behavioural, measured by observation and rating of behaviour, and physiological responses. In animals we are currently reliant on the latter two of these approaches.

Self-reporting human pain scales

The VAS is the scale of choice in adults and children over 5 years of age for measuring pain intensity. It has proven to be reliable and valid, simple and quick for the patient to use, and minimally intrusive (after all, human patients wouldn't be over keen on an observer popping round to handle, manipulate and encourage them to trot around the ward every few hours). The VAS has also been used in people to try and gauge the nature of the pain, by asking patients to rate the unpleasantness of their experience. The scale end points are labelled 'not bad at all' to 'the most unpleasant feeling imaginable'. By asking patients to rate themselves before and after analgesic treatment, or to rate the percentage change they feel in the pain using a VAS, a numerical measure of analgesic effectiveness can be taken. Another version of the

VAS, the visual analogue thermometer (VAT) has been developed for children and people with perceptual-motor problems or difficulty comprehending a VAS. This is basically a white cardboard strip, with a black opening 10cm long running across it left to right, the ends of which are labelled 'no pain' and 'unbearable pain'. The patient moves a red line along the opening, operated by a tab, to the point that corresponds to the intensity of their pain.

Faces scales are a form of self-reporting scale used in children between the ages of around 3 to 12 years to measure pain intensity. They consist of a series of faces, drawings or photos, expressing increasing amounts of pain or distress. Each face is assigned a score reflecting its order within the scale; children are asked to choose the face that shows or matches how they themselves are feeling. Fig 4.7[16] is the Oucher scale, a variant of the faces scale, which is very well validated and shown to be sensitive.

However, all these scales discussed above are unidimensional; they only measure pain intensity, but give no idea of the nature of the pain, or how it's making the patient feel overall. It would be like describing a painting only in terms of its brightness, with no reference to colour, texture of the paint, subject matter or how pleasing to the eye it is.

The McGill Pain Questionnaire (MPQ) was developed in the 1970s to assess the multidimensional nature of pain, and is now one of the most frequently used self-rating pain scales in humans, having proven to be reliable, valid and consistent. The scale was originally formulated by asking groups of students and physicians to classify words into categories that described different aspects or qualities of a painful experience. Three categories of words were established and within each category, words that described the different levels of intensity of each quality were established.

1. *Sensory qualities* – words that described the type of pain being experienced, in terms of the properties of the pain.
   For example, thermal – the different levels of intensity of this sensory quality go from hot, burning, scalding, and up to searing.
   For example, constrictive pressure – the different levels of intensity of this sensory quality go from pinching, pressing, gnawing, cramping, and up to crushing.

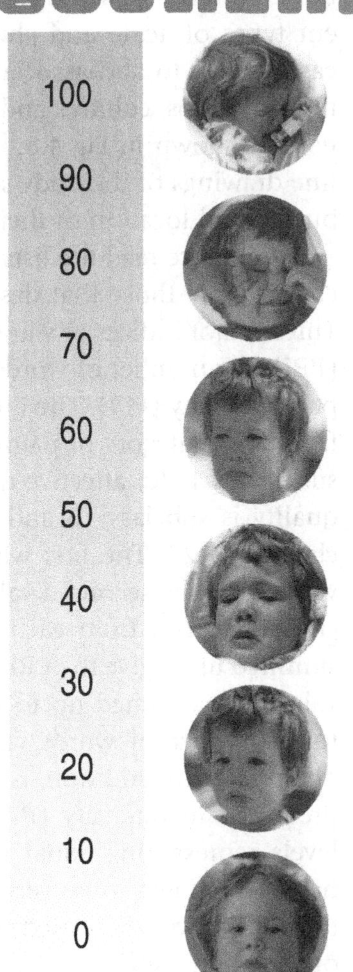

Figure 4.7
The Caucasian version of the Oucher scale, developed and copyrighted by Judith E. Beyer, RN, PhD, 1983. (From McGrath P, Unruh AM. Measurement and assessment of paediatric pain. In: Wall PD, Melzack R, eds. Textbook of pain, 4th edn. Edinburgh: Churchill Livingstone; 1999: 371–384[16], reproduced with permission.)

2. *Affective qualities* – words that describe how the patient feels as a result of the pain.
   For example, fear – the different levels of intensity of this quality go from fearful, frightful, and up to terrifying
   For example, tension – the intensity is described as either tiring or exhausting.
3. *Evaluative* – words that describe the subjective overall intensity of the total pain experience.
   For example, anchor words – ranging from mild, annoying, discomforting through to horrible, unbearable and excruciating.

This early work established a 'language of pain' for the questionnaire, providing a meaningful vocabulary for different types of acute and chronic pain, which patients could easily relate to and associate with across different socioeconomic groups, cultures and nationalities. The final questionnaire is shown in Fig 4.8.[17] The questionnaire also contains line drawings of the body so the patient can show the distribution and location of their pain.

Patients are read the lists of descriptor words and asked to choose only those that describe their pain at that moment. Three major indices or values are taken: the pain rating index (PRI), the number of words chosen (NWC), and the present pain intensity (PPI). The PRI is the sum of all the rank scores from each category of pain quality. The sensory qualities are subclasses 1–10, affective qualities are 11–15, the evaluative quality is subclass 16 and miscellaneous qualities are subclasses 17–20. The first word listed in each subclass has a value of 1, the second a value of 2, etc. After the patient has chosen a word from each relevant subclass, the values are summed up to give the PRI for each category, and then all the values are summed up to give a total PRI, the PRI(T). The total number of words chosen (NWC) is also calculated. The patient, in addition, is asked for an overall score of their present pain intensity (PPI) on a scale of 1 to 5, the five levels representing equal intervals on the scale. The MPQ has been shown to be very reliable, validated and is proven to be sensitive when used to assess mild pain (more so than other scales) and changes in pain after analgesic intervention.[17] Of great interest has been the demonstration that the MPQ can discriminate between different types of pain, even different types of headache such as cluster headaches and migraines.

Another interesting finding from the use of the MPQ is the fact that there seems to be remarkable consistency in the choice of words by patients suffering the same or similar pain syndromes. It would be useful to bear these characteristic pain descriptors in mind when treating veterinary patients with comparable diseases, to provide more insight into their potential suffering. Table 4.6 lists some study results[17] that found descriptors characteristic of some human pain syndromes (only those relevant to animals have been included).

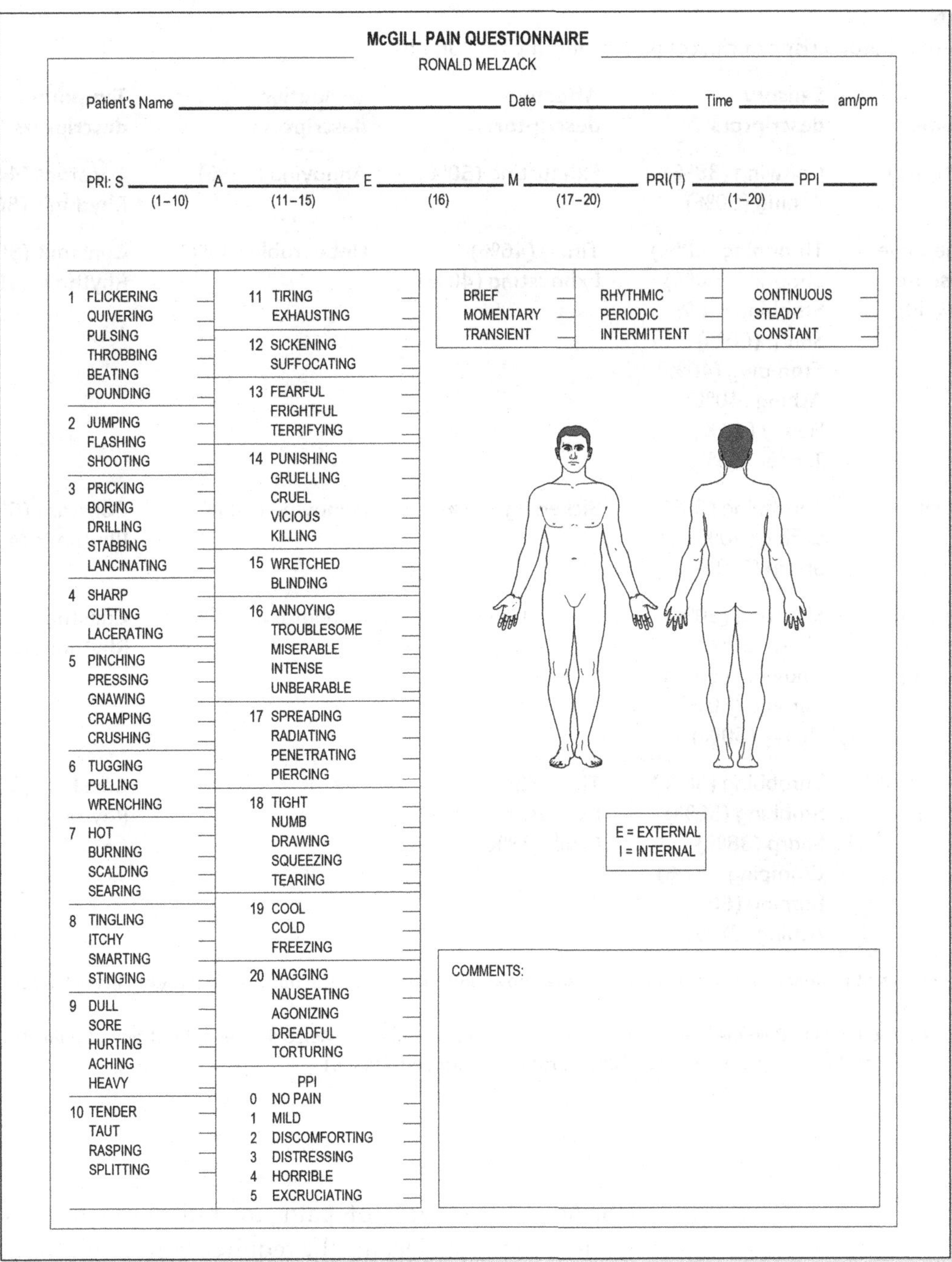

McGILL PAIN QUESTIONNAIRE

RONALD MELZACK

Patient's Name ______________ Date ________ Time ________ am/pm

PRI: S ______ (1–10) A ______ (11–15) E ______ (16) M ______ (17–20) PRI(T) ______ (1–20) PPI ______

1 FLICKERING — QUIVERING — PULSING — THROBBING — BEATING — POUNDING —	11 TIRING — EXHAUSTING —
2 JUMPING — FLASHING — SHOOTING —	12 SICKENING — SUFFOCATING —
3 PRICKING — BORING — DRILLING — STABBING — LANCINATING —	13 FEARFUL — FRIGHTFUL — TERRIFYING —
4 SHARP — CUTTING — LACERATING —	14 PUNISHING — GRUELLING — CRUEL — VICIOUS — KILLING —
5 PINCHING — PRESSING — GNAWING — CRAMPING — CRUSHING —	15 WRETCHED — BLINDING —
6 TUGGING — PULLING — WRENCHING —	16 ANNOYING — TROUBLESOME — MISERABLE — INTENSE — UNBEARABLE —
7 HOT — BURNING — SCALDING — SEARING —	17 SPREADING — RADIATING — PENETRATING — PIERCING —
8 TINGLING — ITCHY — SMARTING — STINGING —	18 TIGHT — NUMB — DRAWING — SQUEEZING — TEARING —
9 DULL — SORE — HURTING — ACHING — HEAVY —	19 COOL — COLD — FREEZING —
10 TENDER — TAUT — RASPING — SPLITTING —	20 NAGGING — NAUSEATING — AGONIZING — DREADFUL — TORTURING —
	PPI: 0 NO PAIN — 1 MILD — 2 DISCOMFORTING — 3 DISTRESSING — 4 HORRIBLE — 5 EXCRUCIATING —

BRIEF —	RHYTHMIC —	CONTINUOUS —
MOMENTARY —	PERIODIC —	STEADY —
TRANSIENT —	INTERMITTENT —	CONSTANT —

E = EXTERNAL
I = INTERNAL

COMMENTS:

Figure 4.8
The McGill Pain Questionnaire. The descriptors fall into four major groups: sensory, 1–10; affective, 11–15; evaluative, 16; miscellaneous, 17–20. The rank value for each descriptor is based on its position in the word set. The sum of the rank values is the pain rating index (PRI). The present pain intensity (PPI) is based on a scale of 0–5. (From Wall PD, Melzack R, eds. Textbook of pain, 4th edn. Edinburgh: Churchill Livingstone; 1999:409–426, reproduced with permission.)

Table 4.6
Descriptors characteristic of clinical pain syndromes in humans

Pain syndrome	Sensory descriptors	Affective descriptors	Evaluative descriptors	Temporal descriptors
Arthritic pain n = 16	Gnawing (38%) Aching (50%)	Exhausting (50%)	Annoying (38%)	Constant (44%) Rhythmic (56%)
Degenerative disc disease pain n = 10	Throbbing (40%) Shooting (50%) Stabbing (40%) Sharp (60%) Cramping (40%) Aching (40%) Heavy (40%) Tender (50%)	Tiring (46%) Exhausting (40%)	Unbearable (40%)	Constant (80%) Rhythmic (70%)
Toothache n = 10	Throbbing (50%) Boring (40%) Sharp (50%)	Sickening (40%)	Annoying (50%)	Constant (60%) Rhythmic (40%)
Cancer pain (metastatic carcinoma) n = 8	Shooting (50%) Sharp (50%) Gnawing (50%) Burning (50%) Heavy (50%)	Exhausting (50%)	Unbearable (50%)	Constant (100%) Rhythmic (88%)
Phantom limb pain n = 8	Throbbing (38%) Stabbing (50%) Sharp (38%) Cramping (50%) Burning (50%) Aching (38%)	Tiring (50%) Exhausting (38%) Cruel (38%)		Constant (88%) Rhythmic (63%)

The percentages of patients who chose each word are shown in brackets, n = the number of patients in each pain syndrome group

(From Melzack R, Joel K. Pain measurement in persons in pain. In: Wall PD, Melzack R, eds. Textbook of pain, 4th edn. Edinburgh: Churchill Livingstone; 1999:409–426, reproduced with permission.)

Behavioural measures of pain in humans

Behavioural measures of pain are only used in preverbal infants and people lacking the required communication skills to use self-reporting pain scales, as the patient's self-report is considered the most valid measure of a pain experience. This is because of all the same difficulties encountered in interpreting changes in behaviour associated with pain in animals, e.g. some people are naturally more stoic and remain calm

Table 4.7
Postoperative pain measure for parents

Did your child:
Whine or complain more than usual?
Cry more easily than usual?
Play less than usual?
Not do the things he/she normally does?
Act more worried than usual?
Act more quietly than usual?
Have less energy than usual?
Refuse to eat?
Eat less than usual?
Hold the sore part of his/her body?
Try not to bump the sore part of his/her body?
Groan or moan more than usual?
Look more flushed than usual?
Want to be close to you more than usual?
Take medications when he/she normally refuses?
One point for each 'Yes' answer
Six or more points suggest clinically significant pain

(From McGrath P, Unruh AM. Measurement and assessment of paediatric pain. In: Wall PD, Melzack R, eds. Textbook of pain, 4th edn. Edinburgh: Churchill Livingstone; 1999:371–384, reproduced with permission.)

despite their true subjective feelings, children's behavioural responses to pain change as they develop (seriously ill neonates may have substantially different responses than healthy individuals of the same age) and behaviours such as crying and facial expression can be associated with other states such as anxiety or hunger.

Measures of acute pain in neonates utilise changes in facial expression, including brow bulging, squeezing eyes shut, deepening of the nasolabial furrow, open mouth and crying. Other scales look at gross body movements, like limb kicking and position, withdrawal and tensing of the torso, which can vary according to age. Behavioural measures of longer lasting pain are less well developed. There is a scale called the Postoperative Pain Measure for Parents,[17] that has been shown to be both very sensitive and specific in detecting clinically significant pain (Table 4.7). This human scale is worth considering as a rough guide for questions to ask owners of animals at postop checks.

Another pain assessment tool used in paediatric medicine that may be potentially useful on the veterinary side for focussing owners' attention when taking a history is the Non-Communicating Children's Pain Checklist[16] (Table 4.8).

Physiological measures of pain in humans

As seen in animals, physiological changes are generally unreliable as sole measures of pain because they are influenced by so many other factors. In humans, heart rate, sweating, transcutaneous oxygen, and the stress response (e.g. plasma cortisol levels), electromyographic activity, cortical evoked potentials and electrodermal activity are considered valid measures; less so are respiration, endorphins and blood pressure.[16,17] An increase in heart rate associated with pain is the most widely used physiological measure in children. Transcutaneous oxygen is generally reduced in neonates subject to painful procedures. Sweating of the palms has been shown to be a sensitive indicator of pain in babies, in fact there is even a palmar sweat index in use, although it also reflects general distress not just pain. The stress hormones are increased with painful stimuli in infants, but again can't be taken as being specific to pain because responses vary with drugs, baselines and age amongst many other factors. Another problem is that the physiological changes associated with pain often habituate or wane as the pain becomes more chronic.

Two composite scales using both behavioural and physiological measures have been established and are used clinically in paediatric medicine.[16] These are the Premature Infant Pain Profile (PIPP) and the COMFORT scale. The PIPP uses six measures (the values of which vary according to the age of the patient), these are behavioural state, change in heart rate, changes in oxygen saturation, brow bulge, eye squeeze and nasolabial furrow. The COMFORT scale is used in paediatric intensive care, and uses eight measures: alertness, calmness, respiratory response, physical movement, blood pressure, muscle tone and facial tension. Just the implementation of recording measurements of pain in children at regular intervals during hospitalisation has been shown to decrease pain by improving pain management.[16] The adoption of any basic pain assessment system in veterinary practice would hopefully result in similar improvements, just by highlight-

Table 4.8
The non-communicating children's pain checklist

Items and areas of the checklist
Vocal
Moaning, whining and whimpering
Screaming/yelling
A specific sound or vocalisation for pain, 'word' cry, type of 'laugh'
Please describe
Eating/sleeping
Eats less, not interested in food
Increase in sleep
Decrease in sleep
Social/personality
Not co-operating, cranky, irritable, unhappy
Less interaction, withdrawn
Seeks comfort or physical closeness
Difficult to distract, not able to satisfy or pacify
Facial expression of pain (cringe, grimace)
Furrowed brow
Change in eyes, including squinching of eyes, eyes wide opened wide, eyes frown
Turn down of mouth, not smiling
Lips pucker up, tight, pout or quiver
Clenches, grinds teeth, chews, thrusts tongue
Activity
Not moving, less active, quiet
Jumping around, agitated, fidgety
Body and limbs
Floppy
Stiff, spastic, tense, rigid
Specify body part/limbs
Gestures to or touches part of body that hurts
Protects or favours or guards part of body that hurts
Flinch or moves body part away, sensitive to touch
Moves body in specific way to show pain (head back, arms down, curls up, etc)
Physiological
Shivering
Change in colour, pallor
Sweating, perspiring
Tears
Sharp intake of breath, gasping
Breath holding

(From McGrath P, Unruh AM. Measurement and assessment of paediatric pain. In: Wall PD, Melzack R, eds. Textbook of pain, 4th edn. Edinburgh: Churchill Livingstone; 1999:371–384, reproduced with permission.)

ing the presence of pain in patients and the need for its treatment.

PROBLEMS WITH PAIN SCORING

Even if there was a fully validated reliable pain scale available, accuracy will always be limited by human observer bias. Humans' assessment of pain will inevitably be influenced by personal experience. Anybody who has had the misfortune of undergoing a painful surgical procedure will always have greater empathy with an animal in a similar situation and probably give them a higher pain score. The placebo effect will come into play if we administer an analgesic that we expect to work, and it is then likely that the next pain score given will be lower even if it's a borderline response. Assessors rarely like to give pain scores that are at either extreme of a scale; people are very reluctant to say an animal is in no pain at all or that they are observing the worst possible pain. This leads to the clustering of pain scores in the middle of a scale in most studies using several observers, which may not be a true reflection of the patient's level of pain.

Anthropomorphic behavioural signs of pain, particularly vocalisation, may be given greater weighting by an observer than more subtle signs. Vocalising animals would then end up with higher pain scores than another patient just showing a hunched appearance, when in fact hunching may reflect a more severe level of pain. Finally, the ability of humans to discriminate between lots of different levels of pain, even in themselves, is questionable. Previous studies[2] have found that adults using 100-point pain scales most accurately self-report only 11–21 levels of pain, and children self-report 6 levels of pain. Studies of accident and emergency department doctors have shown it takes an 18 mm change on a 100 mm VAS before they acknowledged a 'little more' or a 'little less' pain in the patient. Force plate studies on dogs with hip lameness found observers could not distinguish a change in weight bearing of less than 15%, which suggested that at most, only six levels of lameness could be detected by a human observer (although I wouldn't rush to tell an orthopaedic surgeon about this particular finding!).

IDEAL PAIN SCALES

An ideal pain scale for animals and humans is one that not only detects the presence or absence of pain, but can also measure the magnitude of its severity, i.e. intensity, the nature of the pain (e.g. throbbing, burning,) its location, and how it makes the patient feel in terms of suffering and the impact on their quality of life (e.g. sickening, exhausting, terrifying, agonising). An ideal pain scale would also be able to assess acute and chronic pain of visceral, somatic and neuropathic origin, in different species and age groups. Measures should have equal intervals between values on the scale. The scale should be reliable, sensitive and validated. Versatility is also important; this means the scale could just be picked up and used in a few seconds by any untrained observer and this would allow it to be rapidly adopted by the profession for everyday use to evaluate pain and response to analgesic treatment. The ultimate goal of an ideal pain scale would be to ensure that any pain in a patient is detected and the scoring system indicates to the vet the appropriate type and amount of analgesic treatment. Further scoring then determines the degree of pain relief and indicates the need for any further analgesia and the timings of repeat doses.

The way forward for developing pain scales in animals would appear to be a multidimensional approach, where several aspects of behaviour and physiological measures are used to assess the overall pain experience. This would include behaviour when undisturbed by an observer, behaviour with observer interaction and during gentle activity, and the inclusion of physiological measures. Owner assessment is also an invaluable source of information, especially for chronic pain. Other simple objective measures can be taken from owners such as sleep patterns, feeding behaviour and activity levels. It's likely that to maintain accuracy, pain scales need to be adapted for different species and ages, acute and chronic pain and for the particular surgical procedure being undertaken. Anticipated levels of pain, based on the degree of tissue injury may also provide a good baseline to consider when using a scoring system. It is also important to be aware on a personal level of the potential for observer bias when embarking on pain scoring patients.

Box 4.6	Top tips for pain scoring animals
	■ Ideally, the same knowledgeable person, responsible for pain management should score an animal throughout its time in the practice. ■ Remember to get a baseline for each patient wherever possible by making an assessment preop, or pre-pain, when the animal is considered to be in a normal state. ■ Make serial evaluations at regular intervals, preop, and postop or before and after analgesic therapy, until a full recovery is made. Pain can fluctuate and worsen over a short period of time. ■ Remember to record all pain scores in the patient's notes ■ Repeat reassessments should be made after analgesic therapy to determine response to treatment, whether additional analgesia is required and the timing of repeat doses to avoid a pain 'breakthrough'. ■ Handle and interact with the patient, carefully manipulate the painful area and encourage the patient to move around to make a more complete assessment. ■ Incorporate physiological measures into pain assessment, such as heart rate, respiratory rate, blood pressure, pupil size. Mechanical threshold testing in particular; cortisol, adrenaline and β-endorphin levels may be useful but are not realistic in a practice setting. ■ Take a thorough history from the owner (using questionnaires to direct the information) to help assess chronic pain.

REFERENCES

1. Lascelles L, Waterman A. Analgesia in cats. In Practice 1997; April:204
2. Hardie EM. Recognition of pain behaviour in animals. In: Hellebrekers LJ, ed. Animal pain. The Netherlands: Van Der Wees; 2000:51–71
3. Dobromylskyj P, Flecknell PA, Lascelles BDX, et al. Pain assessment. In: Flecknell P, Waterman-Pearson A, eds. Pain management in animals. London: Saunders; 2000
4. Conzemius MG, Hill CM, Sammarco JL, et al. Correlation between subjective and objective measures used to determine severity of postoperative pain in dogs. J Am Vet Med Assoc 1997; 210(11):1619–1621
5. Mathews KA. Pain assessment and general approach to management. In: Vet Clinics of North America: Small Animal Practice 2000: 30(4):729–755
6. Fox SM, et al. The effects of ovariohysterectomy plus different combinations of halothane anaesthesia and butorphanol analgesia on behaviour in the bitch. Res Vet Sci 2000; 68(3): 265–274
7. Holton LL, Scott EM, Nolan AM, et al. Comparison of three methods used for the assessment of pain in dogs. J Am Vet Med Assoc 1998; 212(1):61–66

8. Lascelles BDX, Cripps PJ, Jones A, et al. Efficacy and kinetics of carprofen, administered preoperatively or postoperatively for the prevention of pain in dogs undergoing ovariohysterectomy. Veterinary Surgery 1998; 27:568–582
9. Lascelles BDX, Cripps P, Mirchandani S, et al. Carprofen as an analgesic for postoperative pain in cats: dose titration and assessment of efficacy in comparison to pethidine hydrochloride. Journal of Small Animal Practice 1995; 36:535–541
10. Grisneaux E, Pibarot P, Dupuis J, et al. Comparison of ketoprofen and carprofen administered prior to orthopaedic surgery for control of postoperative pain in dogs. J Am Vet Med Assoc1999; 215(8):1105–1110
11. Firth AM, Haldane SL. Development of a scale to evaluate postoperative pain in dogs. J Am Vet Med Assoc 1999; 214:651–659
12. Reid J. Assessment and scoring pain. Proceedings of a Schering Plough Animal Health Pain Management Seminar. May 2003, Derby, UK
13. Innes JF. How to measure efficacy of treatments for osteoarthritis. ECVS Proceedings July 2003; 12th Annual Scientific Meeting, Glasgow, Scotland, UK
14. Hielm-Bjorkman AKH, Kuusela E, Liman A, et al. Evaluation of methods for assessment of pain associated with chronic osteoarthritis in dogs. J Am Vet Med Assoc 2003; 222(11): 1552–1558
15. Wiseman ML, Nolan AM, Reid J, Scott EM. Preliminary study on owner-reported behaviour changes associated with chronic pain in dogs. Vet Record 2001; 149: 423–424
16. McGrath P, Unruh AM. Measurement and assessment of paediatric pain. In: Wall PD, Melzack R, eds. Textbook of pain, 4th edn. Edinburgh: Churchill Livingstone; 1999: 371–384
17. Melzack R, Joel K. Pain measurement in persons in pain. In: Wall PD, Melzack R, eds. Textbook of pain, 4th edn. Edinburgh: Churchill Livingstone; 1999: 409–426

CHAPTER 5 THE PHYSIOLOGY OF PAIN

DEFINITION OF PAIN AND NOCICEPTION

The International Association for the Study of Pain defined pain as being 'an unpleasant sensory or emotional experience associated with actual or potential tissue damage or described in terms of such damage'. Nociception refers to just the sensory or physiological process involved in a painful experience, it is the detection or recognition of damaging or potentially damaging stimuli, which provides the animal with information related to any tissue damage. The term pain relates to how the overall experience makes the animal feel emotionally as well as physically.

The difference between nociception and pain is analogous to having the knowledge that the piece of cake you're about to eat contains an obscenely generous amount of double chocolate fudge brownie bits compared to the actual feeling of mood-enhancing delight as you consume it. Strictly speaking, nociception can be measured by looking at neurone electrical or chemical activity and could reasonably be assumed to be proportional to pain, although as discussed in previous chapters, quantifying the emotional component of pain in non-verbal animals is fraught with difficulties.

Going back to the cake analogy, the nutritional content of the cake can be measured, and the chocolate content can often be proportional to the ensuing deliciousness, but the actual feelings when you eat the cake can be affected by previous memories, or knowledge that the cake was made especially for you by a loved one, or even spoilt by the fact you're on a diet and that that was your fourth piece today, i.e. the overall emotional experience is a very individual one. It's just as impossible to quantify 'happiness' as it is to quantify 'unpleasantness' in different individuals. The emotional component of pain is rustled up in the highest centres of the brain as a result of many inputs from elsewhere in the central nervous system (CNS) (the brain and spinal cord) and body.

Nociception involves pain receptors (nociceptors) and nerve fibres in the periphery, spinal cord and brain. It consists of three processes termed transduction, transmission and modulation:

1. Transduction – the conversion of the noxious stimulus into an afferent nerve impulse, (an impulse that travels towards the CNS) at the peripheral nociceptor.
2. Transmission – the propagation or carriage of the nerve impulse through the peripheral nervous system, towards the CNS.
3. Modulation – this is the adjustment or dampening down of afferent impulses in the pain pathway by the body's own in-built analgesic system. When the CNS receives pain signals it sends efferent messages (impulses that travel in a direction away from the CNS) back down the spinal cord. Within the spinal cord these efferent signals modify further transmission of pain impulses from nociceptors. This is because the CNS signals cause the release of endogenous opioids and other neurotransmitters, which actually inhibit the processing of pain impulses.

The last step in the overall pain pathway is 'perception'. This entails the integration of information from the nocicep-

Box 5.1 **The pain pathway**

Nociception

The physiological component of pain, comprising:

a. Transduction — conversion of a noxious stimulus into a nerve impulse by nociceptors
b. Transmission — the carriage of impulses along nociceptor fibres to the CNS
c. Modulation — the inhibition of pain signals in the CNS by the body's in-built analgesic system

Perception

The overall conscious, emotional experience of pain, produced by the integration of nociceptor information, plus many other CNS and body inputs in the cerebral cortex.

tor pathway in the cerebral cortex of the brain with other inputs (e.g. from memories, learnt experiences, etc), to produce the conscious, subjective, emotional experience of pain. Having an understanding of nociception and the anatomy and physiology of the pain pathway allows a logical approach to pain management and the use of analgesic drugs, i.e. by interrupting the pain pathway at one or more points and/or enhancing the inherent analgesic system of modulation.

THE PAIN PATHWAY

Transduction

The nociceptive pathway starts with specialised primary sensory neurones, pain receptors (nociceptors) located throughout the body in the skin, peritoneum, pleura, periosteum, subchondral bone, joint capsules, blood vessels, muscles, tendons, fascia and viscera. Nociceptors are actually free nerve endings that respond to mechanical, thermal or chemical stimuli that may potentially or actually cause tissue damage. These stimuli cause ion channels to open in the nociceptor free nerve ending, which triggers an impulse (action potential) to be sent along the nerve fibre. These impulses can be in a continuous form or in bursts and the more intense or greater the noxious stimuli, the faster the rate of firing.

The fibres of nociceptors run to the spinal cord and end in the cell bodies of the fibres, which sit in the dorsal root ganglia. There are two types of nociceptor, Aδ fibre and C fibre, classified according to their type of fibre and stimulus that they respond to. Aδ type nociceptors respond to thermal or mechanical noxious stimuli and the impulses generated travel down their high-speed large diameter myelinated axons (at 5–30 m/s) and signal a sharp stinging or pricking sensation. This is sometimes referred to as 'first pain' and is well localised and transient, lasting only as long as the stimulus is activating the nociceptor. These Aδ type nociceptors are involved in the withdrawal reflex response. C type nociceptors detect a variety of noxious mechanical, chemical and intense hot or cold thermal stimuli. C type nociceptors have smaller diameter unmyelinated fibres that conduct impulses more slowly (at 0.5–2 m/s) to the spinal cord. Impulses from C type nociceptors intensify the pain signalled by the Aδ type ones and are responsible for a dull longer lasting pain that's more diffuse (i.e. a slow burning sensation) and persists after the noxious stimulus has stopped. This is sometimes referred to as 'second' or 'slow pain'. C types become increasingly important as a source of nerve impulses to the CNS if the noxious stimulus persists. Both types of nociceptor have a high threshold, and will therefore not be activated by low intensity innocuous (non-painful) stimuli. This compares with Aβ fibre mechanoreceptors that have a low threshold and are activated by innocuous stimuli such as touch, pressure, vibration and joint movement. Aβ mechanoreceptors have large rapidly conducting myelinated fibres that transmit innocuous tactile sensations at 30–70 m/s to the spinal cord.

Transmission

The cell bodies of Aδ and C nociceptors sit in the dorsal root ganglia of the spinal cord. The nociceptor neurones are often referred to as the 1st order neurones of the nociceptive pathway. Their cell bodies extend axons into the grey matter of the dorsal horn of the spinal cord and synapse with 2nd order neurones. These 2nd order neurones are of varying types and have different functions; they include:

1. Interneurones that are both excitatory and inhibitory, involved in local processing and modulation of pain signals.
2. Neurones extending over multiple spinal segments that are part of reflex arcs. They stimulate efferent fibres that cause muscle contraction, producing a simple motor withdrawal response.
3. Interneurones that project to sympathetic reflex arcs in the region of the initial injury that leads to the release of noradrenaline and local cardiovascular changes such as vasoconstriction.
4. Projection neurones that have axons ascending up the spinal cord into the fore and midbrain. There are three subtypes of these 2nd order projection neurons:
   a. Nociceptive-specific (NS) 2nd order neurones, which receive input from Aδ and C nociceptor fibres only, and are therefore only activated by noxious stimuli. These

neurones are arranged somatotopically in the spinal cord, i.e. in a way that maps the location of their inputs from around the body. Thus they respond to stimuli from discrete topographic areas of the body.

b. Wide dynamic range (WDR) 2nd order neurones. These receive input from Aδ and C fibres and also Aβ fibre mechanoreceptors. Their inputs converge from large areas of the body and originate from both somatic and visceral tissue (i.e. they have a large receptive field).
c. Complex neurones, which receive and integrate inputs from both somatic and visceral tissue.

All types of 2nd order neurones are interactive, and are involved in the initial modulation, processing and integration of pain information that will contribute to the animal's overall organised pain response. Projection neurones that ascend within the spinal cord to the brain form several tracts; the three most important are:

1. Spinothalamic tract – This is the most prominent nociceptive pathway in the spinal cord and it ascends to the thalamus (in the forebrain). One set of these neurones in this tract, which have received inputs from small discrete receptive fields in the periphery, are thought to be involved in the conscious localisation and characterisation of painful stimuli. Another set of neurones that have larger more diverse receptive fields are involved in the emotional reaction to the pain and overall response (changes in behaviour, autonomic stimulation).
2. Spinoreticular tract – Neurones in this tract reach the reticular formation in the brain stem and some will reach the thalamus. These neurones are also implicated in the perception of pain that leads to emotional reactions such as depression, anxiety and suffering. The reticular formation is also thought to be part of the brain responsible for level of sleep and consciousness. Therefore increased reticular formation stimulation from noxious inputs can overcome sleep and general anaesthesia (this explains the 'lightening' of an anaesthetised animal during a painful part of a surgical procedure). It is also an important area for descending modulatory pathways, which inhibit impulse transmission at spinal cord synapses.

3. Spinohypothalamic tract – a more recently discovered ascending nociceptive pathway that seems to contain neurones projecting directly to the hypothalamus in the forebrain. This is an additional route for activating an animal's response to pain as well as the associated neuroendocrine and autonomic changes (i.e. the stress response).

Perception

It is difficult to say at exactly what level within the CNS a nociceptive input becomes perceived as pain and causes feelings of suffering. The most likely level is up in the forebrain and cerebrum. Many different parts of the brain have been identified as being involved in nociception and pain perception.

Medulla oblongata, pons and midbrain

These structures are in the brainstem that connects the spinal cord to the cerebrum. They contain the centres for respiration, control of heartbeat, cranial nerve nuclei and long motor and sensory tracts running down to and up from the spinal cord. They contribute to nociception via connections to the reticular formation and periaqueductal grey matter (PAG).

Reticular formation

This is a network of fibre tracts and nuclei that extends from the spinal cord throughout the brainstem extending into the thalamus and hypothalamus. The reticular formation receives information from many other parts of the brain, and as mentioned earlier, is concerned with alertness, direction of attention to external events, sleep and has major effects on the sensory and motor systems. It can mediate sensory, motor and autonomic functions, which are all interconnected within the formation allowing overall activity to be unified. It sends out connections to the spinal cord, other motor and sensory nuclei in the brainstem, the hypothalamus, thalamus and the cerebral cortex. The reticular system seems to be critical to integration of the pain experience – nociceptive inputs have a profound effect on reticular neuronal activity. Neurones ascending from the reticular formation mediate the affective (emotional) and motivational aspects of pain as they project to the thalamus and limbic system. (The motivational aspect of pain is the initiation of purposeful action and movement by the animal in response to the pain.)

Periaqueductal grey matter (PAG) This is a core of grey substance in the midbrain. It is a major centre for integration for homeostatic control. Ascending projections carrying sensory nociceptive information extend from the PAG up to both the thalamus and hypothalamus. It also has an important role in descending modulation of pain (see later).

Hypothalamus This sits immediately above the pituitary gland in the forebrain. The hypothalamus integrates and processes information about the nervous and hormonal systems of the body. It receives information relating to hormone levels, physical and mental stress, the emotions, and the need for physical activity, and then responds by prompting the pituitary gland appropriately.

Thalamus This constitutes two masses either side of the midline in the forebrain. The thalamus receives sensory inputs from the spinal cord, midbrain, eyes, ears and the cerebral cortex. It is the collecting, coordinating and selecting centre for almost all sensory information, except olfactory (smell), received by the body and then sends on information up to the cerebral cortex amongst other places. It plays a key role in nociception and pain; its nuclei receive inputs that mediate both the sensory-discriminative aspects of pain (the type and nature of the pain) and inputs that contribute to the affective dimension of pain.

Limbic system This is part of the cerebrum, and is concerned with unconscious and autonomic functions such as respiration, body temperature, hunger, thirst, wakefulness, sexual activity plus their associated emotional reactions. Diseases of the limbic system in humans can cause emotional disturbances and instability such as aggression, depression, anxiety, spasmodic laughing and crying, violence and diminished sex drive. Its involvement in pain perception mediates aversive drive, and therefore influences the motivational component of pain and determines purposeful behaviour in response to pain.

Cerebral cortex The cerebral cortex, made up of layers of masses of nerve cell bodies, is the grey outer layer of the cerebral hemispheres that performs the higher neurological functions and is involved in memory and learning. This is where an animal's anticipation, learning, and associations from painful experiences are processed and established, sometimes referred to as the cognitive aspect of pain. The cortex is able to regulate and adjust the cognitive and aversive affective (unpleasant emotional) aspects of pain and to mediate increasingly complex behaviour patterns.

Modulation and descending control

Animals have an intrinsic analgesic system that inhibits ascending pain messages and their perception, via descending signals. This pain control or modulation system has four tiers:

1. The cortex and thalamus
2. PAG
3. The rostral medulla and pons of the brainstem
4. The dorsal horn of the spinal cord.

The PAG receives descending signals from the cortex, amygdala (area of cerebrum associated with memory) and thalamus, and is also modified by inputs from the medulla, reticular formation and spinal cord. The PAG is packed with opioid neurotransmitters and receptors thought to be involved in its antinociceptive activity (inhibition of pain). Stimulation of the PAG and release of endogenous opioids leads to outflow back down to the rostral ventromedial medulla (and also up to the thalamus, hypothalamus, and limbic system). Descending nociceptive inhibition arising from the PAG passes into the medulla of the brainstem, which contributes to antinociception and opioid analgesia. The descending inhibition then enters the spinal cord.

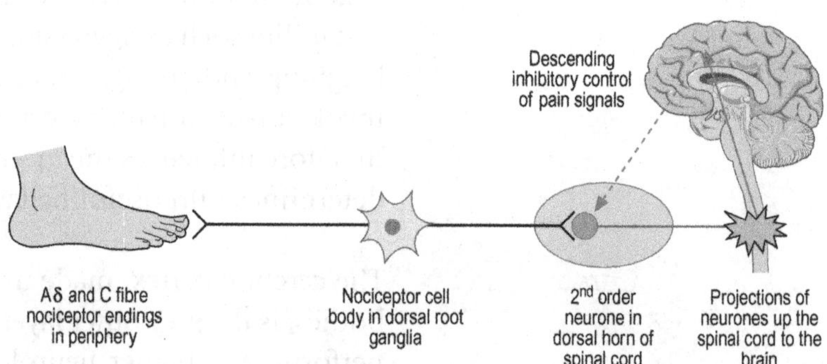

Figure 5.1
The simplified pain pathway.

The last level of modulation is within the dorsal horn of the spinal cord itself. Here, there is not only integration of afferent nociceptive information from around the body but just as much local modulation of ascending messages. There are many neurotransmitters in the spinal cord that will inhibit transmission of nociceptive impulses locally and also fine tune descending control from the brain.

THE GATE THEORY

Modulation of pain signals in the spinal cord by descending messages from the brain, and local inhibition (or excitation) by connecting interneurones, is sometimes referred to as 'gating' or the gate theory, famously discovered by Melzack and Wall in 1965. They proposed that the signal passed up to the brain in the pain pathway is a summation, or the net outcome of excitatory and inhibitory inputs in the spinal cord. A typical 2nd order dorsal horn neurone sat in the grey matter of the spinal cord may receive inputs from Aδ and C fibre nociceptors, and Aβ fibre mechanoreceptors, plus excitatory and inhibitory interneurones that are themselves connected to Aδ, C and Aβ fibres as well as descending neurones from the brain (Fig 5.2). (Aβ fibre mechanoreceptors have low thresholds and are activated by innocuous stimuli such as touch, pressure, limb movement and vibration.)

If the dorsal horn neurone receives pain signals from Aδ and C nociceptor fibres, they cause the neurone to fire, and this is exaggerated by the local excitatory interneuron, but it's

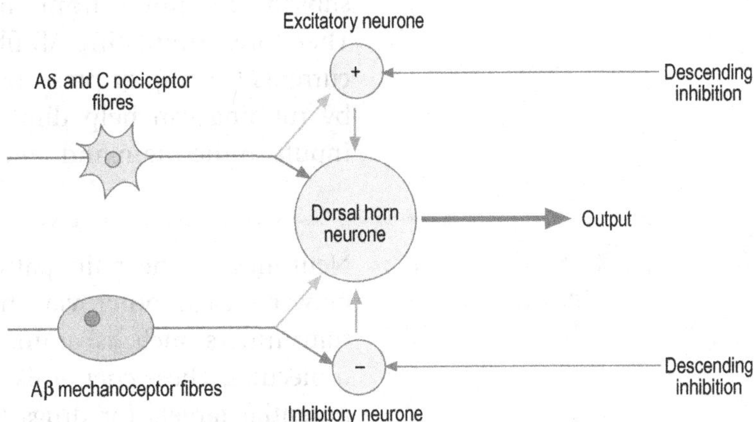

Figure 5.2
Modulation or gating of pain signals in the spinal cord. (From Wall P. Pain: the science of suffering. London: Phoenix; 1999:50, reproduced with permission.)

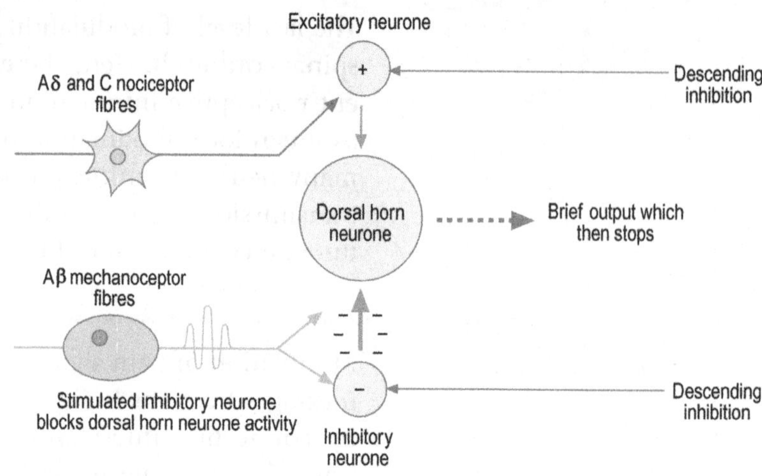

Figure 5.3
Innocuous stimuli are able to transiently block pain signals by closing the gate on noxious inputs in the dorsal horn. (After Wall PD, Melzack R, eds. Textbook of pain, 4th edn. Edinburgh: Churchill Livingstone 1999, p 51.)

also adjusted by descending control. The final signal sent up to the brain is the result of all these different influences. For example, if a dog is distracted by the lure of a squirrel, the brain may send down significant descending inhibition of the pain signal from a cut pad, and the squirrel still gets chased at that particular moment until the pain signals become more overwhelming. The gate theory also helps explain how rubbing a painful area, acupuncture and TENS (transcutaneous electrical nerve stimulation method of pain relief) can produce analgesia. If the dorsal horn neurone only receives inputs from Aβ fibres, it will just fire briefly before being switched off by an inhibitory interneurone connected to the Aβ fibre. This 'closing of the gate' then transiently blocks any subsequent inputs from the Aδ and C nociceptor fibres. Therefore, stimulating Aβ fibres by applying small electrical currents (TENS), or pressure from an acupuncture needle, or by rubbing can help diminish Aδ and C nociceptor fibre inputs to the brain and relieve pain (Fig 5.3).

NEUROTRANSMITTERS INVOLVED IN NOCICEPTION

Neurones in the pain pathway communicate information between each other via chemical signalling using neurotransmitters such as amino acids and other neuropeptide molecules. These chemicals and their receptors provide more potential targets for drugs to provide analgesia therapeutically. Neurotransmitters involved in pain transmission and modulation are classed as excitatory and inhibitory. These chemicals are produced, stored and released in the terminals of afferent nerves entering the spinal cord and interneurones in the dorsal horn. Examples of important excitatory neurotransmitters that facilitate nociceptive transmission include glutamate, aspartate (excitatory amino acids) and substance P, neurotensin, vasoactive intestinal peptide, calcitonin gene-related peptide and cholecystokinin (neuropeptides). Aspartate and glutamate also seem to be important excitatory mediators in the cortex and thalamus.

Neurotransmitters involved in descending inhibition of the pain pathway include GABA (gamma-aminobutyric acid), glycine, serotonin, dopamine, noradrenaline, acetylcholine and histamine, which all affect the overall excitability of the thalamocortex structures. In the PAG, endogenous opioids play a large role in descending modulation, these include endorphins, enkephalins and dynorphins. In the dorsal horn there are dense concentrations of GABA, opioids, glycine, serotonin, noradrenaline, which all produce inhibition of nociceptive transmission. Just to really demonstrate the complexity of the pain pathway, one neurone can contain several different neurotransmitters in its ending, the release of one neurotransmitter can have multiple actions in a given region of the CNS, and a single neurone can be influenced by many transmitters.

SENSITISATION

Once the pain pathway has been stimulated it can show changes in the way it responds to further painful stimuli, i.e. the pain pathway has plasticity. These changes result in the pain pathway responding more vigorously to painful stimuli, so the animal feels relatively more pain for the same noxious stimuli than before the changes (hyperalgesia), and previously non-painful stimuli may now feel painful (allodynia). This phenomenon is called sensitisation of the pain pathway and is a result of changes in the periphery called peripheral sensitisation, and changes up in the CNS called central sensitisation or wind-up.

Peripheral sensitisation

Under normal conditions out in the periphery Aδ and C fibre nociceptors all have a relatively high threshold, and if a noxious stimulus reaches or exceeds this threshold the nociceptor is activated and sends an impulse off down its nerve fibre to the spinal cord. This threshold is fairly consistent between different individuals and species. Innocuous stimuli such as touch or pressure would not reach the high threshold of a nociceptor and therefore would not elicit a pain response. However, they would be detected by another set of sensory neurones in tissue, the Aβ fibre mechanoreceptors that have a low threshold and respond to innocuous stimuli such as pressure, touch and vibration. So for example, if you dropped a banana on your toe, this would not be enough to stimulate a nociceptor, but it would elicit a response from a mechanoreceptor. The mechanoreceptor sends an impulse off to the spinal cord where it's relayed up to the brain and you would just be made aware of something touching your toe, but it's not painful (Fig 5.4).

If, however, you replaced the banana with a hefty 10kg pineapple, then that would exceed the threshold of nociceptors in the toe. The nociceptors would fire an impulse off to the spinal cord, where it's adjusted and finally sent up to the brain where you would consciously perceive pain (Fig 5.5).

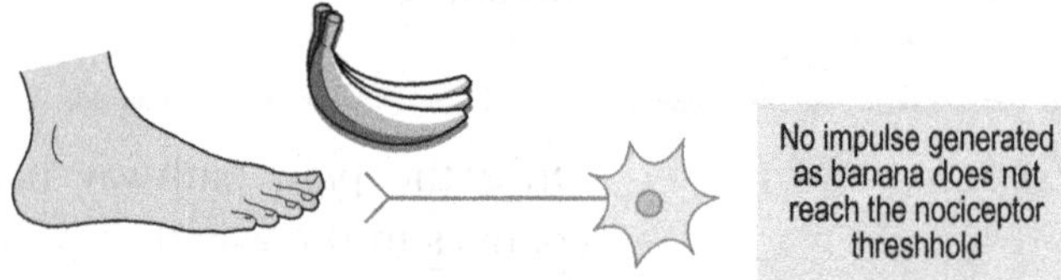

Figure 5.4
A non-painful stimulus (a banana) will not elicit a pain response.

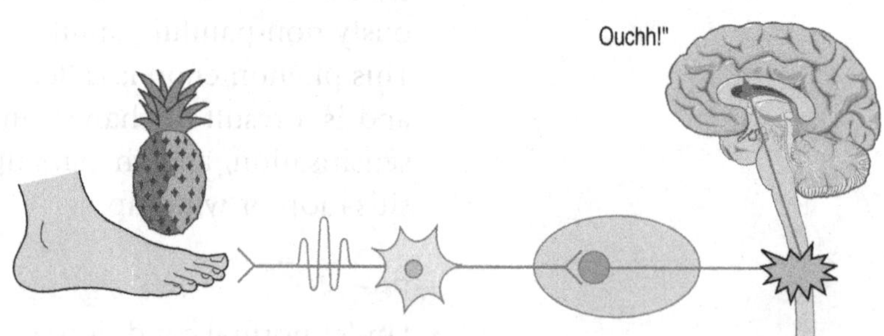

Figure 5.5
A 10kg pineapple exceeds the threshold of a nociceptor and elicits a pain response.

Whenever tissue is damaged by noxious stimuli, such as a speeding pineapple, then inflammation will ensue. The damaged cells in the area of injury will generate and release many different chemicals, mediators and modulators of inflammation. These chemicals are responsible for producing the four cardinal signs of inflammation in the damaged tissue – heat, swelling, redness and pain. Initial effects include vasodilation and leakage of proteins and fluid from capillaries. The chemicals also attract inflammatory cells into the area, macrophages, neutrophils, mast cells and lymphocytes that release more inflammatory mediators, and all these chemicals form what's known as a sensitising soup in the damaged tissue and adjacent surrounding area.

The sensitising soup contains hydrogen and potassium ions, enzymes such as proteases, cyclo-oxygenase 2 (COX-2), nitric oxide synthase (NOS) and prostaglandins, cytokines (e.g. interleukin-1, interleukin-6, tumour necrosis factor TNF), growth factors (nerve growth factor NGF), histamine, bradykinin, serotonin and noradrenaline. The soup not only directly stimulates nociceptors in the area, eliciting pain, but it also lowers the threshold of nociceptors, i.e. sensitises the nociceptors. This means the nociceptors now respond more vigorously to further noxious stimuli (hyperalgesia), and will generate an impulse in response to previously non-painful stimuli that are now able to reach the new low threshold (allodynia) (Fig 5.6).

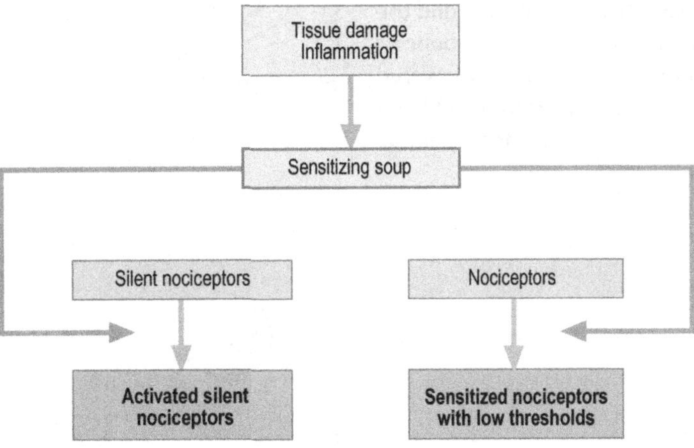

Figure 5.6
Peripheral sensitisation.

More recently there has been the discovery of another set of receptors in the periphery called 'silent nociceptors' (unmyelinated C fibres) that don't seem to respond to any stimuli at all under normal conditions. However, once they are exposed to a sensitising soup in inflamed tissue they become activated and start vigorously discharging impulses to the spinal cord and contribute to peripheral sensitisation. Activated silent nociceptors may respond to both innocuous and noxious stimuli. The area of tissue damage that's affected by peripheral sensitisation is sometimes referred to as the zone of primary hyperalgesia. It's also thought that sympathetic nerve activity in the region may also contribute or augment peripheral sensitisation.

Going back to the fruit analogy. Once the pineapple has been dropped and the toe damaged, inflammation and a sensitising soup will stimulate local nociceptors and lower their threshold. If you drop the pineapple a second time, it will far exceed the new low nociceptor threshold, eliciting a greater response than on the first occasion and resulting in you feeling relatively more pain. If you now drop the banana on the long-suffering toe, this stimulus will be able to reach the new lowered threshold of the sensitised nociceptor and result in a pain response (Fig 5.7).

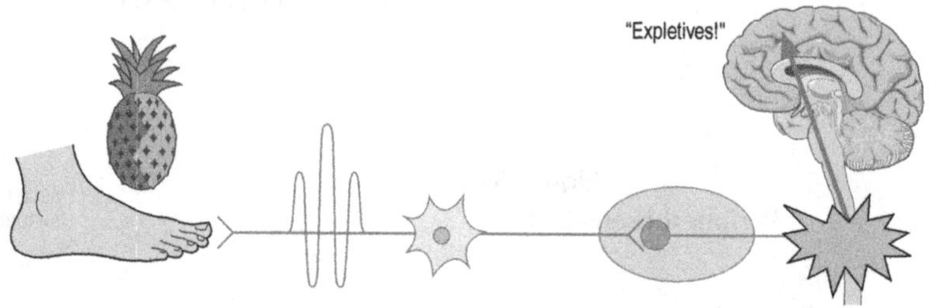

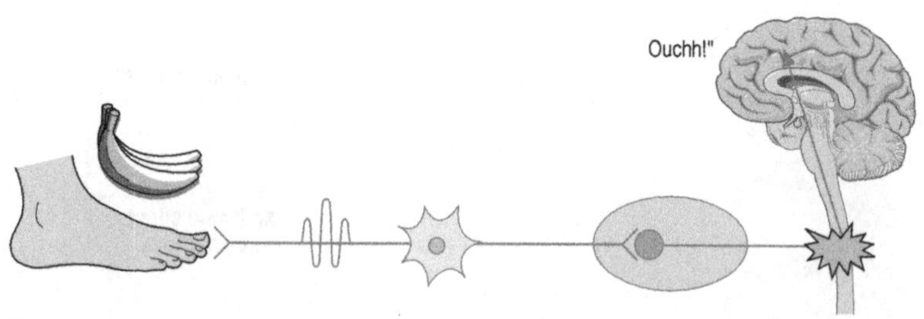

Figure 5.7
Peripheral sensitisation. A noxious stimulus (the 10 kg pineapple) elicits a greater response from the sensitised nociceptor and the previously non-painful banana now reaches the new lowered nociceptor threshold and feels painful.

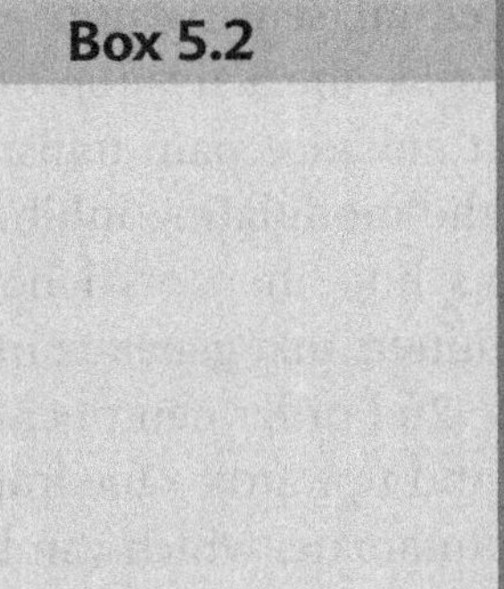

Box 5.2 **Peripheral sensitisation**

1. Nociceptor threshold is lowered by a sensitising soup generated in damaged inflamed tissue; this results in:
   - A noxious stimulus eliciting a greater response from the nociceptor, producing relatively more pain
   - A previously non-painful stimulus being able to reach the new lowered nociceptor threshold and eliciting a pain response.
2. Silent nociceptors are activated and elicit pain signals in response to both noxious and innocuous stimuli.

Central sensitisation or wind-up

If the neurones of the pain pathway up in the brain and spinal cord receive a bombardment of incoming painful impulses from the periphery, they too show changes in activity resulting in the amplification or an exaggeration of further painful inputs and recruitment of innocuous afferent signals. These changes are called central sensitisation and contribute to both hyperalgesia and allodynia. Central sensitisation is also responsible for what's known as secondary hyperalgesia, where an increased sensitivity to noxious stimuli occurs outside the immediate area of tissue damage (where nociceptor thresholds are unchanged).

When neurones in the dorsal horn of the spinal cord receive many afferents from the nociceptor Aδ and C fibres they become hyperexcitable, their thresholds drop and they start firing with greater duration and magnitude up to the brain. This means further pain inputs to the spinal cord are effectively exaggerated en route to the brain, and will persist after the nociceptor input from the periphery has actually stopped. There is also a change in the receptive field of spinal cord neurones in the pain pathway. Inputs from Aβ fibres that detect innocuous mechanical stimuli are recruited by sensitised dorsal horn neurones and are processed as pain signals, therefore generating pain. Dorsal horn neurones, e.g. wide dynamic range (WDR) 2nd order neurones, can receive inputs from large areas of the body. If they are hyperexcitable, they will amplify inputs from tissue outside the damaged area leading to secondary hyperalgesia.

The exact mechanisms of central sensitisation are very complex and numerous and involve the activation of chemical signalling mechanisms that enhance pain transmission and changes that also depress the modulating inhibition of pain signals. Nociceptive inputs into the dorsal horn will cause the release of neurotransmitters that generate impulses by causing depolarisation in the 2nd order neurones, propagating pain messages onwards and upwards. One important excitatory neurotransmitter is glutamate, which can bind to AMPA receptors (amino methylisoxazole proprionic acid), and NMDA receptors (N-methyl-D-aspartate) causing depolarisation of the next neurone. Initially, glutamate is unable to bind NMDA receptors as they are blocked by a magnesium ion. Once a pain signal has entered the dorsal horn, glutamate binds its AMPA receptor and this not only continues the pain signal, but also displaces the magnesium ion stuck on the NMDA receptors. This means the next time a pain impulse enters the dorsal horn both AMPA and NMDA receptors are available for binding glutamate, making the neurone with the receptors even more likely to depolarise, i.e. it becomes sensitised. It seems that incoming pain signals can also lead to increased synthesis of neurotransmitters and an upregulation in the numbers of their receptors, changes which would all contribute to the amplification of subsequent pain afferents.

Such changes can occur within minutes and hours of an initial pain stimulus. Just some of the neurotransmitters thought to be important in inducing central sensitisation include glutamate, substance P and BDNF (brain derived neurotrophic factor); the local release of prostaglandins and nitric oxide NO in the spinal cord are also implicated. Severe injuries and types of pain involving nerve damage can eventually cause the release of growth factors in the dorsal horn that result in sprouting of neurones and the formation of new synapses and 'rewiring'. It is thought that the degree of changes associated with central sensitisation probably depends on the intensity and duration of the initial painful stimulus, and that they should return to normal after the original injury resolves. However, central sensitisation can persist beyond the duration of healing of the original injury and lead to chronic pain syndromes (see later).

Box 5.3	Central sensitisation
	A bombardment of painful afferents cause changes in dorsal horn neurones in the pain pathway: ■ Neurones become hyperexcitable and exaggerate further painful inputs ■ Neurones start processing innocuous inputs from Aβ fibres as pain signals

Box 5.4	Sensitisation
	Sensitisation of the pain pathway produces hyperalgesia and allodynia. 1. Hyperalgesia – Increased or heightened pain response to a noxious stimulus. Results from: ■ Peripheral sensitisation, where nociceptors respond more vigorously to noxious stimuli ■ Central sensitisation, where hyperexcitable dorsal horn neurones exaggerate incoming nociceptor signals and fire with greater magnitude and duration up to the brain. 2. Allodynia – A previously non-painful stimuli now feels painful. Results from: ■ Peripheral sensitisation, where innocuous stimuli can now reach the new lowered threshold of nociceptors and elicit a pain signal (and silent nociceptors become activated) ■ Central sensitisation, where inputs from Aβ fibre mechanoreceptors, signalling innocuous stimuli like touch, are now processed as pain signals by dorsal horn neurones.

Duration of sensitisation

The changes in the pain pathway seen in sensitisation, both peripheral and central, would be expected to revert back to normal as the original tissue injury and inflammation resolves. However, the exact duration of sensitisation is unknown and probably varies according to the nature, intensity and duration of the initial noxious stimuli. If pain is established a long time, it takes a long time for the changes in the pain pathway to go back to normal. This makes sense if you consider that sensitisation can eventually lead to genes for the expression of receptors and neurotransmitters involved in pain transmission to be switched on and upregulated, and neurones to sprout and form new synapses, etc. It would be useful to ascertain when there are still significant changes present in the pain pathway, as this would help establish guidelines for the duration of postop analgesia, something that is still very much a topic for debate.

There has been some early work done, mainly in large animals, looking at the duration of sensitisation.[1] One study looked at dairy cows with mild and severe unilateral mastitis and used mechanical threshold testing on the hindlimbs (innervated by the same spinal segment as the udder) as a measure of sensitisation resulting from the mastitis, i.e. the pressure of a skin probe applied to the hindlimb at which the cows showed a pain response. In the cows with mild mastitis, changes in the mechanical threshold of the hindlimbs were reduced on the affected side for 7 days. This sensitisation started to fall off from 4 days. The sensitisation in cows with severe mastitis lasted up to 20 days. Another study on sheep undergoing exploratory laparotomy found changes in the pain pathway were back to normal by 7 days postop. Mechanical threshold testing has been used in lame sheep to demonstrate sensitisation of the pain pathway.[2] Sheep with chronic lameness were treated, and then assessed (with threshold testing) 2 weeks after the end of treatment when they were no longer clinically lame. In sheep that had had severe lameness, the mechanical threshold was still significantly lower than the control group with no history of lameness. It took up to 3 months after the end of treatment for the threshold to return to normal.

TYPES OF PAIN

Pain is often referred to as being physiologic or pathologic, depending on the state of the nervous system, and is also classified according to the tissue of origin (somatic, visceral or neuropathic) and duration (acute or chronic). Classification of pain in this way, and its analogy in human patients, enables a better understanding of the probable nature and characteristics of the pain being experienced by animals, who are unable to describe it. It also helps to indicate the most appropriate or effective type of analgesic therapy to use.

Physiologic and pathologic pain

Pain that is detected and processed by the pain pathway under normal conditions (before any sensitisation has occurred) is often referred to as physiologic pain. This is the pain that is produced by intense noxious stimuli that reach the high threshold of nociceptors, warning the animal of potential tissue damage and evoking reflex and avoidance behaviour. It serves as a protective mechanism as part of normal body defences. The intensity of physiologic pain is closely related to the intensity of the stimulus; it's well localised, transient and the pain pathway is able to provide information on the nature, location, duration, and intensity of the noxious stimuli. Innocuous stimuli do not normally evoke a pain response as they can only reach the low threshold of Aβ mechanoreceptors, and signal touch or pressure, etc.

Physiologic pain is processed in the spinal cord and descending inhibition will often suppress the signals. These mechanisms probably evolved to alert the animal to potential tissue damage but then allow the animal to escape from noxious stimuli and get away from danger. If the noxious stimulus is intense enough or causes any tissue damage, an inflammatory reaction is set off and peripheral sensitisation will occur. This results in a barrage of nociceptive signals reaching the spinal cord, resulting in central sensitisation. From an evolutionary perspective, sensitisation and increased pain perception forces the animal to rest and avoid both noxious and innocuous stimuli (such as lying on an open wound) that could cause further trauma and delay healing.

Pathologic or clinical pain is where significant tissue damage has occurred (usually during surgery) and the noxious stimulus is therefore ongoing and sensitisation of the pain pathway, hyperalgesia and allodynia are major features of the pain – so it can be elicited by Aβ fibres as well as Aδ and C fibres. Pathologic pain outlasts the stimulus, spreads to non-damaged areas and does not serve any useful function in a clinical setting (see Chapter 2). The aim is to minimise its occurrence in the first place by minimising sensitisation, and then to treat it as effectively as possible to optimise the patient's recovery. Pathologic pain can arise from injury to various types of tissue and can be classified into inflammatory pain (somatic and visceral) or neuropathic pain (involving damage to the nervous system itself), and also whether it is acute (recently occurring) or chronic (long lasting).

Somatic pain

Somatic pain arises from the stimulation of nociceptors in the skin and superficial muscles, joint structures, etc. that are frequently subject to external stimuli that can potentially cause tissue damage. These somatic nociceptors are numerous and respond to mechanical damaging stimuli, inflammatory mediators and other chemicals and thermal stimuli (hot and cold) as described earlier. Pain from somatic tissues is usually highly localised and it hurts at the site of the noxious stimulus. It tends to be of a sharp stabbing nature and if it radiates, the pain probably follows the distribution of the somatic nerve. Somatic pain is usually constant, although it can be periodic. Humans very rarely report nausea associated with somatic pain, unless there is bone involvement. Somatic pain can further be divided into superficial pain resulting from stimulation of nociceptors in the skin and deep pain arising from underlying structures like muscles, joints, tendons, periosteum and ligaments.

Visceral pain

Visceral pain arises from the stimulation of nociceptors located in abdominal or thoracic organs, and has quite different characteristics to somatic pain. Visceral nociceptors will rarely be exposed to the same sort of external stimuli as somatic ones but are more commonly subject to disease processes that don't necessarily cause tissue destruction. They are far more sensitive to ischaemia, inflammatory chemicals and distension (or stretch) than mechanical or thermal stimuli. Examples where such stimuli arise include ischaemia of the myocardium in people, inflammation of the bladder in cystitis or pancreatitis, and distension of the gastrointestinal tract. The threshold for visceral pain may be determined by the area of visceral tissue (and number of nociceptors) affected, rather than the intensity of the noxious stimuli at any one point. This means that a localised mechanical stimulus, such as a small bowel perforation, may feel less painful than mild stretching of the whole liver capsule.

Visceral nociceptors are more sparsely distributed than somatic ones, their afferent fibres branch widely and converge on the dorsal horn over a wide area (over a number of segments), which may explain why visceral pain is poorly localised and diffuse. Visceral pain tends to be dull and vague and may feel like a cramping or gnawing pain that fluctuates. It is more often periodic than constant and can build to peaks of pain. Humans often suffer from nausea and vomiting associated with visceral pain. The other characteristic feature of visceral pain is that it can be 'referred'; it can create the perception that the painful stimulus is originating from muscle or skin rather than viscera. Referred pain is thought to be due to the fact that both somatic and visceral nociceptive afferent fibres converge on the same dorsal horn neurones, and are also conveyed up to the brain in the same tracts. Pain signals originating from visceral receptors could be processed in the CNS as pain from the body surface nociceptors that share dorsal horn neurones. Although there is much less evidence, it does seem that visceral nociceptors are subject to peripheral sensitisation during inflammation in a similar way to somatic nociceptors.

Neuropathic pain

This is the pain generated by direct damage to peripheral nerves or the CNS. It results in several distinct types of hyperalgesia and allodynia due to both abnormalities in peripheral pain afferents and abnormal processing of pain inputs in the spinal cord and brain. If a peripheral nerve is cut or damaged it generates a massive aberrant input of nociceptor signals into the spinal cord. This results in intense excruciating pain and also produces a long lasting type of central sensitisation (involving NMDA receptors, glutamate and substance P). A few days after the nerve injury a second form of abnormal peripheral afferent signals develop: the injured nerve fibres and associated cell bodies in the dorsal root ganglion start firing spontaneously (ectopic discharges). This ectopic discharge is chronic and seemingly leads to excitation of other types of neighbouring sensory fibres (such as mechanoreceptors and sympathetic nerves). The proximal stump of severed nerves form benign swellings made up of a mass of nerve fibres, called neuromas, which are also capable of ectopic discharge.

Damaged C fibre nociceptors and neuromas are known to develop a new set of receptors, adrenoceptors, on their endings that will generate pain impulses when activated by adrenaline, released by adjacent sympathetic nerves. This results in what's known as 'sympathetically maintained pain', which contributes to driving the chronic neuropathic pain and adds to the severe allodynia and hyperalgesia arising from these peripheral changes.

As described earlier, central sensitisation will result from a barrage of incoming pain afferents to the CNS, which will be massive and persistent in the case of nerve fibre trauma. Central sensitisation contributes to the hyperalgesia and allodynia seen in neuropathic pain, but there are other unique central changes associated with this type of injury. The terminal ends of Aβ mechanoreceptors sprout branches that form new synapses with nociceptor neurones in the dorsal horn (Aβ mechanoreceptors normally terminate in deeper layers of the spinal cord than the Aδ and C nociceptors, which reside in more superficial layers). Sympathetic nerve fibres also sprout new connections with dorsal root ganglion cells, which is another mechanism for abnormal activation of nociceptive neurones. There may also be a loss of inhibition of pain signals in the spinal cord, again contributing to hyperalgesia. This could arise if Aβ mechanoreceptor fibres are severed (causing a loss of sensation in the innervated tissue) based on the Gate theory. Without Aβ fibre inputs, dorsal horn neurone output to the brain, in response to Aδ and C fibre inputs, will be uninhibited, and there will be no blocking or gating of these signals. Another loss of inhibition may arise by the release of an endogenous opioid antagonist, cholecystokinin (CCK), and a corresponding increase in the number of its receptors, in response to peripheral nerve injury. This effect would reduce descending inhibition that's mediated by opioids.

Neuropathic pain can be very severe and unresponsive to treatment. It is characterised in humans by spontaneous or persistent burning sensations, with a shooting quality, unusual tingling, crawling, or electrical sensations, combined with a loss of normal sensitivity to heat, etc. There is hyper-

Table 5.1
Comparison of different types of pain, as reported in human patients

Factors	Somatic pain	Visceral pain	Neuropathic pain
Radiation	May follow distribution of somatic nerve	Diffuse	Abnormal, may be 'shooting'
Character	Sharp and definite	Dull and vague, may be colicky, cramping, squeezing, etc	Burning, tingling, crawling or electrical sensations
Relation to stimulus	Hurts where the stimulus is, associated with external stimuli	May be referred to another area, associated with internal stimuli	May be referred, associated with external stimuli but of prolonged duration, and can also be spontaneous
Time relations	Often constant, sometimes periodic	Often periodic and builds to peaks, sometimes constant	Spontaneous, can be persistent or paroxysmal
Associated symptoms	Nausea usually only with deep somatic pain owing to bone involvement	Often nausea, vomiting, sickening feeling	Severe allodynia combined with loss of normal sensation (foci of numbness) Self-mutilation in animals

(After Cousins M, Power I. Acute and postoperative pain. In: Wall PD, Melzack R, eds. Textbook of pain, 4th edn. Edinburgh: Churchill Livingstone; 1999:447–491, with permission.)

algesia and severe allodynia (hyper-responsiveness to even very gentle mechanical stimuli such as bending of hairs); prolonged pain duration and referred pain with abnormal radiation can also be a feature. Obviously these signs are hard to diagnose in an animal, but self-mutilation may be a sign of neuropathic pain. It's very difficult to treat and often has a poor response to opioids. Table 5.1 summarises and compares what's known about the characteristics of visceral, somatic and neuropathic pain.

Phantom limb pain and stump pain

Humans that have sadly lost a limb often report that they can still feel the missing body part and a range of sensations arising from it, including severe pain in some patients. This has been termed phantom pain and is thought to be a particularly severe form of neuropathic pain resulting from the severing of large nerve trunks that innervated the limb. There is no reason to believe that some animals don't also experience the same pain as a consequence of similar surgery or trauma. The exact incidence of phantom pain in people is unknown but recent studies report rates of between 60% and 80%,[3] and the onset in the vast majority of sufferers was within the first 7 days after limb loss. It seems that phantom pain can gradually diminish over time (surveys suggest 1–5 years in people which is a huge proportion of a cat or dog's life). The nature of the pain, generally speaking, is reported as being intermittent, with bouts occurring daily or weekly, and lasting for up to a few hours. The words most often used to describe phantom limb pain are shooting, pricking and boring (and less commonly, stabbing, burning, throbbing or squeezing). It's mainly localised in the distal part of the missing limb, such as the foot or toes in leg amputees. There are some cases where humans report that their phantom pain resembles pain experienced in the body part before amputation (preamputation pain).

Stump pain occurs in almost all human amputees immediately after surgery, but a significant number will still report it months or years afterwards. Stump pain is more common in patients who are also suffering from phantom limb pain.[3] Descriptions of this stump pain include pressing, squeezing, burning, stabbing or throbbing. Pressing on the stump,

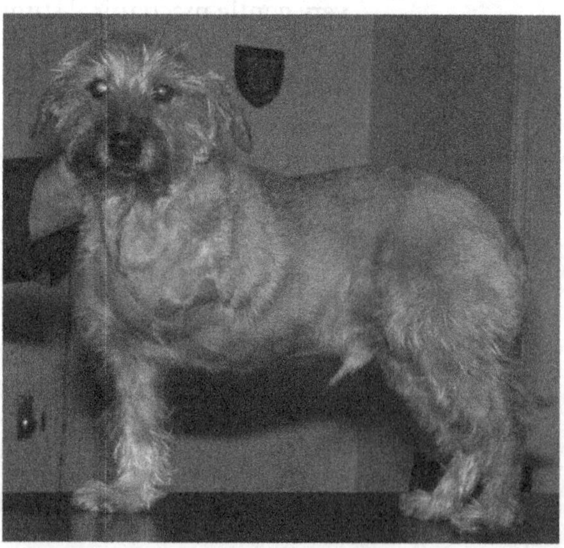

Figure 5.8
Phantom limb pain may well affect animals as well as humans after amputation.

which can show areas of intense hyperalgesia and allodynia, can trigger the pain for hours. Phantom limb pain and stump pain are thought to be a result of a huge barrage of pain signals from the severed nerves innervating the lost limb causing a vast amount of central sensitisation and the chaotic reinnervation of stumps by neuromas in the periphery. There is some evidence to suggest that there is reorganisation of neuronal activity up in the cortex and thalamus of the brain – this could help explain the resulting phantom limb image and pain perception in patients. Again, as is often the case with chronic pain syndromes, treatment is often limited in its effectiveness. One study in human patients found that the use of preop epidural local anaesthetics and opioids did reduce the incidence of postop phantom pain, but subsequent studies did not repeat the findings.[3]

Acute pain

Pain is often classified according to its duration. Acute pain typically arises from tissue trauma (most commonly postop surgical pain) or inflammation and lasts for the duration of the healing process. It can be of mild to severe intensity, and is most intense 24–72 hours after the initial tissue injury. Acute pain is associated with the stress response (sympathetic over-activity and the release of stress hormones) and usually responds well to analgesic therapy. Acute recurrent pain can arise if there is repeated exposure to a noxious stimulus or acute inflammation.

Chronic pain

Chronic pain is arbitrarily defined as pain lasting for more than 3–6 months. Chronic pain involves sensitisation of the pain pathway (as described above) and these changes in the pain pathway of the nervous system typically produce pain that persists beyond the healing of the original injury or after removal of the noxious stimulus. The pain itself is not only exaggerated in duration but also in amplitude. It can occur spontaneously or can be provoked by an external stimulus (noxious or innocuous in nature). Common examples of chronic pain syndromes in small animals are osteoarthritis, cancer and postamputation pain and it's important to realise that the sensitisation of the pain pathway actually becomes part of the disease process itself, contributing to patient morbidity, suffering and reduced quality of life. Unfortunately chronic pain is notoriously difficult to treat and often requires multiple therapies. Chronic pain is sometimes referred to as pathologic pain in some texts.

THE NEUROMATRIX THEORY OF PAIN

The neuromatrix theory of pain has recently been proposed to help explain the occurrence of phantom limb pain and chronic pain syndromes in people who are often characterised by severe pain associated with little or no discernable injury or pathology.[4] We have no means of making a definitive diagnosis of such states in animals (albeit a response to analgesic therapy) but we cannot rule out their existence. The theory also provides some explanation for why chronic psychological and physical stress is often associated with chronic pain in humans, and points to new forms of treatment (see Chapter 10).

The theory suggests that pain is produced by a characteristic pattern of nerve impulses, generated by a widely distributed network of interconnected neurones in the brain. The structure of this network of neurones (the neuromatrix) is probably genetically determined and modified during life from the sensory inputs it receives. It processes all the incoming information from our environment and experiences and produces a constant outflow of nerve impulse patterns (neurosignatures) that are converted into a constantly changing stream of awareness in the brain. The neurosignature patterns may also activate movement, behavioural programmes and homeostatic mechanisms as well as overall perception. Neurosignature patterns may be triggered by sensory stimuli but importantly, they may also be generated independently of them and in the absence of any sensory input. This would explain how a missing limb might still be perceived in every way, despite the brain not actually receiving any sensory information from the periphery.

The theory suggests that the neuromatrix is the primary mechanism that generates the neural pattern that produces pain. Its output pattern is determined by multiple influences that converge on the neuromatrix, of which the peripheral sensory input is only a part. These influences include input from the areas of the brain associated with learning, past experience, personality, anxiety and level of attention. Visual, vestibular, visceral and somatic inputs, autonomic and hypothalamic-pituitary-adrenal system information, the immune system, and endogenous opioids are just some of the other influences thought to contribute to outflow patterns generated by the neuromatrix. Hence stress can potentially have quite an impact on the outflow of pain neurosignatures.

PAIN PATHWAY PHYSIOLOGY AND ANALGESIC THERAPY

An understanding of the anatomy and physiology of the pain pathway and its plasticity during sensitisation have led to the establishment of two very important principles of effective pain management in practice, those of pre-emptive analgesia, and multimodal analgesia. Both these approaches are discussed in detail below.

Pre-emptive analgesia

As detailed earlier, stimulation of the pain pathway results in sensitisation, whereby the pain pathway responds more vigorously to further painful stimuli, or to previously non-painful stimuli, so that relatively more pain is then experienced. Once sensitisation has been established, pain is much more difficult to control because the pathway is generating huge pain signals in response to both noxious and normally innocuous stimuli, and literally firing at the slightest touch. This means far more analgesic drugs are required to dampen down the pain signals, and adequate pain relief may not even be possible. If initial stimulation of the pain pathway is reduced or blocked then less sensitisation occurs, and the subsequent pain will be much easier to control. This means that if analgesic drugs are given before any pain is experienced, i.e. pre-emptively, then once tissue damage does occur the pain pathway already has a block applied to it, so there is less firing of the pain pathway, less sensitisation developing, and the ensuing pain is easier to control.

The commonest clinical situation where this pre-emptive effect can be applied is before surgery. During surgery there is massive stimulation and firing of the pain pathway as tissue is cut, crushed and traumatised, etc. The only difference with general anaesthesia (compared to an awake animal) is that there isn't the conscious 'ouch' at the end of the pain pathway when all the signals reach the brain. Once the animal comes round from anaesthesia, there will be an enormous degree of sensitisation of the pain pathway postop if there hasn't been any analgesia provided, and the patient will be in intense pain and discomfort. Sensitisation is an integral part of postop pain. Therefore it makes sense to give analgesics preoperatively wherever possible, to reduce initial stimulation of the pain pathway during surgery and minimise sensitisation, which will result in much less postop pain that's easier to control. In a nutshell, pain should be prevented wherever possible, rather than waiting for it to occur before treating it.

To be most effective, pre-emptive analgesia should aim to reduce initial stimulation of nociceptors, by blocking inflammation and the formation of the sensitising soup and blocking noxious inputs into the CNS. Chapters 6, 7 and 8 discuss the different classes of analgesics that can be used pre-emptively to achieve these effects. The greater the surgical trauma that's expected, then the more preoperative analgesia should be administered. Obviously, further postoperative administration of analgesics is still commonly needed even with pre-emptive analgesia, but the pain should be easier to control.

The advantages of preoperative administration of analgesia compared to postoperative were demonstrated in a study[5] that looked at bitch spays, comparing groups of dogs given preoperative analgesia in the form of carprofen (Rimadyl®), a non-steroidal anti-inflammatory drug (NSAID) with a group given postoperative carprofen. A third group were not given any analgesia, so that the full effects of sensitisation could be evaluated. NSAIDs work by helping to block inflammation and the formation of the sensitising soup, thereby reducing stimulation and peripheral sensitisation of nociceptors. They are also considered to have a central action, blocking COX 2, a chemical mediator thought to play a role in transmission of pain up the spinal cord and central sensitisation. Pain was assessed for up to 20 hours postoperatively using a DIVAS pain scale (and mechanical threshold testing – see under 'Sensitisation' Chapter 3). At all the time points when pain was assessed, the dogs that did not receive any analgesia were experiencing the most pain, whilst those that received carprofen preoperatively were experiencing the least

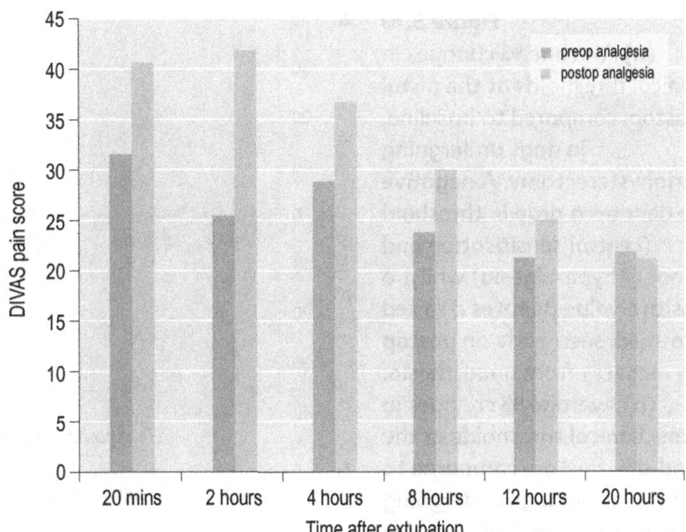

Figure 5.9 DIVAS pain scores for dogs undergoing ovariohysterectomy given preop carprofen, compared with a group given postop carprofen analgesia. (After Lascelles BD, Jones A, Waterman-Pearson AE. Efficacy and kinetics of carprofen, administered preoperatively or postoperatively, for the prevention of pain in dogs undergoing ovariohysterectomy. Veterinary Surgery 1998; 27: 568–582, reproduced with permission.)

pain of all the groups (Fig 5.9). The study concluded that preop administration of carprofen had a greater analgesic effect than postop administration in the early postoperative period. Therefore the timing of analgesic administration is important to optimise the control of postop pain.

The advantages of preop administration have also been demonstrated for pethidine, a μ-opioid agonist with a short duration of action of up to 2 hours.[6] In this study, 40 dogs undergoing ovariohysterectomy were divided into three groups. One group received pethidine analgesia preop, another group received pethidine postop and the third group received no analgesia. Pain was assessed before anaesthesia (to gain a baseline value for each dog) and then from 20 mins postop to 20 hours postop. Two measures of pain were used, a subjective VAS score, and an objective measure using mechanical nociceptive threshold testing at the wound site on the ventral abdomen and at the distal tibia (pinnae and the distal radius).

Although the dogs receiving postop pethidine had the lowest VAS pain scores for the first 2 hours postop, the dogs that had preop pethidine had the lowest pain scores from 2 to 20 hours postop. The dogs that had no pain relief started to show the effects of central sensitisation by 8 hours postop; their mechanical thresholds at the distal tibia notably dropped. This effect was significantly prevented by the preop administration of pethidine but not by postop

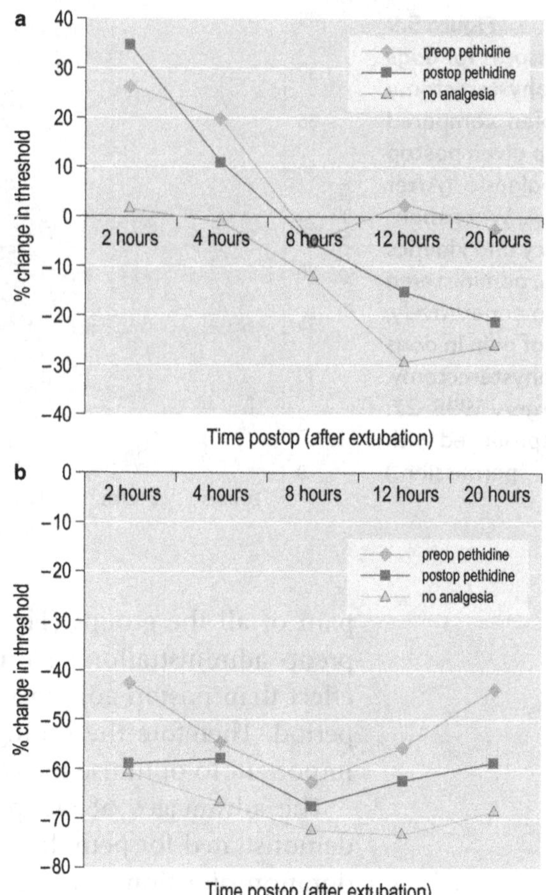

Figure 5.10 **(a)** Average % changes in mechanical thresholds at the distal tibia postop, compared to baseline, in dogs undergoing ovariohysterectomy. A negative value denotes a drop in threshold (central sensitisation and secondary hyperalgesia) whilst a positive value denotes a raised threshold, seen early on postop during recovery from anaesthesia. **(b)** Average % changes in mechanical thresholds at the wound site, postop, compared to baseline, in dogs undergoing ovariohysterectomy. The negative values denote a drop in threshold (hyperalgesia).

administration. At the wound site, mechanical thresholds dropped in all three groups within 1 hour postop as hyperalgesia developed. However, this hyperalgesia was least in the preop pethidine group (Fig 5.10). The study found that pethidine was an effective analgesic when used postoperatively to control pain in the immediate postop period (the first 2 hours). However, the administration of preop pethidine resulted in significantly less pain in the later postop period, probably due to the blocking of noxious signals entering the CNS during surgery, and therefore preventing central sensitisation. Ideally, the best results would be obtained from the administration of both pre- and postop pethidine.

Preoperative analgesia often reduces the dose of anaesthetic drugs used periop and results in a smoother anaesthetic with noticeably less twiddling of the vaporiser required, particularly when the patient is subject to a very painful stimuli (such as pulling on ovarian stumps in a bitch spay). A recent study[7] looked at the effects of preop administration of both carprofen and butorphanol (an opioid partial agonist-antagonist with a mild analgesic and sedative action) on the amount of isoflurane required to anaesthetise dogs when a pain stimulus was applied to the tail. A towel clamp was applied around the tail for 60 seconds under anaesthesia, and the MAC (minimum alveolar concentration) of isoflurane determined after preop carprofen, preop butorphanol, or both preop carprofen and preop butorphanol together, compared with a control group that received no analgesia. Preop carprofen alone produced a 6.4% reduction in MAC, preop butorphanol alone produced a 20.2% reduction in MAC, and when the two drugs were both given preop, there was a 29.5% reduction in MAC. Although these reductions in MAC were not all statistically significant, the findings strongly suggest preop analgesia has a potential benefit in reducing the amount of subsequent inhalant anaesthetic agent and hence the cardiovascular depressant effects of these drugs on the patient.

Chapter 2 discussed the detrimental consequences of clinical pain in animals, including the finding that postop pain following surgery in cancer patients can promote metastatic spread (and recurrence) of the tumour. This enhancement of tumour spread can be greatly attenuated by the provision of adequate analgesia. The impact of the timing of analgesic administration, preop compared with postop, has also been investigated.[8]

A study[8] used a particular line of rats inoculated with mammary adenocarcinoma cells (which have a very predictable pattern of spread to the lungs in this experimental model). Initially it was established that surgery without any analgesia resulted in a 2-fold increase in the number of lung metastases, compared to rats that did not undergo any surgery, and that this enhancement of tumour spread was significantly reduced by administration of morphine both preop and postop. However, rats that received morphine preop appeared to derive greater benefit from the analgesia, compared to rats receiving morphine postop. Rats given

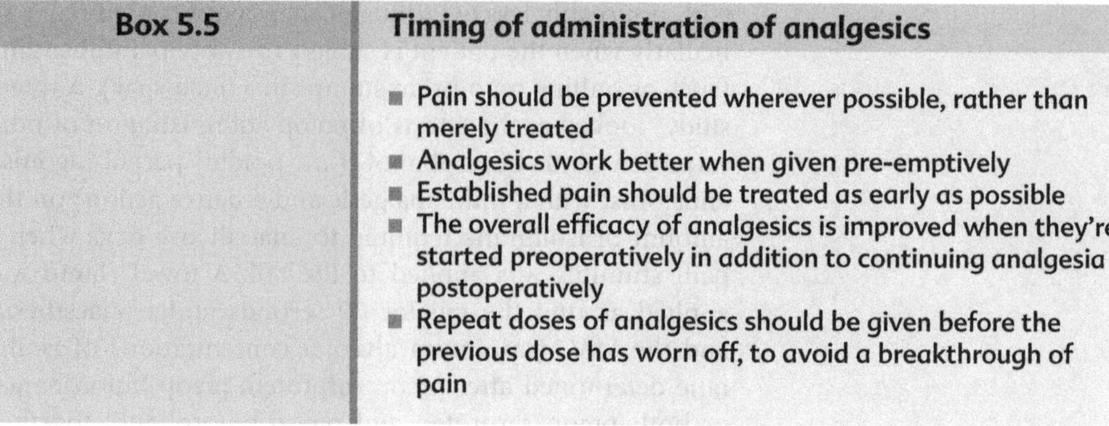
Box 5.5 **Timing of administration of analgesics**

- Pain should be prevented wherever possible, rather than merely treated
- Analgesics work better when given pre-emptively
- Established pain should be treated as early as possible
- The overall efficacy of analgesics is improved when they're started preoperatively in addition to continuing analgesia postoperatively
- Repeat doses of analgesics should be given before the previous dose has worn off, to avoid a breakthrough of pain

morphine preop showed a 65–70% reduction in lung metastases, whilst those receiving postop morphine only showed a 50% reduction in lung metastases. These findings support the suggestion that preop administration of morphine analgesia is key in optimising its beneficial effects on reducing the increase in metastatic spread of tumours associated with surgical pain. It's important to emphasise that continuation of analgesia postoperatively is also essential to minimise the detrimental effects of pain, but that the overall efficacy of analgesia is improved by starting it pre-emptively.

It's not always possible to get analgesics on board before tissue trauma occurs, patients may already be in great pain after a road traffic accident or other trauma by the time they arrive for treatment. It's still very beneficial to administer analgesia as soon as possible as the degree of central sensitisation will be greater the longer the initial pain continues. Some drugs can be used to try and reverse central sensitisation after it has developed, such as ketamine (see Chapter 8).

The principle of pain prevention can be applied to analgesic protocols longer term, where patients need to receive repeated doses of analgesics to maintain pain relief. If dosing intervals are too long, the pain pathway will be allowed to start firing in response to the ongoing noxious stimulus, and a degree of sensitisation will follow every time there is a breakthrough in pain relief, so the pain becomes increasingly difficult to control. As a result, larger doses of drugs may be required. Ideally, analgesic drugs should be administered

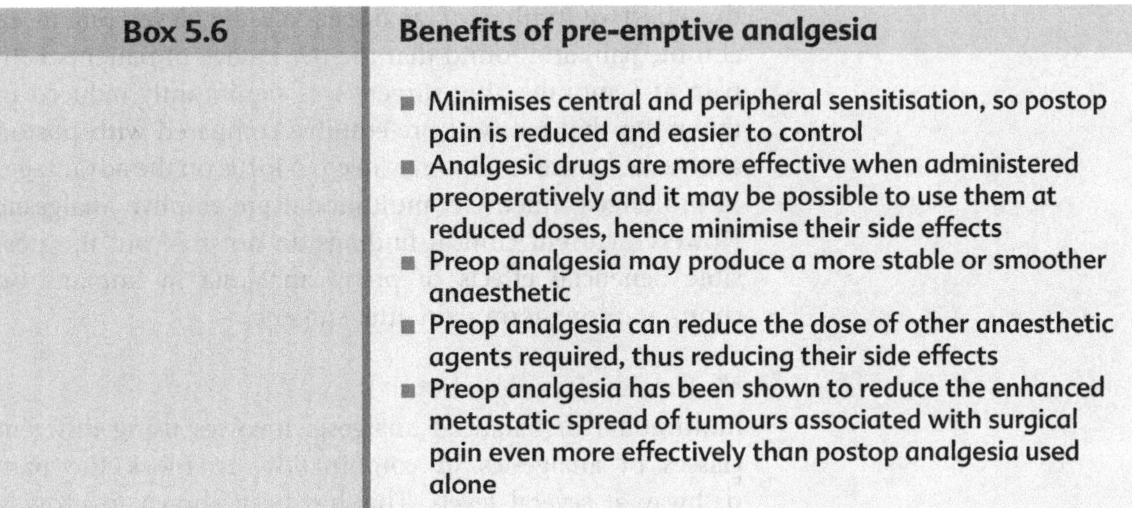

Box 5.6 **Benefits of pre-emptive analgesia**

- Minimises central and peripheral sensitisation, so postop pain is reduced and easier to control
- Analgesic drugs are more effective when administered preoperatively and it may be possible to use them at reduced doses, hence minimise their side effects
- Preop analgesia may produce a more stable or smoother anaesthetic
- Preop analgesia can reduce the dose of other anaesthetic agents required, thus reducing their side effects
- Preop analgesia has been shown to reduce the enhanced metastatic spread of tumours associated with surgical pain even more effectively than postop analgesia used alone

before the previous dose has worn off to avoid any breakthrough pain (with care taken to avoid overdoses).

Pre-emptive analgesia in human patients

Strangely enough the pre-emptive effect of analgesics has not yet been clearly demonstrated clinically in human patients, despite a wealth of experimental evidence of its potential benefits, as seen in animals.[9] A recent article reviewed 80 clinical trials in people to see if pre-emptive administration of NSAIDS, opioids, local anaesthetic blocks and NMDA antagonists lead to better postop pain relief in the first 24 hours than postop administration (measured by pain scoring). The authors cited several possible flaws in the analysis of the available data such as insensitivity of pain scoring to low intensity pain and small differences in pain intensity and the use of perioperative opioids in both treatment groups in some trials. The review found that timing of analgesia did not influence the quality of postop pain control, whatever the type of pre-emptive analgesia.

The negative findings could be due to inadequate levels of analgesia, too low or too high noxious stimulation during surgery that either results in insignificant sensitisation, or overwhelming sensitisation despite analgesic blockade, or insufficient duration of treatment to prevent subsequent sensitisation. The beneficial effects may have been more measurable after 24 hours. One trial that was included looked at the effect of timing of analgesia on the development of chronic pain and found that the percentage of patients with pain at 6 months after surgery was significantly reduced in the group that received pre-emptive compared with postop analgesia. Future studies may need to focus on the advantages of prolonged, intensive, multimodal pre-emptive analgesia. However, current clinical findings do not rule out the possible beneficial effects of preop analgesia in humans on short- and long-term pain after surgery.

Multimodal analgesia

Multimodal or balanced analgesia involves using different classes of analgesics in combination, to block the pain pathway at several levels. This has been shown to provide better analgesia than using one drug by itself, even at high doses. The reason that the multimodal approach is more effective is probably because the pain pathway is so complex and involves many different neural mechanisms, neurotransmitters and receptors in the periphery and up in the spinal cord and brain. It's therefore unlikely that one drug would be able to effectively block such a diverse array of activities and provide completely effective pain relief.

Added to this is the fact that clinical pain usually comprises more than one type of pain, such as visceral and somatic pain, and neuropathic and inflammatory components. There is often simultaneous acute and chronic pain, and a degree of central and peripheral sensitisation present. Taking all this into account, it will require several different types of analgesic drug, acting at different points along the pain pathway with various mechanisms of action, to alleviate pain most effectively. For example, a NSAID will act peripherally to reduce inflammation and nociceptor output to the spinal cord. This can be combined with an opioid, which acts centrally to reduce nociceptive inputs to the brain, and also a local analgesic which blocks specific nerve pathways en route to the spinal cord. The mechanisms of action of the major classes of analgesics are discussed in Chapters 6, 7 and 8 in further detail. It's generally accepted that combining different types of analgesics gives a synergistic effect, i.e. the resulting analgesia is better than the individual drug actions added together. Another advantage of the synergism seen with the multimodal approach is that drugs can be used at

Box 5.7 **Benefits of multi-modal analgesia**

- **The resulting analgesia is better than using individual drugs alone at high doses**
- **Analgesics may be used at lower doses, thereby reducing potential side effects**
- **Helps avoid gaps in pain relief caused by slow onset of action, and varying durations of action of individual analgesic drugs**

lower doses, thereby reducing the risk of their potential side effects.

Using combinations of different classes of analgesics is also useful to avoid gaps in analgesia, by overcoming some of the problems arising due to varying onsets and duration of actions of drugs. For example, if an opioid given preop only lasts 2 hours, there could be a gap in analgesia postop before a repeat dose of opioid is given (after all it's very difficult to determine exactly when an analgesic has stopped having an effect), particularly if the repeat dose has a slow onset of action. If, however, a NSAID has been given preop as well, this may last for 24 hours, and prevent any pain breakthrough in the immediate postop period, even when the opioid wears off.

Multimodal analgesia in humans

Multimodal analgesia is currently recommended for effective postoperative pain relief in human medicine.[10] Single analgesics alone, either opioids or NSAIDs, are not considered able to provide effective pain relief for most moderate to severe pain, and are associated with the risk of side effects such as nausea, vomiting, sedation or bleeding in people. By combining opioids with NSAIDs and local anaesthetics, synergistic analgesia is achieved and lower total doses of analgesics are used, with fewer side effects. So for example, a human patient undergoing major surgery would receive the following periop analgesia: infiltration of the wound with local anaesthetic, a peripheral nerve block with local anaesthetic, an epidural using both an opioid and local anaesthetic, a systemic NSAID and a systemic opioid. This protocol provides at least five different blocks on the pain pathway and should result in very effective analgesia.

Key principles of pain management based on the physiology of the pain pathway

1. **Pain should be prevented wherever possible, rather than just treated.**
2. **Animals should ideally emerge from anaesthesia pain free.**
3. **Analgesics must be provided pre-emptively or as early as possible after a noxious stimulus, at an adequate dose, to minimise sensitisation and postop pain. Analgesia should also be continued postoperatively.**
4. **Repeat doses of analgesics must be administered at the correct dosing intervals to try and avoid pain breakthrough and minimise sensitisation, to achieve effective pain relief.**
5. **Multimodal analgesia, using combinations of different classes of analgesics together, provides better analgesia than using individual drugs alone, even at high doses.**

REFERENCES

1. Nolan A. The pathophysiology of pain. Proceedings of the AVA Autumn Meeting, Dunblane, Scotland. 5–7 September 2001
2. Waterman-Pearson A. Pain and analgesia – have things really changed? Proceedings of the AVA International Scientific Meeting, Chester, England. 6–7 December 2001
3. Staehelin Jensen T, Nikolajsen L. Phantom pain and other phenomena after amputation. In: Wall PD, Melzack R, eds. Textbook of pain, 4th edn. Edinburgh: Churchill Livingstone; 1999:799–814
4. Melzack R. Pain and the Neuromatrix in the brain. Journal of Dental Education 2001; 65(12):1378–1382
5. Lascelles BD, Jones A, Waterman-Pearson AE. Efficacy and kinetics of carprofen, administered preoperatively or postoperatively, for the prevention of pain in dogs undergoing ovariohysterectomy. Veterinary Surgery 1998; 27:568–582
6. Lascelles BDX, Cripps PJ, Jones A, Waterman AE. Postoperative central hypersensitivity and pain: the pre-emptive value of pethidine for ovariohysterectomy. Pain 1997; 73: 461–471
7. Ko JCH, Lange DN, Mandsager RE, et al. Effects of butorphanol and carprofen on the minimal alveolar concentration of isoflurane in dogs. J Am Vet Med Assoc 2000; 217(7): 1025–1028
8. Page GG, McDonald JS, Ben-Eliyahu S. Preoperative versus postoperative administration of morphine: impact on the neuroendocrine, behavioural and metastatic-enhancing effects of surgery. British Journal of Anaesthesia 1998; 81:216–223
9. Moiniche S, Kehlet H, Dahl JB. A qualitative and quantitative systematic review of pre-emptive analgesia for postoperative pain relief. Anesthesiology 2002; 96(3): 725–741
10. Jin F, Chung F. Multi-modal analgesia for postoperative pain control. Journal of Clinical Anaesthesia 2001; 13: 524–539

FURTHER READING

Dyce KM, Sack WO, Wensing CJG. Textbook of veterinary anatomy. Philadelphia: WB Saunders; 1987

Muir WM, Woolf CJ. Mechanisms of pain and their therapeutic implications. J Am Vet Med Assoc 2001; 219(10):1346–1356

Lamont LA. Tranquilli WJ, Grimm KA. Physiology of pain. In: Vet Clinics of North America: Small Animal Practice 2000; 30(4): 703–728

Wall PD, Melzack R, eds. Textbook of pain, 4th edn. Edinburgh: Churchill Livingstone; 1999

Wall P. Pain: the science of suffering. London: Phoenix; 1999

Flecknell P, Waterman-Pearson A, eds. Pain management in animals. London: Saunders; 2000

CHAPTER 6 THE OPIOID ANALGESIC DRUGS

OPIATES AND OPIOIDS

Opioids have been used for pain relief for over 2000 years and are still considered one of the most potent and safest classes of analgesic. Opiates are drugs derived from opium, such as morphine and codeine, whilst the term opioid is used for all drugs acting on opioid receptors, in a similar way to morphine, and include the opiates. Opioids are sometimes referred to as narcotic analgesics because of their ability to cause drowsiness (narcosis) in humans and some species of animals. Opioid receptors are found in the spinal cord and brain associated with the pain pathway, and are also generated or expressed out in the periphery in inflammatory conditions.

Three types of opioid receptor have been identified – mu (μ), kappa (κ) and delta (δ). These receptors have been reclassified as OP3 (μ), OP2 (κ) and OP1 (δ) and more recently an orphan opioid receptor, called ORL1 has also been identified.[1] However, the rest of this book will still use the more widely used traditional mu, kappa and delta nomenclature. Animals and humans have their own endogenous opioids, including enkephalins and endorphins, which have different selectivities for each receptor type and can produce analgesia or hyperalgesia depending on the relative quantities and conditions under which they're released. These peptides are also involved in learning and memory in the brain.

Opioid drugs work by acting on opioid receptors to produce analgesia, sedation and euphoria to varying degrees depending on:

1. The receptor types they bind, i.e. selectivity
2. The affinity the drug has for a receptor

3. The effect the drug exerts at the receptor, i.e. agonist activity versus antagonist activity.

Opioids can have activity at more than one type of receptor, and their selectivity will help predict their main effects. Opioids that are selective agonists at mu receptors, such as morphine, tend to produce the best analgesia. Opioids with high affinity for receptors are slowly released from them and tend to have a longer duration of action such as buprenorphine (6–8 hours). Opioids can act as full agonists, antagonists or partial agonist/antagonist at receptors, and this is one way in which they are classified. Agonists will produce a maximal response from binding the receptor, partial agonists can only produce a partial response no matter how high the dose of the drug, and antagonists will bind a receptor but not produce any effect. Partial agonists/antagonists produce a partial response at the receptor, but have a 'ceiling effect', where the response cannot be increased further above a given dose. In fact the response may diminish as an antagonistic effect kicks in at higher doses, resulting in a bell-shaped dose–response curve (Fig 6.1).

Table 6.1 shows the selectivity and effects of commonly used opioids on each receptor type. From the table it can be seen that morphine has high selectivity for mu receptors, and acts as an agonist, producing great analgesia. It also binds kappa and delta receptors but to a much lesser extent. Buprenorphine binds mu receptors selectively as well, but only acts as a partial agonist, so the expected level of analgesia is significantly less than morphine. Naloxone acts as a selective antagonist at mu receptors and is used to reverse the effects of other opioids (e.g. in cases of overdose). The main effects of opioids are analgesia, sedation and

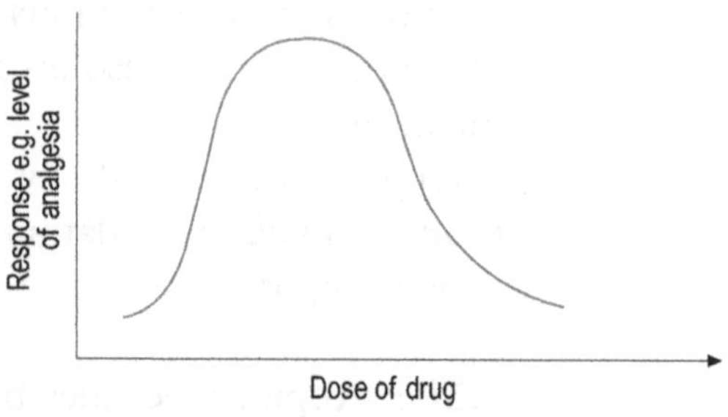

Figure 6.1
Example of a bell shaped dose–response curve for a partial agonist/antagonist opioid.

Table 6.1
Selectivity and activity of common opioids

	Receptor selectivity			
	μ	κ	δ	Receptor activity
Morphine	+++	+/–	+/–	Agonist
Pethidine	++	–	–	Agonist
Fentanyl	+++	–	–	Agonist
Buprenorphine	+++	++	+/–	Partial agonist
Butorphanol	++	++	–	Mixed agonist/antagonist
Nalbuphine	+	++	+	Mixed agonist/antagonist
Naloxone	+++	+	+	Antagonist

(From Lascelles BDX. Clinical pharmacology of analgesic agents. In Hellebrekers LJ, ed. Animal Pain. The Netherlands: Van Der Wees 2000:85–116, reproduced with permission.)

euphoria. They have minor effects on the respiratory and cardiovascular systems and the gastrointestinal tract as detailed below.

ACTION OF OPIOIDS

Analgesia

Opioids produce analgesia by blocking the transmission of nociceptive signals up to the brain by acting on receptors located at the level of primary afferent nociceptors in the spinal cord. Opioids seem to reduce the excitability of these dorsal horn neurones by causing postsynaptic neurone hyperpolarisation. They also act at higher centres in the brain to block pain transmission and to increase the amount of descending inhibition on the pain pathway. When opioids activate their receptors it inhibits the presynaptic release, and postsynaptic response to, excitatory neurotransmitters (e.g. acetylcholine, substance P) from neurones involved in nociception. Opioids with agonist activity at mu receptors will produce analgesia, the degree of which depends on the level of selectivity and amount of agonist activity.

Drugs that are pure agonists at mu receptors, e.g. morphine, fentanyl, give a higher level of analgesia than the partial agonists, e.g. buprenorphine, or agonists/antagonists, e.g. butorphanol. These latter drugs have a ceiling effect for analgesia, as mentioned above. Kappa selective agonists cause too much dysphoria in humans to be clinically useful, whilst delta agonists and partial agonists are currently being investigated as they may have fewer side effects than mu agonists.[1] Opioids not only reduce the perception of pain but also the associated psychological stress in humans. They have been shown to have a significant pre-emptive effect in animals (see Chapter 5) and synergism with NSAIDs and local anaesthetics. Therefore it's recommended that opioids be given preop or as early as possible and in combination with other classes of analgesic for optimum pain relief. An important point to note when using opioids for ongoing analgesia is that the dose needs to be titrated with the pain experienced in each individual. Patients should be assessed at regular intervals and further opioids administered if indicated; the average durations of action should really be used just as a guideline, not an absolute period of time.

Opioid receptors seem to have a clinically significant presence in the periphery in inflamed tissue and are expressed on nerve endings and inflammatory cells. If low doses of opioids are injected locally into inflamed tissue they produce analgesia (but effects are not obvious in normal tissue). An experimental model in dogs with induced arthritis found a very high density of opioid receptors (mu) present in articular and periarticular tissue of acutely inflamed joints and a 50-fold increase in morphine binding sites in the synovial membranes.[3] Studies have reported that intra-articular opioids can provide very effective analgesia in joints. Intra-articular morphine after stifle surgery has been shown to reduce the need for systemic analgesia postoperatively and is as efficacious as epidurally administered morphine.[4,5] The potential for side effects with local opioids seems very low,[4] and a recent paper found no significant changes in synovial fluid or joint tissue histology after intra-articular injection of an opiate, methadone.[6]

Opioids such as morphine can also be given epidurally alone or in combination with local anaesthetics to provide excellent long-lasting analgesia of caudal body parts (see Chapter 7). Epidurally administered opioids are thought to diffuse across the meninges (membranes covering the spinal cord and brain) into the spinal cord and block pain transmission at the level of the dorsal horn. It's thought they act presynaptically to inhibit the release of substance P, an important pain pathway neurotransmitter. They may also act postsynaptically to hyperpolarise neurones, so they are less likely to fire. Segmental analgesia occurs following epidural morphine; there is more profound analgesia of a more rapid onset at spinal regions close to the site of injection than those further away. Time to maximum analgesia after epidural morphine is 30–60 minutes. Local and epidural administration of opioids not only seems to prolong their duration of action compared to systemic administration but can also reduce side effects and anaesthetic requirements. Epidural morphine can provide analgesia for up to 24 hours for perianal or hindlimb surgery, laparotomy or even thoracotomy (as morphine will spread cranially after epidural administration).

When opioids are combined with local anaesthetics for epidurals there is significant synergy, resulting in better, longer-lasting analgesia.[7] The only drawback is that motor function is usually lost with the inclusion of local anaesthetics. Complications of epidural opioids are relatively few in the dog. Urine retention may occur with morphine or fentanyl, possibly due to bladder muscle weakness or depression of the urine-voiding (emptying) reflex. Some dogs will need manual expression or catheterisation to empty the bladder. Significant respiratory depression and vomiting is unlikely in animals with this route of administration of morphine. Oddly, localised pruritus around the epidural injection site of morphine has been seen in dogs. Ideally, preservative-free preparations of opioids should be used for epidurals to avoid any chemical damage to the spinal cord.

Sedation

Opioids produce sedation in humans and dogs (less so in cats) and a decrease in spontaneous motor activity (i.e. movement). When given pre-emptively they can reduce the amount of subsequent anaesthetic requirements, and are often used routinely for premedication for this reason. Their pre-emptive analgesic effect is a result of greatly reducing central sensitisation, as they protect the CNS from the barrage of incoming afferent pain signals during surgery. This benefit

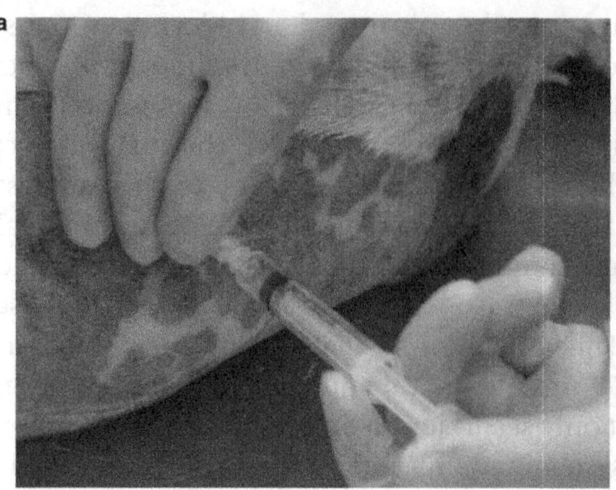

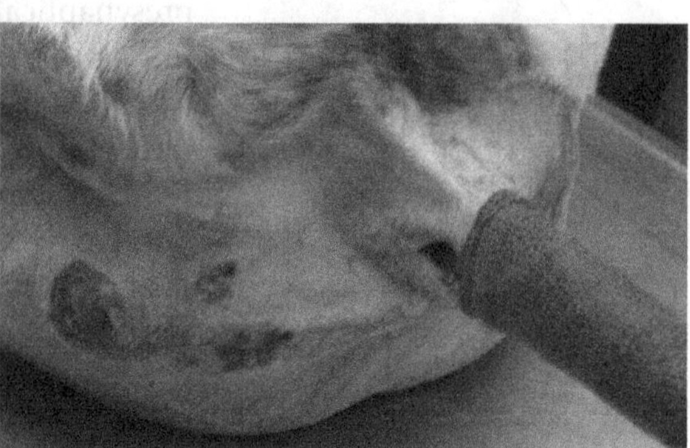

Figure 6.2
Epidural morphine can provide excellent analgesia for perianal and hindlimb surgery, without loss of motor function.

Box 6.1	Actions of opioids
	■ Analgesia – Primarily in CNS – Some local peripheral effect ■ Sedation ■ (Euphoria)

usually far outweighs the increased postop sedation that may occur with their use.

Euphoria

Mu receptor agonists can cause euphoria in people, and it's thought animals experience similar effects. Kappa receptor activity in contrast causes dysphoria. The euphoric effect is thought to help relieve anxiety and stress in patients that are in unfamiliar surroundings, and helps facilitate handling.

SIDE EFFECTS OF OPIOIDS

Respiratory depression

The respiratory depression is caused by opioids reducing the responsiveness of the brain stem to levels of CO_2, which is the primary stimulation for respiration (the hypoxic stimulus to breathing is unaffected). They also depress the centres that regulate respiratory rhythm. In general, respiratory rate may be slowed but tidal volume unchanged. However, dogs may pant after opioid administration, particularly with higher doses of morphine or pethidine and if they are not already in pain. Panting is not related to an effect on the respiratory centre but is a response to the opioid resetting the thermoregulatory centre in the brain 1–3 degrees Fahrenheit below normal, so the dogs pant to lower their temperature. Panting may also be a result of the release of histamine causing a degree of pulmonary oedema.[2]

Primates are far more susceptible to the respiratory depression caused by opioids than other species and clinically it's rarely seen in dogs and cats. The exception to this is with the use of the very potent opioids fentanyl and alfentanil, used in animals intraoperatively to provide profound analgesia, which usually require the patient to be ventilated. Partial agonists produce less respiratory depression and there may be a ceiling to this effect, just as there is with their analgesia. If respiratory depression does occur (this is more likely at high doses, in combination with other depressive agents, or in animals not in pain) then the opioid can be reversed with naloxone, an opioid antagonist, although this also reverses the analgesia. Alternatively, a respiratory stimulant can be used, such as doxapram – repeat dosing may be needed as it has a short duration of action (10–20 min).

Cardiovascular effects

Generally most opioids have little effect on the cardiovascular system. Morphine, fentanyl and alfentanil can cause bradycardia (slow heart rate) and a mild hypotension if injected rapidly intravenously. The bradycardia is due to action on receptors in the brain stem that inhibit sympathetic tone to the heart. It can be reversed by giving antimuscarinics such as atropine. The hypotension can be due to a central effect on the vasomotor centre, and occasionally by histamine release. It can be avoided by slow intravenous (i.v.) injection or using the intramuscular (i.m) route instead. Venous tone tends to be reduced which makes the drugs useful for cases with congestive heart failure, as it effectively reduces preload on the heart. Pethidine is contraindicated i.v and should only be given i.m. as it causes a lot of histamine release, resulting in hypotension in dogs and cats. Pethidine has been reported to reduce myocardial contractility but it's debatable as to whether this is clinically significant.[1,2] Etorphine, an opioid used in combination with methotrimeprazine (known as 'small animal immobilon'), causes pronounced hypotension and bradycardia in dogs.

Gastrointestinal effects

Opioids initially cause a period of gastrointestinal hypermotility with an increase in rhythmic contractions but peristalsis is reduced. This is then followed by GI stasis that can result in constipation. Opioids also increase smooth muscle and sphincter tone, including biliary and pancreatic ducts, thereby inhibiting pancreatic secretions and increasing pressure in the common bile duct. Therefore opioids should not be used in cases of pancreatitis or biliary stasis. Pethidine is the only exception as it has a spasmolytic action and does not cause spasm of ducts, so it is indicated as an analgesic in these conditions. Morphine and closely related opiates can also cause vomiting by stimulating the chemoreceptor trigger zone, particularly in pain-free animals. Defecation often accompanies opioid-induced vomiting. It's well worth considering these two potential side effects when designing premedication protocols; a near at hand supply of clean bedding might be an essential prerequisite.

Antitussive effect

Opioids with activity at mu and kappa receptors have an antitussive (cough suppressant) effect, by depressing the cough centre in the medulla of the brain. There is a poor correlation between analgesic properties and the antitussive effect – butorphanol and codeine are both good cough suppressants even at doses below those required for analgesia.

Excitation

There is a myth that opioids cause mania or excitation in cats, based on some work done in 1925, which used massive overdoses of morphine in cats (100 times more than current recommendations). At clinically correct doses morphine does not cause excitation in cats. However, it's probably best to avoid i.v. administration in cats as temporary overstimulation of the CNS can be seen (although this may be hard to diagnose in the typical tortoise-shell that is not altogether sold on the idea of receiving veterinary attention in the first place!). Excitation and dysphoria are reported to be possible after administration of opioids in all animals, particularly at very high doses, but it's very rarely seen clinically and is thought to be less likely in animals already in pain.[8] The risk of excitation can be reduced by the concurrent administration of acepromazine. Naloxone, a pure antagonist, can be given in severe cases of excitation, or a partial antagonist such as butorphanol (which avoids some of the antianalgesic effect that will result from using naloxone).

Urinary tract

Opioids can increase the bladder sphincter tone, making it more difficult for some patients to pass urine. It's worth regularly palpating the bladder of hospitalised patients on opioid treatment to check they're not retaining urine.

Tolerance and dependence

Tolerance to a drug is where bigger and bigger doses are needed to achieve the same effect, i.e. the drug becomes less effective as repeated doses are given. Acute tolerance has been seen in pain-free laboratory animals after large doses of opiates but it's not seen clinically in animals given pre-emptive opioids. Dependence on a drug is the need to continue receiving it after previous exposure, to prevent the development of an abstinence syndrome; this phenomenon has not been reported in animals.

Ceiling effect of partial agonists and agonist/antagonists

Early work has led to the theory that the partial agonists and agonist/antagonists, e.g. buprenorphine and butorphanol respectively, have a bell-shaped dose–response curve, so that increasing doses above a certain point (the ceiling) actually leads to reduced analgesia (see Fig 6.1). It's also thought that these opioids can reverse the analgesia of

Box 6.2 Main side effects of opioids

NB The risk of side effects of opioids rarely outweighs the benefits of the analgesia they will provide.

- **Vomiting**
- **Gut stasis (constipation)**
- **Respiratory depression**
- **Ceiling effect with partial agonists/antagonists**
- **Antitussive effect**
- **Histamine release**

pure mu opioid agonists if they are given at the same time. Traditionally this has led to the reluctance of vets to give pure mu agonists after partial ones, and the withholding of early repeat doses of the partial agonists, which will inevitably lead to suboptimal pain relief in some patients. At the moment, the basis of these assumptions is being questioned as more recent work suggests that clinical doses of buprenorphine in cats and dogs may be hundreds of times below the doses that start to antagonise the analgesia of earlier doses.[2] Similarly for butorphanol, a mixed agonist/antagonist, recent work suggests that analgesic response may not be dose related and there appears to be no ceiling effect seen in cats given a large range of doses.[9] The concern about antagonism of pure mu agonists has also become controversial. Current thinking is that buprenorphine can be used at higher than recommended doses and more frequently in the dog and cat. Occasionally the analgesia may still be inadequate (as with any protocol) and the further administration of a pure mu-agonist does appear to produce analgesia.[2]

PHARMACOKINETICS AND METABOLISM

Generally the opioids are well absorbed from the gut but due to extensive first pass metabolism in the liver they have poor bioavailability (only a small amount of the dose actually makes it into the bloodstream) when given orally. Bioavailability is good from subcutaneous or intramuscular injection. Intravenous injection is only advisable with some of the opioids and should be done slowly to avoid histamine release. Rectal administration of opioids such as morphine is used in humans, but since the absorption via this route is no better than oral administration, there is no point using it in dogs unless it's the only option available (thankfully). As previously discussed, epidural administration helps prolong the duration of opioid analgesia and reduce side effects, and the transdermal route is also used for very lipophilic opioids like fentanyl which can be administered via a skin patch (see below). The main route of opioid metabolism is usually via the liver; they undergo glucuronidation and demethylation and the metabolites are excreted in bile. Some opioid metabolites have analgesic activity themselves. The plasma half-life of opioids seems to be a poor predictor of their clinical duration of action, probably because it's more dependent on the affinity and release time of the opioid from receptors and the fact that elimination from CSF (cerebrospinal fluid) can take longer than plasma elimination.[8]

CONTRAINDICATIONS

In animals that already have respiratory depression, opioids are best avoided as any further depression may become clinically significant. However, if the respiratory impairment is associated with thoracic or upper abdominal pain, e.g. fractured ribs or thoracotomy cases, then the alleviation of pain using opioids like morphine will more than compensate for any respiratory depression caused by the drug itself and respiration will actually be improved.

Opioids can also increase intracranial pressure. This effect is a consequence of respiratory depression, which results in raised arterial carbon dioxide levels and this will cause an increase in cerebral blood flow and intracranial pressure. Therefore in patients with head injuries it's better to avoid opioids until a diagnosis and full assessment has been made and arterial carbon dioxide is regulated by controlled ventilation. Similarly in patients with higher centre or brain stem trauma, drugs that depress the CNS such as opioids should be used with great caution, and respiratory depression closely monitored.

Due to significant hepatic clearance, extra care is recommended when using opioids in very young or very old animals or those with reduced hepatic blood flow (due to other drugs, hepatic shunts or disease).

DRUG INTERACTIONS

In human patients it's been recognised that there can be a severe interaction between opioids, particularly pethidine and pentazocine, and the monoamine oxidase inhibitor (MAO) selegiline used for the treatment of depression. There are also reports of reactions between fentanyl and other MAO drugs. Reactions include pyrexia, coma, rigidity, severe hypertension, seizures and delirium.[8,10] Selegiline is sometimes used in dogs for behavioural disorders or the treatment of pituitary-dependent hyperadrenocorticism. Although there are no reports of reactions in animals the concurrent use of opioids and MAO drugs in veterinary patients should be avoided if possible. However, if opioids are necessary, morphine would appear to be the drug of choice, but it's suggested that a test dose be given initially and if no adverse effects are seen, subsequent doses can be carefully titrated. Amitraz is another type of MAO used in pets topically or impregnated into collars to treat various ectoparasites.

INDIVIDUAL OPIOID DRUGS

Morphine

Morphine, a pure mu agonist, was first isolated in 1806 and is considered the 'gold standard analgesic'; it is still the drug of choice for severe pain. There is no ceiling effect so increasing the dose of morphine will increase the analgesia. Morphine is widely distributed around the body and rapidly cleared. The half-life in dogs is short, approximately 1 hour, and nearer 3 hours in cats. It has poor bioavailability when administered orally or rectally but is almost completely absorbed from the intramuscular route. Morphine can produce significant histamine release if given rapidly i.v. Therefore it must be given slowly and in small quantities via this route in dogs (and in addition be diluted for i.v. use in cats). Morphine can be given i.m. s.c. and can also be used epidurally, intra-articularly and as a continuous i.v. infusion. The duration of action in dogs is 2–4 hours, and in cats up to 6–8 hours. Morphine can cause vomiting in both cats and dogs (particularly in pain-free animals) so it may not be wise to use it after ocular or gastric surgery. Panting and bradycardia may well be seen in pain-free dogs when morphine is given on its own. The drug is also thought to inhibit the urine-voiding reflex (as well as increasing sphincter tone) so patients can have reduced urination after administration.

Diamorphine, more commonly known as heroin, is synthesised from morphine, and has no activity until it has been metabolised into morphine. As an analgesic it has no advantages at all over morphine.

Papaveretum

This is a mixture of purified opium alkaloids including morphine. It has similar analgesic and sedative effects as morphine and is also known as omnopon. It is only licensed for human use.

Pethidine

Pethidine (or meperidine), a pure mu agonist, is less potent than morphine but also causes less sedation and vomiting. It's even more likely to cause histamine release if given i.v. and it is difficult to achieve effective plasma levels if administered s.c., so pethidine should always be administered i.m. It has a rapid onset of action, (within 10–15 mins) which is useful for acute trauma cases, but a short duration of 1–2 hours. Its short duration limits its use postoperatively and for long-term pain management. Pethidine has an atropine-like structure that gives it an anticholinergic effect. This results in pethidine having a unique antispasmolytic action on the gut and is therefore the only opioid indicated in cases of acute pancreatitis or biliary disease. It also means it's a very useful analgesic after intestinal surgery and in cats with urolithiasis. Currently pethidine injection 50 mg/ml is licensed i.m. for both cats and dogs (and horses) in the UK.

Fentanyl

This is a pure mu agonist with a very fast onset of action, within 2–5 mins after i.v. injection and a very short duration of action of only 5–20 minutes depending on the dose. It's given as an i.v. bolus, or as intermittent boluses, or as an infusion intraoperatively. The infusion time is limited to less than 2 hours, as fentanyl has a relatively long elimination half-life and will start to accumulate. Fentanyl maybe useful postop as a short-term pain relief measure whilst other longer acting opioids are given time to take effect. It's also a potent respiratory depressant and its use is generally restricted in animals under general anaesthesia to those that can be mechanically ventilated. Bradycardia is also seen with this opioid, which can be avoided by the concurrent use of an antimuscarinic drug. Fentanyl is not yet available on its own as a licensed veterinary product in the UK.

Fentanyl skin patches

Fentanyl can be absorbed through the skin (it is highly lipid soluble) and more recently has started to be used in veterinary medicine in the form of transdermal skin patches designed for chronic pain relief in human cancer patients. The skin patches (Durogesic®) contain a reservoir of fentanyl in an alcohol cellulose gel released to the skin through a membrane that controls the rate of delivery. They come in three sizes that release fentanyl at different rates (25 μg/h, 50 μg/h and 100 μg/h for 72 hours). Great care must be taken with these patches, as children removing them from pets and applying them to themselves can easily go into respiratory arrest. In practice it would be prudent to restrict their use to hospitalised inpatients only.

The patches, designed for humans, come in several sizes and the dose can be reduced for veterinary patients by leaving sections of the patch covered so that only a quarter or half of the patch is stuck to the skin. Do not cut the patches as this can result in accidental human exposure. The patches can theoretically be applied anywhere on the animal but most studies use the lateral thorax or preferably between the shoulder blades to avoid interference from the patient. Before applying the patch the skin should be shaved and cleaned with water and allowed to dry. Do not use soaps or detergents as any residues may stop the patch sticking and increase the risk of a skin reaction. Once the site has been prepared the patch is applied and held firmly in place for 2 minutes. It's advisable to cover the patch with a bandage and label it with the time of application and size of the patch. Care must be taken to ensure the patch doesn't become inadvertently warmed up as this will greatly increase the dose of fentanyl delivered, so ensure the patient is not lying on a heat pad (cases of fatalities have been recorded in human patients in this circumstance).[11]

Once the patch is applied it takes up to 24 hours before peak blood levels are reached in cats and dogs (other analgesics may therefore be required meantime) then plasma levels seem to stay fairly constant, providing analgesia for at least 72 hours or more until the patch is removed. Blood levels decay relatively slowly after patch removal (2–12 hours in dogs) because it's thought there is a reservoir of fentanyl in the dermis that continues to be absorbed.[11] The disposal of the patches is also of concern, as they contain a controlled drug (see Appendix). There does seem to be variation between individuals (and even for the same individual given replacement patches) in the absorption and metabolism of fentanyl in this delivery form, and care should be taken to reassess each patient because some may need additional opioids if they are responding poorly to the patch.

Alfentanil

Alfentanil is a related opioid to fentanyl and is only given by i.v. injection, producing very fast-acting short duration analgesia of only 2–5 minutes. Essentially it is used as an infusion to provide intraop analgesia in small animals and will reduce the amount of inhalation anaesthetic agent required. It can be used preop to help induce anaesthesia in combination with other induction agents. Like fentanyl it will also produce significant respiratory depression and bradycardia (premedication with antimuscarinics such as atropine or glycopyrrolate is recommended).

Methadone

Methadone is another mu agonist that has a similar analgesic effect to morphine but does not cause histamine release so can be given i.v. if a rapid onset of analgesia is required. It causes less sedation than morphine and vomiting is not seen as often. Its duration of action is longer than morphine in humans but this hasn't been confirmed in animals, and is thought to last up to 4 hours in dogs and up to 6 in cats (there is some variation in these times from different studies). It can be administered i.v., i.m., or s.c.

Oxymorphone

Although commonly used in the USA this mu agonist is not available as a veterinary product in the UK. It has similar properties and duration of action to morphine, but does not cause histamine release and can be given i.v., i.m. or s.c. Respiratory depression can be seen if it's used during anaesthesia and it does produce sedation.

Hydromorphone

This is another mu agonist not widely used in the UK, but referred to in American texts. It produces more sedation than oxymorphone but is shorter acting. Hydromorphone can be given by all parenteral routes as histamine release does not seem to be a problem.

Buprenorphine

Buprenorphine is a partial mu agonist, rather than a full mu agonist; hence it doesn't produce the same degree of analgesia as a full agonist such as morphine. It slowly associates with the receptors resulting in a slow onset of action: 30–60 minutes. However, because it also slowly dissociates from its receptors it rather usefully has a relatively long duration of action for an opioid: 4–8 hours in dogs and cats. Buprenorphine has a particularly high affinity for its receptors making it difficult to displace, so opioid antagonists cannot easily reverse its actions. It's currently licensed for use in the dog only (i.m. route) in the UK and is widely used for the treatment of mild to moderate pain. Some work has been done recently looking at the oral administration of the injectable liquid preparation of buprenorphine in cats using absorption through the buccal mucosa as route of administration (which avoids first-pass hepatic metabolism occurring after absorption from the gut).[12] The study found that bioavailability of buprenorphine in cats was 100% via the oral mucosa and the pharmacokinetics were the same as for i.v. or i.m. injection. If the efficacy of this technique is confirmed it would provide a very owner- and patient-friendly way to continue repeat doses of a potent opioid analgesic longer term in cats.

Butorphanol

Butorphanol is a mu antagonist and kappa agonist and is thought to provide only a short duration of mild analgesia. Studies suggest analgesia only lasts between 30 minutes and 2.5 hours in cats and dogs when used for postop pain.[1,2] It appears to be more effective as a sedative (especially in combination with acepromazine) and as an antitussive than an analgesic. It is currently licensed for use in cats, dogs and horses in the UK.

Nalbuphine

This is a mixed agonist/antagonist, acting as an antagonist at mu receptors, a partial agonist at kappa receptors and an agonist at delta receptors. It tends to cause dysphoria rather than euphoria but produces minimal sedation and respiratory depression, although it's known to be painful on injection. Analgesia lasts for up to 2 hours.

Pentazocine

This is another mixed kappa agonist and mu antagonist considered to be short acting. It can be given to dogs and cats but has been reported to produce marked ataxia when used i.v. at higher doses in cats.

Codeine

Codeine is licensed in combination with paracetamol in a tablet form for dogs only in the UK (Pardale-V Tablets®). Codeine is a prodrug, it has no activity itself until it has been metabolised. About 10% of the dose in humans is converted into morphine in the liver, accounting for it's mild analgesic effect. Unfortunately it's ineffective in some human patients because they do not have the liver enzymes necessary for codeine metabolism, although it's unknown if the same is true in small animals. It is also used for cough suppression and may well cause constipation.

Naloxone

Naloxone is an opioid antagonist used to reverse opioid agonists and partial agonists by displacing them from their receptors (but has no effect itself), usually in the event of side effects or overdose and toxicity. It can reverse the analgesia of the opioid as well as side effects and so care must be taken to ensure the patient isn't suddenly left without any other pain relief on board, precipitating a severe stress response. To help avoid this situation, start at a low dose (it may be necessary to dilute) and give the naloxone slowly, just until the unwanted opioid effects are reversed. Naloxone has a short duration of action of 30–60 minutes, so repeat doses are usually necessary.

FUTURE DEVELOPMENTS IN OPIOID ANALGESIA

Sufentanil

This is another member of the fentanyl-like group of opioids, with even greater analgesic potency. It's used in humans as an i.v. bolus, infusion or epidurally and intrathecally. It has similar respiratory and cardiovascular effects as fentanyl. Its use in veterinary medicine is not yet widely reported.

Remifentanil

This is a mu opioid agonist recently introduced on the human side for intraop infusion. It has a similar structure and effects as fentanyl (short acting, rapidly cleared) and so may be found to be useful in veterinary patients in the future.

Oral morphine

Some recent studies have looked at the use of a sustained release morphine preparation given orally to dogs. Bioavailability was fairly low at 20%, absorption was slow over 6 hours and the half-life suggested that twice daily dosing at 2–5 mg/kg maybe appropriate.[11] Further work needs to be done to assess the efficacy and safety of this form of morphine in dogs, but it may have a potential use in managing chronic pain conditions such as cancer (see Chapter 11).

Buprenorphine transdermal skin patches

Transdermal skin patches containing buprenorphine have recently been licensed for moderate to severe cancer pain in humans (Transtec®). They are available in three sizes delivering buprenorphine at 35 μg/h, 52.5 μg/h and 70 μg/h over 72 hours in humans. It's probably only a matter of time before these are studied in veterinary patients. They may prove to be very useful in general practice as buprenorphine is subject to less stringent controlled drug regulations than fentanyl.

Key points about opioid analgesics

1. Opioids are amongst the safest and most effective analgesics.
2. Morphine is still considered the 'gold standard' analgesic and more often than not the most suitable drug for severe pain.
3. Opioids primarily block pain at the end of the pain pathway by acting on receptors in the spinal cord and brain. Receptors are also expressed peripherally in inflamed tissue such as joints.
4. Opioids produce analgesia, sedation and euphoria to varying degrees.
5. Pure mu agonists such as morphine provide the most effective analgesia compared to partial mu agonists or mixed antagonists.
6. The main side effects are respiratory depression, vomiting, gut stasis, the risk of histamine release and an antitussive effect.
7. The risk of opioid side effects rarely outweighs the benefits of the analgesia that they provide.
8. Opioids should be avoided in cases of non-pain-related respiratory depression, and head injuries until a full patient assessment is made and the animal can be closely monitored.
9. Opioid agonists can be reversed using antagonists such as naloxone.
10. The main route of opioid metabolism is via the liver.
11. Most opioids are governed by strict controlled drug regulations (see Appendix).

REFERENCES

1. Nolan AM. Pharmacology of analgesic drugs. In: Flecknell P, Waterman-Pearson A, eds. Pain management in animals. London: Saunders; 2000:21–52
2. Lascelles BDX. Clinical pharmacology of analgesic agents. In: Hellebrekers LJ, ed. Animal pain. The Netherlands: Van Der Wees; 2000:85–116
3. Keates HL, Cramond T, Smith MT. Intra-articular and peri-articular opioid binding in inflamed tissue in experimental canine arthritis. Anaesth Analg 1999; 89(2):409–415
4. Day TK, Pepper WT, Tobias TA, et al. Comparison of intra-articular and epidural morphine for analgesia following stifle arthrotomy in dogs. Vet Surg 1995; 24(6): 522–530
5. Sammarco JL, Conzemius MG, Perkowski SZ, et al. Postoperative analgesia for stifle surgery: a comparison of intra-articular bupivacaine, morphine or saline. Vet Surg 1996; 25(1): 59–69
6. Jones TA, Hand WR, Ports MD, et al. An evaluation of the histological effects of intra-articular methadone in the canine model. AANAJ 2003; 71(1):51–54
7. Campoy L. Epidural and spinal anaesthesia in the dog. In Practice 2004; 26(5):262–269
8. Papich MG. Pharmacologic considerations for opiate analgesic and NSAIDs. Vet Clinics of North America: Small Animal Practice 2000; 30(4):815–837
9. Lascelles BDX, Robertson SA. Use of thermal response to evaluate the antinociceptive

effects of butorphanol in cats. Am J Vet Res 2004; 65(8):1085–1089

10. Pascoe PJ. Problems of pain management. In: Flecknell P, Waterman-Pearson A, eds. Pain management in animals. London: Saunders; 2000:161–177
11. Pascoe PJ. Opioid analgesics. Vet Clinics of North America: Small Animal Practice. 2000; 30(4):757–772
12. Robertson S.A, Taylor P.M, Sear J.W. Systemic uptake of buprenorphine by cats after oral mucosal administration. Vet Record 2003; 152:675–678

APPENDIX Controlled Drug Regulations

The opioids are classed as controlled drugs (CD) as they are capable of being abused by humans, and so there are stricter controls applied to them than for other prescription-only medicines (POM). Under the Misuse of Drugs Regulations 1985, all controlled drugs are divided into five groups or schedules, in decreasing order of stringency of control (Table A6.1).[A1]

Veterinary surgeons are not allowed to prescribe or possess Schedule 1 controlled drugs – these include cannabis, LSD and other hallucinogenic drugs. The majority of the opioids that are suitable for more severe pain, pure mu agonists, are classed as Schedule 2 drugs. Partial agonists and antagonists,

Table A6.1
Classification of opioids into controlled drug schedules

Schedule	Opioids
Schedule 1	
Schedule 2	Morphine Papaveretum Pethidine Fentanyl Methadone Alfentanil Remifentanil
Schedule 3	Buprenorphine Pentazocine
Schedule 4	
Schedule 5	Codeine (in preps with small amounts)
Non CD opioids (POM only)	Butorphanol Naloxone

Table A6.2
Example of the information that must be recorded for purchase of a schedule 2 CD made by the practice

Date supply received	Name and address of supplier	Amount obtained	Form of drug supplied
21/12/04	Smiths Wholesalers 22 Storage Street Newtown Notts NG99 1ZX	2 × 10 ml	Morphine injection

(After British Veterinary Association Code of Practice on Medicines. London: Publications BVA; 2000, reproduced with permission.)

more suitable for mild to moderate pain, are usually classed as Schedule 3. The regulations and record keeping for obtaining a supply of each type of CD, writing a prescription or dispensing them directly in the practice are summarised below.

Schedule 2 opioids

To purchase a supply, the requisition or order form must be signed by the vet and they also need to put their full name, address, professional qualifications and specify the total amount of drug to be purchased and the reason for its use. Every time a purchase is made of a schedule 2 CD, it must be recorded in a register, as shown in Table A6.2.[A1]

Whenever a dose is used in the practice, comprehensive records must be kept in a register, which should have separate sections for each particular controlled drug, e.g. a section for morphine, another for pethidine, etc. Table A6.3 details the information that must be recorded for every dose within 24 hours of its use. Entries need to be made in ink and should not be changed – if they are, a note must be made as to the date and reason for the change. Registers must be kept for 2 years after the date of the last entry.

Schedule 2 CDs must be kept in a locked cabinet that can only be opened by a vet or somebody with their authority. These drugs can only be disposed of in the presence of a person authorised by the Secretary of State (a Police Officer or Home Office Inspector).

If a vet decides to write a prescription for a schedule 2 opioid, rather than dispense it directly, the prescription must take the form of the usual POM prescription but must in addition be handwritten by the vet and include the form,

Table A6.3
Example of the information required for recording each dose of schedule 2 CD used in a practice

Date on which transaction was effected (i.e. date drug given)	Name and address of person supplied (pet and owner name)	Particulars as to licence or authority of person supplied to be in possession	Amount supplied	Form of drug given
21/12/04	Mrs Brown's dog, Max. 11 Meadows Drive Hayton, Notts DN22 4AR	Direct administration (i.m. inj)	50 mg (1 ml)	Pethidine injection

(After British Veterinary Association Code of Practice on Medicines. London: BVA Publications; 2000, reproduced with permission.)

strength and total quantity of drug to be dispensed (in both numbers and words).

Schedule 3 opioids

The same regulations apply to these opioids as schedule 2 when it comes to obtaining them from a supplier, and writing a prescription. However, there is no requirement to record each drug purchase in a register or record each dose as it's used. Schedule 3 opioids must also be kept in a locked cabinet, and invoices of purchases kept for 2 years.

Schedule 5 opioids

These drugs are exempt from the CD regulations detailed above apart from the retention of invoices for 2 years.

REFERENCE

A1 British Veterinary Association Code of Practice on Medicines. BVA Publications: London; 2000

CHAPTER 7

THE NON-STEROIDAL ANTI-INFLAMMATORY ANALGESIC DRUGS (NSAIDS)

INTRODUCTION

The NSAIDs are analgesics that block the pain pathway both peripherally and centrally; in addition they are also anti-inflammatory and antipyretic (reduce a fever). They comprise of two groups of weak organic acids: carboxylic acids (e.g. aspirin, carprofen) and the enolic acids (e.g. phenylbutazone, meloxicam). The history of the NSAIDs started with Hippocrates back in 440–377 BC, who noted the analgesic and antipyretic properties of extracts of the bark of the willow (*Salix alba*). This started to be used for mild pain in the 1st century, and fast forwarding to the 19th century, the active ingredient salicylic acid was isolated and started to be synthesised. However, it was found to be very bitter and often irritant to the stomach and so in 1857 an altogether better version, a derivative called acetylsalicylic acid, now known as aspirin, was produced. Aspirin is still the most commonly used non-prescription drug in the world, but its mechanism of action, and those of the other NSAIDs was not actually elucidated until 1971.

NSAIDs inhibit the production of a group of inflammatory mediators, the prostanoids, which are responsible for sensitising nociceptors in damaged tissue. Centrally they inhibit the transmission of pain signals in the spinal cord (and possibly the brain) and reduce a fever. One of their main advantages is a much longer duration of action compared to opioids, most of them providing 24 hours or more analgesia, but NSAIDs are also associated with a range of potential side effects that can restrict their use and give rise to several contraindications which clinicians must be aware of. They can be very useful analgesics for the control of acute and chronic moderate to severe pain, and some compare favourably to opioids in terms of the level of analgesia they can provide.

Combinations of opioids and NSAIDs, which block the pain pathway by different mechanisms, seem to have a synergistic effect and can provide excellent analgesia suitable for the treatment of moderate or severe pain, particularly if they are used pre-emptively. NSAIDS with a preoperative license, and hence a suitable safety profile, have been shown to have a significant pre-emptive effect in veterinary patients and can reduce both peripheral and central sensitisation.[1,2] It's important to realise that not all NSAIDS are the same; there is a lot of variation in individual drug safety profiles. Not only that, but susceptibility to the side effects of NSAIDs varies between species. Cats and dogs are both more susceptible to their adverse effects than humans, so data on NSAIDs from one species cannot always be extrapolated to another. For example, ibuprofen used at human dose rates in dogs can produce severe toxic effects; similarly, aspirin used at canine dose rates in cats can be toxic.

NSAIDS AND THE INFLAMMATORY PATHWAY

When tissue is damaged the injured cells release a cascade of chemicals that form an inflammatory or sensitising soup that produces local changes in the surrounding tissue. These changes include vasodilatation of arterioles, increased permeability of capillaries and venules, migration of white blood cells into the area and stimulation of nociceptors. This results in the four cardinal signs of inflammation – heat, redness, swelling and pain. The purpose of this acute inflammatory response is to mobilise the body's immune system against the noxious stimulus causing the tissue injury, remove it from the site of damage and repair the tissue. If the inflammatory stimulus persists then chronic inflammation ensues. One major pathway in the generation of inflammatory mediators is the arachidonic acid cascade.

When cells are damaged an enzyme in the cell membrane called phospholipase A_2 becomes activated and in turn activates and releases another membrane-bound substance, arachidonic acid. Arachidonic acid is then converted into many different inflammatory mediators (termed eicosanoids) by various enzymes. One such enzyme, cyclo-oxygenase (COX), converts arachidonic acid into the prostanoids, comprising the prostaglandins (PGE_2, PGD_2, and PGF_2), prostacyclin PGI_2 and thromboxane A_2 (TXA_2). The prostanoids have many inflammatory activities (particularly vasodilatation and oedema formation) but they also play a key role in the pain associated with inflammation. The prostaglandins and prostacyclin sensitise nociceptor endings to other mediators in the inflammatory soup such as histamine and bradykinin, which directly stimulate nociceptors causing pain, i.e. prostanoids are in part responsible for hyperalgesia and peripheral sensitisation. Prostaglandins cause pyrexia (a fever) by acting on the thermoregulatory centre in the hypothalamus. Thromboxane A_2 is generated by COX enzyme present in platelets and is involved in platelet aggregation. Another enzyme, 5-lipoxygenase (LOX), converts arachidonic acid into the leukotrienes, a group of mediators that are more involved in attracting and activating white blood cells into the area of tissue damage as well as other inflammatory changes. The arachidonic acid cascade is summarised in Fig 7.1.

NSAIDS primarily block COX and inhibit the production of inflammatory prostanoids, thereby relieving pain and inflammation and reducing pyrexia. A new class of NSAIDs has just been developed called 'dual inhibitor NSAIDs' as they block both COX and 5-LOX enzymes. The corticosteroids inhibit the arachidonic acid cascade higher up, at the level of phospholipase A_2, and inhibit the formation of both prostanoids and leukotrienes.

COX 1 AND COX 2 ENZYMES

A few years ago it was discovered that there were two forms of the COX enzyme, rather unimaginatively called COX 1 and COX 2. COX 1 is considered constitutive, i.e. it's present at fairly constant levels all the time and is responsible for producing prostaglandins involved in normal housekeeping duties in various tissues. These housekeeping prostaglandins increase local blood flow in the gastric mucosa and are

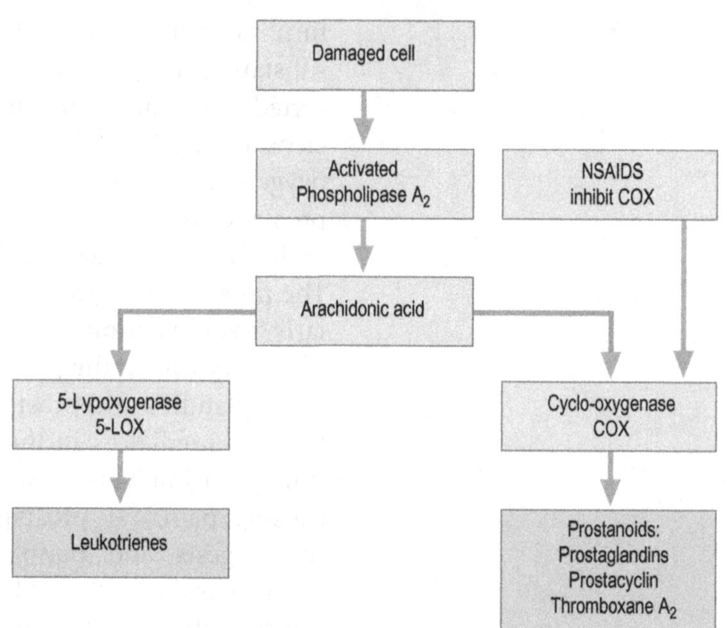

Figure 7.1
The arachidonic acid cascade.

involved in the production of mucus and bicarbonate that protect the stomach lining against its own acid secretions. Housekeeping prostaglandins generated by COX 1 play an important role protecting the kidney against ischaemic damage in the event of a drop in systemic blood pressure. Hypotension will cause the sympathetic nervous system and the renin–angiotensin system to kick into action resulting in vasoconstriction that will bump blood pressure back up. In this scenario there is the release of housekeeping prostaglandins just in the kidneys that cause a localised vasodilatation. This maintains blood flow to the kidney cells, protecting the renal tissue from ischaemic damage under these conditions. COX 1 present in platelets is responsible for the formation of thromboxane A_2 required for normal platelet aggregation and clotting. It therefore becomes clear that if a NSAID significantly inhibits COX 1 and housekeeping prostaglandins there is a potential risk of gastric ulceration, reduced blood clotting and renal damage, which are the classic side effects associated with NSAIDs.

COX 2 is considered inducible; in most tissues it's only generated during inflammation and is responsible for the production of inflammatory prostaglandins, whose actions are described above. Inhibition of COX 2 is how NSAIDs exert their therapeutic effects. Fig 7.2 summarises the roles of COX 1 and COX 2.

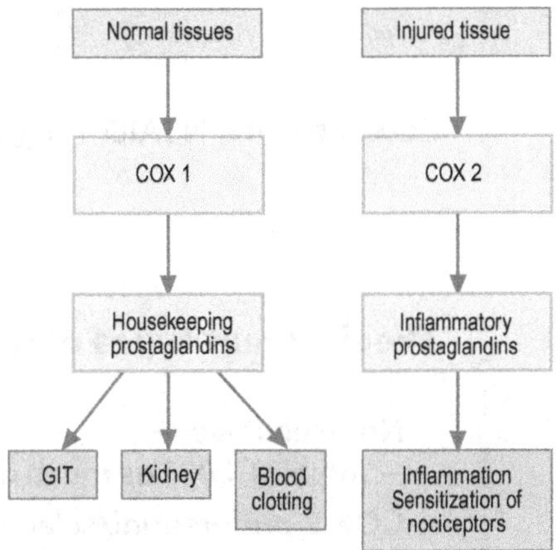

Figure 7.2
The roles of COX 1 and COX 2.

COX RATIOS

Once COX 1 and COX 2 had been discovered, people started looking at how well NSAIDs inhibited COX 2, whilst leaving COX 1 alone, to try and assess their potential efficacy and safety. Studies were done on cell cultures to measure the concentrations of a NSAID needed to get 50% inhibition of each COX enzyme, called the IC_{50} values. Ideally a drug should have a very high IC_{50} for COX 1, so it would require huge amounts of drug before there is any inhibition of housekeeping prostaglandins, whilst also having a low IC_{50} for COX 2, so only a small amount of drug is needed to get a nice anti-inflammatory analgesic effect. Since plain water would have a fabulously high (nudging infinity) IC_{50} for both COX 1 and for COX 2, both values need to be looked at together. Dividing the IC_{50} for COX 1 by the IC_{50} for COX 2, called the COX ratio, does this. If the COX ratio is greater than 1, then the NSAID is inhibiting COX 2 more than COX 1 (i.e. a much greater amount of drug is needed to inhibit COX 1 than COX 2) and such drugs are often termed COX 2-selective or preferential NSAIDs. Conversely, a COX ratio less than 1 indicates COX 1 is inhibited more than COX 2, and the drug is considered non-selective for COX 2. More recently a group of NSAIDs have been developed and launched that inhibit COX 2 hundreds of times more than COX 1 and these NSAIDs are termed COX 2-specific NSAIDs or 'coxibs'. Rather confusingly, some studies calculate COX ratios the other way round, with the IC_{50} for COX 2 divided by the IC_{50} for COX 1.

Box 7.1

COX ratio of a NSAID = IC_{50} for COX 1 / IC_{50} for COX 2

Box 7.2 **The different types of NSAID**

- Non-selective
  - Inhibit COX 1 as much as, or more than COX 2
- COX 2 preferential/selective
  - Inhibit COX 2 more than COX 1
- Coxibs
  - Highly selective for COX 2
  - Sometimes called COX 2 specific
- Dual inhibitors
  - Inhibit both COX and 5-LOX (not necessarily selective for COX 2)

Both COX 2 selective and Coxib NSAIDs can also be termed COX 1 sparing

COX ratios were very much a hot topic a few years ago, however, it's important to realise that different studies report different ratios for the same drugs, and that ratios will vary depending on the cell type and assay systems used in each experiment – there is no standardised way to calculate a COX ratio. They are an in-vitro measurements, and are often calculated from cell lines from species other than those who receive the drug in real life. COX ratios, i.e. NSAID selectivity, do not seem to be consistent between different species and should not be extrapolated. The ratios can be a useful indicator to the potential safety and efficacy of a NSAID, but are by no means the entire story. It is what happens in a real whole animal that is the most valuable and important information. This is becoming increasingly obvious as it has transpired that the roles of COX 1 and COX 2 are not as clear-cut as first thought. Table 7.1 gives a rough guide to the relative COX selectivity of various NSAIDs in veterinary use.

Table 7.1 Approximate COX selectivity of some NSAIDs in veterinary patients (number of + signs indicates increasing activity)

NSAID	COX 1 inhibition	COX 2 inhibition
Aspirin	++++	–
Carprofen	+	+++
Flunixin	+++	+
Ibuprofen	+++	+
Ketoprofen	+++	+
Meloxicam	+	+++
Phenylbutazone	++++	–
Tolfenamic acid	++	++

(From Livingston A. Mechanism of action of non-steroidal anti-inflammatory drugs. Vet Clinics of North America: Small Animal Practice 2000; 30(4):773–781, reproduced with permission.)

OTHER ROLES OF COX 1 AND COX 2

COX 1 is known to be present in many tissues including the stomach, kidney, platelets and reproductive tract. COX 2 is induced at the sites of inflammation in various cell types, such as white blood cells, vascular endothelium, smooth muscle, chondrocytes, fibroblasts and synovial cells, but is found constitutively in the brain and kidneys of some species including the dog. The questions being raised at the moment are whether COX 2 can play a useful role in tissue and if so, is its complete inhibition by NSAIDs such a good idea. Also, could some COX 1 inhibition be helpful if it plays a part in mediating inflammation.

Studies in mice completely deficient in COX 2 suggest that it may help modulate inflammation, and inflammation could be prolonged in the absence of COX 2. Although COX 2 is not normally present in the gastric mucosa it does appear to be expressed when there is gastric ulceration, and plays a role in the repair of the ulcer. Therefore, if gastric ulceration is already present, inhibiting COX 2 could lead to delayed healing of the mucosa.[4] COX 2 is found to be present constitutively in kidneys of dogs and rodents and is thought to be important for normal renal development in neonates and maybe renal homeostasis in adults.[4] In the reproductive tract COX 2 seems to be involved in ovulation, embryo implantation and placental development and parturition.[4]

Recent studies have also been looking at the role of COX 2 in bone healing; findings suggest that inhibition of COX 2 by coxibs and other NSAIDs can lead to delayed fracture healing in animal experimental models.[5] The steps involved in normal bone healing are an inflammatory response, bone resorption and new bone formation. Prostaglandins appear to be involved in all these steps – initial inflammation, an increase in osteoclast activity and bone resorption, and an increase in osteoblast activity and new bone formation. Inhibition or an absence of COX 2 reduces prostaglandin production and is the likely mechanism for NSAIDS to impair fracture healing.[6] Studies have found delays in fracture repairs in mice genetically deficient in COX 2, and as a result of administration of some coxibs and older NSAIDs (given at high doses and/or for extended periods of time) to mice, rats and rabbits. However, despite these findings, COX 2 inhibitors have not proven to be problematic clinically in humans despite very widespread use, and the studies do not reflect the typical doses and durations of NSAIDs used in patients. Therefore the clinical significance of these findings remains unclear and it's important to remember that the benefits of analgesia combined with the short duration of NSAID therapy used in most cases is likely to make an overall adverse effect unlikely.

Some studies on mice deficient in COX 1 suggest it may play a role in the early stages of acute inflammation before COX 2 comes into effect. Such new information coming to light is somewhat changing the focus on NSAID development away from just trying to inhibit COX 2 and spare COX 1.

COX 3

A variant of COX 1 found in large amounts in the cerebral cortex of dogs has recently been named COX 3. It seems likely that there are genetic differences between individuals in the structure of their COX 1 enzyme, COX 3 being one of them. This structural variation probably affects the binding and activity of NSAIDs and could explain why one drug seems to work well in some individuals but not others, and why there is such variation in individual tolerances to NSAIDs.[7]

OTHER MECHANISMS OF ACTION OF NSAIDS

There are thought to be some other non-COX dependent mechanisms of action of NSAIDs, not shared by all the drugs, and their contribution to clinical effects is unknown. Other areas of activity include inhibition of neutrophil chemotaxis (the attraction and movement of white blood cells into inflamed tissue), activation and inhibition of eicosanoids at their receptors, modulation of cytokines (small proteins that regulate cell function and differentiation) and other cell messengers. The non-COX activity of the dual inhibitor NSAIDs and carprofen are discussed below.

Dual inhibitors

If the arachidonic acid cascade is rudely interrupted by NSAIDs at the level of COX, then it's thought that more arachidonic acid is diverted into the 5-LOX part of the pathway, resulting in increased leukotriene production. Leukotrienes cause adherence and activation of leucocytes (white blood cells) to the vascular endothelium of GI tract blood vessels. These leucocytes could cause vascular occlusion and will release their own mediators that can lead to reduced blood flow, local ischaemia, tissue damage and GI ulceration. The idea behind dual inhibitors, e.g. tepoxalin, is to avoid this by blocking both COX and 5-LOX. Any significant advantages of dual inhibitors in a clinical setting (in terms of better analgesia or safety) have not yet been proven, and COX selectivity may not be a feature of these drugs.

PG-sparing NSAIDs

Carprofen is a NSAID that is considered relatively prostaglandin sparing;[8] it seems to be a weak inhibitor of COX, but is still a potent anti-inflammatory and analgesic. The COX inhibition it does have appears to be selective for COX 2 in canine cell studies,[9] but doesn't explain its entire efficacy. It probably works on other parts of the inflammatory pathways, and a recent study suggests it may inhibit a proinflammatory transcription factor, NfκB, that would otherwise activate cells to synthesise a range of substances involved in the inflammatory response (e.g. COX 2, inducible nitric oxide synthase).[10]

ACTIONS OF NSAIDS

Analgesia

Peripherally, NSAIDs reduce the pain associated with inflammation by inhibiting the production of prostaglandins that sensitise nociceptors and nerve endings to other inflammatory mediators, and in doing so they will reduce the development of peripheral sensitisation. There is evidence that prostaglandins act as transmitters of pain signals within the CNS, which is also how NSAIDs are thought to have a significant central analgesic effect. In addition to this it now seems COX 2 is induced within the spinal cord in response to peripheral inflammation, and helps mediate wind-up. This mechanism explains why NSAIDs have been shown to reduce the development of central sensitisation. All these sites of action make NSAIDs very useful for the treatment of acute pain preop and postop, and also chronic pain states where sensitisation is a significant part of the pathology.

Anti-inflammatory effect

Inflammatory prostaglandins not only enhance pain, but they also promote vascular leakage and vasodilatation in damaged tissue. Therefore, NSAIDs will reduce oedema formation, swelling and erythema (redness).

Anti-pyretic

NSAIDS are very effective at relieving a fever by blocking the production of COX 2 and prostaglandins in the brain that are thought to be responsible for pyrexia during inflammation.

Anti-endotoxic

Some NSAIDs such as flunixin are thought to have an anti-endotoxic effect that may be mediated through inhibition of inflammatory pathways other than COX 2. Endotoxins, like those released from bacteria, bind receptors on vascular wall cells and white blood cells. This stimulates a proinflammatory transcription factor, NFκB, that trots off to the cell nucleus and activates the massive production of mediators of endotoxaemia, e.g. COX 2 and inducible nitric oxide synthase (iNOS). Flunixin and carprofen have been shown in-vitro to inhibit this activation,[10] which may be an antiendotoxic mechanism of action and also contribute to their overall anti-inflammatory action.

NSAIDs and cancer

Recent work has found that inhibitors of COX 2 can be useful in the prevention and treatment of certain cancers in humans and animals. COX 2 was first implicated in the development of colon cancer in humans, and it was later found to be over-expressed in other tumours including intestinal, oesophageal, bladder, breast, lung and prostate. COX 2 can be induced in tissue not only by inflammation, but also in response to tumour-promoting growth factors and is known to reduce cell apoptosis (the normal programmed cell death mechanism) that characterises the switch of normal cells into cancer cells. The exact mechanism of action of NSAIDs to prevent and regress tumours is still not completely understood, but may involve COX 2 inhibition, increased apoptosis, antiangiogenic effects (inhibition of new blood vessel growth, necessary to meet the metabolic needs of growing tissue) and activation of immune responses through decreased prostaglandin production or even via pathways independent of COX.

NSAIDs rarely provide a cure for certain cancers but several studies have shown that they can be used as a palliative treatment in animals and can increase mean survival times. It's therefore a therapeutic option that could be considered for cases that have failed to respond to traditional treatment or where there are complicating factors, or where surgery isn't possible, etc. The NSAID that's been studied the most for use in cancer is piroxicam, a good inhibitor of COX 2 in dogs, as this was the one initially found to have an antitumour effect in people. It should be noted that this NSAID is not licensed for animals in the UK, and is not recommended for use in cats. Examples of published work on the use of NSAIDs in veterinary cancer patients are as follows.

A study[11] looked at the use of piroxicam in 34 dogs with transitional cell carcinoma of the bladder (known to express high levels of COX 2). Surgery is usually the treatment of choice, but if the tumour is located at the bladder trigone resection is impossible. Two out of the 34 dogs showed complete remission, whilst a further four had partial remission (a 50% or more reduction in tumour size). Piroxicam suppositories have been used in dogs with rectal polyps and carcinoma. It was shown to significantly reduce the clinical signs and improve the quality of life and in some dogs there was complete remission.[12] It's well known that rectal polyps can progress to carcinomas and the use of NSAIDs in these patients may limit this malignant transformation. Polypoid cystitis in dogs is another benign condition that may become malignant. The use of COX 2 inhibitors such as piroxicam and meloxicam appears to limit the development of malignancy and may help control clinical signs of this disease.[13] Surgical removal is the usual treatment but this may not be possible if the polyps sit near the trigone. NSAIDs could also be used to augment incomplete resection to minimise the risk of recurrence.[13]

Another paper was published looking at piroxicam for the treatment of a range of tumours in 62 dogs.[14] In this trial partial remission was reported in 3 out of 10 dogs with transitional cell carcinoma, 3 out of 5 dogs with squamous cell carcinoma, and 1 out of 3 dogs with mammary adenocarcinoma. Finally, one paper has been published using piroxicam or carprofen for the treatment of prostatic carcinoma in 35 dogs.[15] The vast majority of tumours (regardless of exact tissue origin) were found to express COX 2 (not found in normal prostates) and dogs treated with either NSAID lived significantly longer than dogs not receiving a NSAID. The average survival time of dogs that received carprofen or piroxicam was 6.9 months, compared with only 0.7 months for untreated dogs.

All this recent data suggests NSAIDs may have an important role in the prevention and therapy of a range of cancers in the future.

Side effects of NSAIDs

Side effects of NSAIDs are mainly due to inhibition of housekeeping prostaglandins and include GI ulceration, renal damage, and reduced blood clotting. An idiosyncratic hepatopathy, although very rare, is also seen on occasion which is linked more to NSAID metabolism rather than COX inhibition. A potentially detrimental effect on arthritic cartilage is also an area of concern for some of these drugs. As

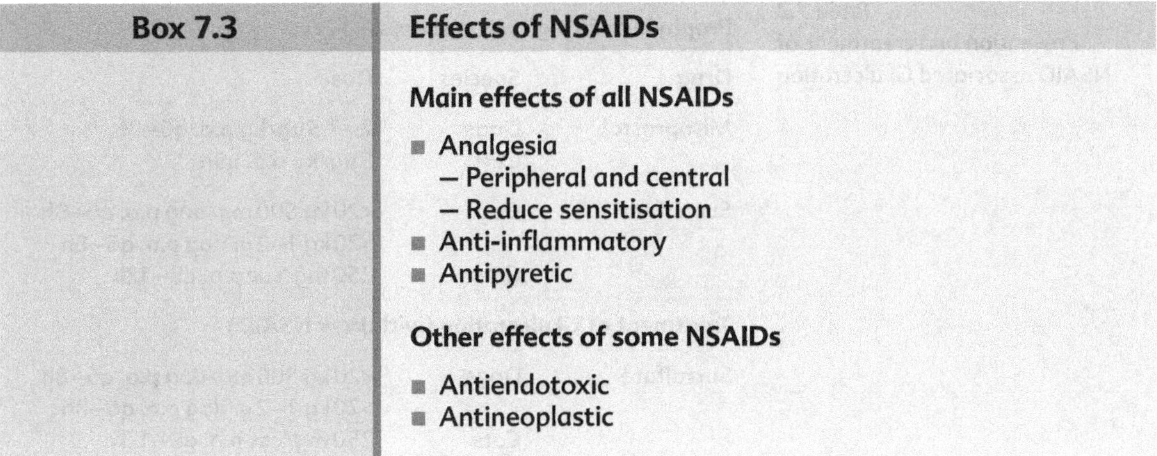
Box 7.3 **Effects of NSAIDs**

Main effects of all NSAIDs

- Analgesia
  - Peripheral and central
  - Reduce sensitisation
- Anti-inflammatory
- Antipyretic

Other effects of some NSAIDs

- Antiendotoxic
- Antineoplastic

already noted, not all NSAIDs are the same and the likelihood and even the nature of side effects does vary between individual drugs; these are discussed later. Generally speaking the COX 2 selective NSAIDs are considered 'safer', but they are still NSAIDs and the potential risks should still be considered when they are used.

GI ulceration

The commonest side effect of NSAIDs is gastrointestinal irritation leading to a range of signs from vomiting right through to ulceration and more rarely a protein-losing enteropathy. The cause is inhibition of the housekeeping prostaglandin PGE_2 that maintains blood flow to the mucosa and helps produce protective mucus secretions. In addition to this, aspirin has a direct irritant effect on the mucosa. The newer COX 2 selective NSAIDs, or the COX 1 sparing NSAIDs as they are sometimes referred to, do seem to reduce the incidence of GI side effects.

Measures can be taken to reduce the likelihood of ulceration in higher risk patients by concurrent administration of misoprostol, a synthetic prostaglandin. Known side effects of misoprostol are diarrhoea, vomiting and abdominal cramps and it must not be used in pregnant animals. Once gastric ulceration is present (and the NSAID has been withdrawn) treatment with either an H-2 receptor antagonist, e.g. ranitidine, or with a proton pump inhibitor, e.g. omeprazole, is recommended – both types of drug work by reducing gastric

Table 7.2
Prevention and treatment of NSAID associated GI ulceration

Drug	Species	Dose
Prophylaxis in high risk patients		
Misoprostol	Dogs Cats	2–7.5 µg/kg p.o. q6–8h 5 µg/kg p.o. q8h
Sucralfate	Dogs Cats	<20 kg 500 mg/dog p.o. q6–8h >20 kg 1–2 g/dog p.o. q6–8h 250 mg/cat p.o. q8–12h
Treatment of GI ulceration (withdraw NSAID)		
Sucralfate	Dogs Cats	<20 kg 500 mg/dog p.o. q6–8h >20 kg 1–2 g/dog p.o. q6–8h 250 mg/cat p.o. q8–12h
Ranitidine*	Dogs Cats	2 mg/kg s.c., p.o. q8–12h 3.5 mg/kg p.o. q12h
Omeprazole*	Dogs Cats	0.5–1.5 mg/kg p.o. q24h (max of 8 weeks) 0.75–1 mg/kg p.o. q24h

*NB use either ranitidine or omeprazole

acid secretion. Sucralfate suspension can also be added; this drug binds to mucosal defects forming a protective barrier against gastric acid. It also accelerates healing of ulcers and stimulates local housekeeping prostaglandin production. Ideally it should be given an hour before food, and other medications need to be administered 1 hour before or 2 hours after sucralfate as it interferes with drug absorption. It's not a specific prophylactic treatment for ulcers but there is a case for using it alongside NSAIDs in high-risk patients. Table 7.2 summarises the prevention and treatment of NSAID induced gastric ulceration. All doses are from the BSAVA Small Animal Formulary, 4th edition (published by the BSAVA).

Renal damage

If an animal is experiencing reduced renal blood flow – due to hypovolaemia, haemorrhage, hypotension, or, not uncommonly, as a consequence of general anaesthesia – then NSAIDs can precipitate renal damage. Housekeeping renal prostaglandins are normally released under these conditions and produce a localised vasodilatation that maintains renal perfusion; NSAID inhibition of this mechanism can lead to ischaemic damage of kidney cells. Carprofen and meloxicam have gained preoperative licenses in the UK, allowing them to be used in healthy patients undergoing general anaesthesia. Since COX 2 is expressed constitutively in the kidney, it is still not established whether it is just COX selectivity that actually confers better renal safety or not.[16] Not all NSAIDs are suitable for periop use because of worries about nephrotoxicity. Using i.v. fluids to maintain blood pressure and renal perfusion, monitoring arterial blood pressure to help avoid hypotension developing, and minimising cardiovascular depressant drugs during anaesthesia can reduce the risk of renal damage. NSAIDs should not be used with other potentially nephrotoxic drugs.

Blood clotting

NSAID inhibition of COX 1 in platelets will block the production of thromboxane A_2, needed for normal platelet aggregation. Aspirin is unique in inhibiting thromboxane A_2 for the lifetime of the platelet, and so is actually used therapeutically as an antithrombolytic. Most NSAIDs do not prolong bleeding times at clinical doses, but they should not be used with other drugs that affect clotting, as theoretically the sum effect could push bleeding times above the normal range.

Idiosyncratic hepatopathy

NSAIDs can very rarely cause an idiosyncratic hepatopathy, a side effect recognised in both humans and dogs. The problem is idiosyncratic, i.e. it is an unpredictable patient-specific characteristic, not dependent on dose or duration of treatment. The current thinking is that some patients have a peculiarity in the way they metabolise the drug, and generate metabolites (acyl glucuronides) that bind covalently to liver and plasma proteins. These altered proteins seem to be antigenic and cause an immune-mediated reaction against the liver, resulting in hepatic toxicosis.[17] An alternative theory is that some patients may form or accumulate metabolites that are directly toxic to heptocytes.[17,18]

There has been one review of cases in dogs that had received carprofen[19] but it's important to realise this rare adverse reaction is possible with other NSAIDs in veterinary use. It mistakenly became associated with just carprofen, as this was by far the most widely used NSAID at the time the cases came to light in the USA. There was also a concern that Labrador retrievers were over represented in the affected population of dogs, but it's now thought that this breed are probably over represented in the population of dogs that receive NSAIDs (usually for osteoarthritis).

The signs of NSAID-induced idiosyncratic hepatopathy in dogs range from raised liver enzymes with no clinical signs, through to jaundice and a potentially fatal acute hepatic crisis. Of the 21 cases reviewed in the USA presenting signs (starting with the most common) were anorexia, vomiting, lethargy, diarrhoea and polydipsia and polyuria. Onset of signs was on average about 19 days after treatment was initiated. Biochemical changes included raised ALT, AST, ALP and total serum bilirubin levels. Increases in ALT levels often exceeded those of ALP. Abdominal radiography and ultrasound were usually unremarkable. Of the dogs that had liver biopsies performed, changes ranged from mild to severe acute hepatocellular injury (multifocal to diffuse hepatic necrosis, with ballooning degeneration of cells and parenchymal collapse) with inflammation and cholestasis. The severity and progression of clinical signs did not correlate to dose or duration of treatment, magnitude of liver enzymes or histological changes.

Treatment entails withdrawing the NSAID as soon as possible and general hepatic supportive treatment (e.g. i.v. fluids, broad-spectrum antibiotics, hepatic support diet) and the vast majority of cases will resolve without long-term problems.

Cartilage effects

Some NSAIDs have been found to increase the breakdown of osteoarthritic cartilage in human and canine studies. Cartilage is made up of cartilage cells, chondrocytes, sat in an extracellular matrix. The matrix is composed of water and large molecules including type II collagen and proteoglycan. These molecules give cartilage its biomechanical properties (stiffness on compression and elasticity). Chondrocytes continually synthesise new proteoglycan and also release enzymes that degrade old proteoglycan. In normal healthy cartilage there is a fine balance between this anabolism and catabolism. Osteoarthritis is characterised by a progressive loss of cartilage proteoglycan; chondrocyte metabolism is switched to a catabolic state so that proteoglycan breakdown exceeds synthesis. It appears that some NSAIDs suppress proteoglycan synthesis in arthritic cartilage, whilst having much less effect on normal cartilage. Aspirin has been shown to promote cartilage degeneration in-vitro and in-vivo in arthritic cartilage of dogs, significantly lowering proteoglycan content.[20] Ibuprofen has also been shown in-vitro to reduce proteoglycan synthesis in canine cartilage. The mechanism appears to be independent of prostaglandin inhibition.

Some work has been done on NSAIDs licensed for long-term treatment of osteoarthritis in dogs. In one experimental study,[21] meloxicam was given to dogs within the first 24 hours after acute joint inflammation was induced in the stifle. At the end of the study the joint cartilage was examined in-vitro and meloxicam was found to have no effect on proteoglycan synthesis. There has been more work published on carprofen's effect on cartilage to date, which has actually suggested a positive rather than a negative or neutral effect on cartilage metabolism. In-vitro work discovered that proteoglycan synthesis was significantly increased in canine arthritic cartilage by carprofen at concentrations found in the synovial fluid of dogs given label doses (4 mg/kg/day).[22,23]

A later in-vivo study,[24] looking at an experimental model of stifle arthritis after cranial cruciate rupture, examined articular cartilage 12 weeks after injury. Dogs administered carprofen from 4 weeks to 12 weeks post injury at either 4.4 mg/kg or 8.8 mg/kg/day were generally found to have smaller and less severe cartilage lesions compared to untreated dogs. The difference was statistically significant for the severity of lesions on the tibial plateau at 4.4 mg/kg/day. More work needs to be done to elucidate the various mechanisms of action of NSAID effects on cartilage and its clinical significance in animals. The next question to answer would be whether there is any extra benefit to using nutraceuticals (preparations containing the building blocks of proteoglycans such a glucosamine and chondroitin) with NSAIDs.

Box 7.4 **The main potential side effects of NSAIDs**

- GI ulceration
- Renal damage
- Reduced blood clotting
- Idiosyncratic hepatopathy

Bone marrow

A very rare side effect of phenylbutazone in animals is bone marrow suppression. This NSAID is no longer used in humans and one of the reasons it was withdrawn was a high incidence of this side effect.

Coxibs and cardiovascular side effects

Very recently on the human side it has emerged that coxibs, as a subclass of NSAIDs, can increase the risk of cardiovascular disease such as heart attacks and strokes in humans following long-term treatment. There is no evidence that the risk persists after treatment is stopped. One coxib, rofecoxib, was withdrawn in September 2004, and further studies are being undertaken on the others that are available on the human market, e.g. celecoxib, valdecoxib. Current advice is that patients with a history of ischaemic heart disease or cerebrovascular disease should not be given coxibs. As yet there is no direct relevance of this on the veterinary side.

PHARMACOKINETICS AND METABOLISM

NSAIDs are well absorbed following oral, s.c., and i.m. administration and become highly protein bound in the plasma (over 99% for some drugs). The half-life of NSAIDs (time taken for blood levels to drop by 50%) has a very poor correlation to duration of analgesia.[1] This is because the drugs accumulate at sites of inflammation, bound up to protein that has leaked out into the inflammatory fluid from the circulation. Hence levels of NSAID remain much higher, for much longer, at sites of tissue damage than they do in the blood.[8] So even NSAIDs with short half-lives can be dosed once daily. Most NSAIDs are metabolised in the liver, and normally the metabolites are inactive and excreted in urine and bile (there may be some enterohepatic recirculation).

Extra care is needed with dosing levels and intervals in cats because they are lacking in the hepatic enzyme glucuronyl transferase that can be needed for NSAID metabolism. As a result, some NSAIDs have a very long half-life in cats and can accumulate to toxic levels if they are given repeat doses before the previous ones have been cleared. Always check the manufacturer's recommendations and avoid extrapolating dose rates of NSAIDs from one species to another.

Neonates (animals under the age of about 6 weeks) may not be able to eliminate drugs as well as adults because of immature renal and hepatic clearance mechanisms, so dose rates of NSAIDs may need to be adjusted in these patients. Geriatric animals are more likely than others to receive long-term NSAIDs, for the treatment of osteoarthritis. This group of patients have a higher incidence of concurrent problems such as renal insufficiency and careful patient assessment and discussion with the owner is important before prescribing NSAIDs. At the end of the day, a risk/benefit assessment needs to be made for each individual patient. The benefit of analgesia and improved quality of life often outweighs the increased risks of using a NSAID. If an animal is in too much pain to get out of its basket and potter round the garden to have a wee without falling over, does it really matter if an analgesic potentially affects life expectancy?

CONTRAINDICATIONS

Due to the increased risk of adverse effects, all NSAIDs are contraindicated in animals with a history of GI ulceration, renal, hepatic or cardiac impairment (cardiac impairment can reduce renal blood flow), or animals suffering from dehydration, hypovolaemia, hypotension or clotting disorders. Animals that are in shock, such as from road traffic accidents, or those at risk from haemorrhage, are not suitable candidates for NSAID administration until they have been suitably stabilised and the circulation supported with i.v. fluid therapy. Opioids may be indicated early on to provide analgesia in the interim.

Theoretically NSAIDs can prolong gestation by inhibiting prostaglandins involved in parturition. As discussed earlier, there is a possibility they can interfere with fertility and embryo implantation as well, so they are contraindicated in pregnancy. Anecdotally however, they do seem to be frequently used in practice in the very short term to provide periop analgesia in caesarean section.

Patients with moderate to severe pulmonary disease are not ideal candidates for NSAID treatment as housekeeping prostaglandins play a part in relaxing bronchial and tracheal muscle to hold airways open, so their inhibition may cause deterioration in these patients.

DRUG INTERACTIONS

NSAIDs should not be used concurrently with corticosteroids as both classes of drug have the potential to inhibit the production of housekeeping prostaglandins and used together, there is a much higher risk of side effects. For the same reason, two different NSAIDs should not be used concurrently in the same patient, and wash-out periods are recommended between changing from one to another. It's advisable not to use NSAIDs with other drugs that are nephrotoxic, or that reduce renal perfusion or blood pressure. NSAIDs may in theory decrease the effectiveness of furosemide and ACE inhibitors as these drugs work by stimulating prostaglandin synthesis to increase renal blood flow. NSAIDs are highly protein-bound in the plasma, so care must be taken when using them with other protein-bound drugs (e.g. phenobarbital) as they can displace each other, resulting in lots of free active drug in the circulation and a higher risk of toxicity.

Although not a drug interaction, it's known that some NSAIDs can slightly lower total thyroxine T_4 levels in dogs. This effect does not cause hypothyroidism but could lead to a misdiagnosis of hypothyroidism if only T_4 is measured. To evaluate thyroid function in dogs receiving NSAIDs, it is prudent to recommend cessation of treatment for 7–10 days before testing, and to include measurement of serum free T4 and TSH (both unaffected by NSAIDs).[25]

INDIVIDUAL NSAIDS FOR VETERINARY USE

Carprofen

Carprofen is generally considered relatively prostaglandin sparing, in that it's a relatively weak inhibitor of COX, and probably exerts effects elsewhere in the inflammatory pathways. The COX inhibition it does have is greater for COX 2 than COX 1 so it is still classed as COX 2 preferential/ selective, and clinically it has a very good safety profile.

Carprofen is licensed in the UK for preop injection in both cats and dogs and is also licensed long-term in dogs. As detailed above, there is evidence that carprofen may have a positive effect on cartilage metabolism in osteoarthritis. Its level of analgesia has been shown to be as effective as pethidine when given pre-emptively to control postop pain. Although it has a short half-life in dogs of approximately 8 hours, it can be given once daily to provide 24 hours of analgesia. The half-life in cats is much longer and quite variable, an average of 20 hours, and the duration of analgesia after a single injection in cats is thought to be 48 hours (up to 72 hours). Studies demonstrate no significant effect on blood clotting times.

Meloxicam

This NSAID is also licensed for preop use in cats and dogs and long-term in dogs. It is classed as COX 2 preferential/ selective. Its half-life in dogs is about 24 hours, and is suitable for once daily dosing. It's available as an oral suspension as well as an injectable form and, like carprofen, it is considered one of the safer NSAIDs and is one of the most widely used NSAIDs in veterinary practice. Studies so far show that it has no detrimental effect on arthritic cartilage.

Tepoxalin

This NSAID is the first dual inhibitor to be launched in the UK for use in dogs. It is licensed for 1 month of treatment as a novel oral preparation, a lyophilisate that melts on contact with moisture in the dog's mouth. It is a good inhibitor of both 5-LOX and COX, although it actually inhibits COX 1 more than COX 2. It has a slightly less stringent warning for use in animals with renal insufficiency; the data sheet just says special care should be taken when treating dogs with marked renal insufficiency.

Ketoprofen

Ketoprofen is not considered selective for COX 2 in dogs as it is a strong inhibitor of COX enzymes and is thought to have some inhibition of 5-LOX. It is a potent anti-inflammatory analgesic, and is licensed for short-term use in the cat and dog and medium to long-term use in the dog at a reduced dose rate. A small animal injection is available but is not licensed for preop use.

Tolfenamic acid

Tolfenamic acid injection is licensed in the UK for use in cats with upper respiratory disease in conjunction with antibiotics as an antipyretic and in dogs for postop pain and inflammation. It is not licensed preop in either species, and tablets are also available. The tablets can be given longer term to dogs, but every 3 days of medication should be followed by 4 days without medication.

Phenylbutazone

This relatively old NSAID is still available for cats and dogs in tablet form, and can be used longer term at reduced dose rates. It is regarded as a classical NSAID and is no longer commonly used first-line because the newer drugs have improved safety profiles.

Cinchophen

This NSAID is available in a combination product with very low doses of prednisolone for dogs. It is often used 3rd or 4th line in cases of end-term osteoarthritis. At the end of treatment, the dose needs to be gradually reduced over time due to the steroid content. It is licensed in the UK for 2 weeks, and then treatment should be stopped for 14 days before restarting the tablets.

Vedoprofen

This is available as an oral gel for dogs in a dosing syringe. It is licensed initially for a month, and then may be given for longer depending on clinical response.

Deracoxib

This is a coxib NSAID licensed for osteoarthritis and postop pain in the USA for dogs. It will be interesting to see in due course whether clinically it is viewed as an improvement on current NSAIDs.

FUTURE DEVELOPMENTS

Therapies

Future uses for NSAIDS, apart from their potential therapeutic effects in cancer, may include the treatment of Alzheimer's in humans. Epidemiological evidence suggests that people receiving NSAIDs for the treatment of osteoarthritis have a lower incidence of dementia. There is also some interest in the use of NSAIDs for the treatment of atherosclerosis, a form of vascular inflammation. Dual inhibitors (NSAIDs blocking both COX and 5-LOX) are being looked at for immune-based inflammatory conditions such as atopic dermatitis.

New NSAIDS

A new group of NSAIDs are being investigated on the human side called nitric oxide releasing NSAIDS, e.g. NO-naproxen.[26] They are basically ordinary NSAIDs with a nitric oxide NO group stuck on the side. When they are given orally the NO group is cleaved, releasing NO into the stomach. NO is a vasodilator that enhances blood flow within the gastric mucosa and helps to prevent NSAID induced ulceration.

Topical NSAIDs are widely used in humans and are regarded as efficacious with a reduced risk of side effects compared to systemic administration, e.g. ibuprofen, ketoprofen. Due to problems with applying topical formulations in the furrier patient, ophthalmic preparations will probably be the most useful ones to consider in veterinary practice.

Key points about NSAIDs

1. NSAIDs inhibit the production of inflammatory mediators in damaged tissue and the transmission of pain signals in the spinal cord.
2. NSAIDs are analgesic, anti-inflammatory and antipyretic.
3. They interrupt the pain pathway and reduce sensitisation both peripherally and centrally.
4. NSAIDs are suitable for moderate to severe (in combination with opioids) acute and chronic pain.
5. Duration of action is often as long as 24 hours.
6. They have the potential for a range of side effects, and safety profiles vary significantly between individual drugs and species. Dosages and safety profiles should not be extrapolated between species.
7. Generally, NSAIDs that are more selective for COX 2 (i.e. COX 1 sparing) are considered safer.
8. Potential side effects include GI ulceration, renal damage, reduced blood clotting and idiosyncratic hepatopathy.
9. NSAIDs have several contraindications and care must be taken with patient selection and assessment before administration.

REFERENCES

1. Lascelles BD, Jones A, Waterman-Pearson AE. Efficacy and kinetics of carprofen, administered preoperatively or postoperatively, for the prevention of pain in dogs undergoing ovariohysterectomy. Vet Surg 1998; 27:568–582
2. Welsh EM, Nolan AM, Reid J. Beneficial effects of administering carprofen before surgery in dogs. Vet Record 1997; 141: 251–253
3. Livingston A. Mechanism of action of non-steroidal anti-inflammatory drugs. Vet Clinics N Am: Small Animal Practice 2000; 30(4): 773–781
4. Jones CJ, Budsberg SC. Physiologic characteristics and clinical importance of the cyclo-oxygenase isoforms in dogs and cats. J Am Vet Med Assoc 2000; 217(5):721–729
5. Seidenberg AB, Yuehuei H, An YH. Is there an inhibitory effect of COX 2 inhibitors on bone healing? Pharmacol Res 2004; 50:151–156
6. Harder AT, An YH. The mechanisms of the inhibitory effects of nonsteroidal anti-inflammatory drugs on bone healing: a concise review. J Clin Pharmacol 2003; 43(8): 807–815
7. Budsberg SC. NSAIDs – quo vadis? Proceedings of the BSAVA Annual Congress, Birmingham 2004
8. McKellar QA, Delatour P, Lees P. Stereospecific pharmacodynamics and pharmacokinetics of carprofen in the dog. J Vet Pharm Ther 1994; 17:447–454
9. Ricketts AP, Lundy KM, Seibel SB. Evaluation of selective inhibition of canine cyclo-oxygenase 1 and 2 by carprofen and other NSAIDs. Am J Vet Res 1998; 59(11): 1441–1446
10. Bryant CE, Farnfield BA, Janicke HJ. Evaluation of the ability of carprofen and flunixin meglumine to inhibit activation of nuclear factor kappa B. Am J Vet Res 2003; 64(2):211–215
11. Knapp DW, Richardson RC, Chan TCK, et al. Piroxicam therapy in 34 dogs with transitional cell carcinoma of the urinary bladder. J Vet Intern Med 1994; 8:273–278
12. Knottenbelt CM, Simpson JW, Tasker S, et al. Preliminary clinical observations on the use of piroxicam in the management of rectal tubulopapillary polyps. JSAP 2000; 41: 393–397
13. Knottenbelt CM. Recent advances in cancer therapy. In: Proceedings of University of Glasgow Faculty of Veterinary Medicine CPD Mini Congress Saturday 31st May 2003, Glasgow.
14. Knapp DW, Richardson RC, Bottoms GD, et al. Phase I trial of piroxicam in 62 dogs bearing naturally occurring tumours. Cancer Chemother Pharmacol 1992; 29:214–218
15. Sorenmo KU, Goldschmidt MH, Shofer FS, et al. Evaluation of cyclooxygenase 1 and cyclooxygenase 2 expression and the effect of cyclooxygenase inhibitors in canine prostatic carcinoma. Vet Compar Oncol 2004; 2(1): 13–23
16. Nolan AM. Pharmacology of analgesic drugs. In: Flecknell P, Waterman-Pearson A, eds. Pain management in animals. London: Saunders; 2000:21–52
17. Boelsterli UA, Zimmerman HJ, Kretz-Rommel A. Idiosyncratic liver toxicity of non-steroidal anti-inflammatory drugs: Molecular mechanisms and pathology. Crit Rev Toxicol 1995; 25(3):207–235
18. Boelsterli UA. Mechanisms of NSAID induced hepatotoxicity. Drug Safety 2002; 25(9): 633–648
19. MacPhail CM, Lappin MR, Meyer DJ, et al. Hepatocellular toxicosis associated with administration of carprofen in 21 dogs. J Am Vet Med Assoc 1998; 212(12):1895–1901
20. Brandt KD. Nonsteroidal anti-inflammatory drugs and articular cartilage. J Rheumatol 1987; 14(Supplement 14):132–133

21. Rainsford KD, Skerry TM, Chindemi P, et al. Effects of the NSAIDs meloxicam and indomethacin on cartilage proteoglycan synthesis and joint responses to calcium pyrophosphate crystals in dogs. Vet Res Commun 1999; 23:101–113
22. Benton HP, Vasseur PB, Gregory A, et al. Effect of carprofen on sulphated glycosaminoglycan metabolism, protein synthesis and prostaglandin release by cultured osteoarthritic canine chondrocytes. Am J Vet Res 1997; 58(3):286–292
23. Schneider TA, Budsberg SC. Plasma and synovial concentrations of carprofen in dogs with chronic osteoarthritis. Vet Comp Orthop Traumatol 2001; 14:19–24
24. Pelletier J, Lajeunesse D, Jovanovic DV, et al. Carprofen simultaneously reduces progression of morphological changes in cartilage and subchondral bone in experimental dog osteoarthritis. J Rheumatol 2000; 27(12):2893–2902
25. Gulikers K, Panciera D. The Influence of Various Medications on Canine Thyroid Function. Compend Continuing Educ 2002; 24(7):220
26. Monck N. NO-naproxen AstraZeneca. IDrugs 2003; 6(6):593–599

CHAPTER 8 OTHER ANALGESIC DRUGS

ALPHA 2 AGONISTS

The alpha 2 agonists are probably more widely regarded as potent sedatives, and often get reserved for intra-cat injection in the half-puma feral nightmare that's taken 2 years to get into a box to bring to the vet. However, they are in fact extremely effective analgesics, particularly useful for the control of periop and postop pain, usually in combination with other analgesics. These drugs act on receptors called alpha 2 adrenoreceptors associated with the sympathetic nervous system in the pain pathway of the brain and spinal cord. Their receptors are also present in the periphery and are responsible for the range of other effects seen with these drugs, most notably the cardiovascular side effects.

The alpha 2 agonists produce analgesia with sedation, anxiolysis (a reduction in anxiety), muscle relaxation and a vast reduction in the doses of any other anaesthetic agents used subsequently (i.e. they are very dose-sparing). An understanding of the cardiovascular changes they produce is important, not least of all to avoid panic setting in when observing the monitoring picture of patients with the untrained eye! Sadly, a misunderstanding of their effects on blood pressure and mucous membrane colour has meant they are sometimes left on the shelf when in fact they can be a very useful analgesic at low doses, particularly as part of the multimodal approach, providing short duration moderate analgesia equivalent to a partial opioid. Due to the fact they do cause changes in the cardiovascular system these drugs are only indicated in otherwise healthy animals. Rather usefully the alpha 2 agonists can be reversed with atipamezole, if their half-life is short enough. Atipamezole does not chemically interact with alpha 2 agonists; it just knocks them off their receptors without having a significant effect itself.

In the CNS the majority of alpha 2 adrenoreceptors sit on the endings of presynaptic neurones; the binding of alpha 2 agonists stops the release of the usual transmitter substance noradrenaline from these nerve endings, reducing sympathetic tone and producing analgesia, sedation, anxiolysis and muscle relaxation. This central effect probably helps maintain a slowed heart rate (bradycardia) as well (see later under cardiovascular changes). Alpha 2 adrenoreceptors are also present out in the periphery, in the walls of small end arterioles and also in the pancreas, liver, kidney and eyes, amongst other places. Outside the CNS the majority of receptors sit on the postsynaptic neurone, and paradoxically, binding by an alpha 2 agonist actually results in increased sympathetic stimulation, producing the other effects associated with these drugs as detailed below.

Just to add a bit of complexity, there is another set of receptors associated with all these neurones called alpha 1 adrenoreceptors; alpha 2 agonists can bind these receptors as well, which opposes some of their therapeutic effects, reducing their potency. Ideally alpha 2 agonists should have very high specificity for the alpha 2 receptors and act as a full agonist at them. Table 8.1 lists the alpha 2 agonists available for small animal use and shows their specificity for the alpha 2 receptors. Most of the information that follows relates primarily to medetomidine, as this is one of the most widely used and extensively studied alpha 2 agonists in small animal practice. More recently, several centres have started looking at medetomidine at very low doses for infusions as an intraop and postop analgesic. It seems these microdoses can provide good quality analgesia whilst minimising cardiovascular changes.

Table 8.1
The relative specificity of alpha 2 agonists at their receptors (binding to alpha 2 receptors results in therapeutic effects)

Drug	Ratio of binding to receptors Alpha 2 : Alpha 1	Type of alpha 2 agonist
Medetomidine	1620:1	Full agonist
Xylazine	160:1	Partial agonist
Romifidine	200:1	Partial agonist

Actions of alpha 2 agonists

Analgesia

There are alpha 2 receptors associated with the pain pathway in the dorsal horn of the spinal cord. Binding of alpha 2 agonists inhibits firing of the primary afferent nociceptors coming into the spinal cord and causes hyperpolarisation of the second order neurones, which makes it harder for them to fire off an impulse. Alpha 2 agonists also activate descending inhibition of the pain pathway by action on receptors higher up in the brain. All these effects produce analgesia equivalent to a partial opioid for about 60–90 minutes duration (figures relate to medetomidine).[1] If the patient is given atipamezole the analgesia is reversed as well as sedation so care must be taken to ensure the patient has another analgesic already on board if pain is still present. Alpha 2 receptors have a similar distribution in the CNS as opioid receptors, even found on the same neurones, and there is great synergy between the two groups of drugs. If an alpha 2 agonist is used with an opioid the analgesia and sedation are very much enhanced, the overall effect being greater than the sum of the two drugs used alone. This allows both drugs to be given at lower dose rates, therefore reducing their potential for side effects. The alpha 2 agonists also have synergistic effects with ketamine, and are often used in combination to provide analgesia and full anaesthesia.

Alpha 2 agonists have been used epidurally to provide analgesia. Xylazine is reported to still produce sedation due to some systemic uptake but the cardiovascular changes are minimal (slight decrease in heart rate and blood pressure).[2,3] Xylazine has a structure similar to lidocaine and it's thought that it may have some local anaesthetic-like activity as well. It provides good analgesia for 1–4 hours without loss of motor function. Medetomidine has also been used for epidurals and can provide 4–8 hours of analgesia. However, the cardiovascular changes are reported to be more marked than with xylazine, with a bradycardia and an increase in blood pressure.[2] Both drugs given via the epidural route for analgesia have an onset time of 5–10 minutes.[3]

Sedation (anxiolysis and muscle relaxation)

Sedation is due to alpha 2 agonists acting on receptors in the CNS, primarily in the area known as the locus cereleus. The drug causes hyperpolarisation of these neurones, inhibiting their firing and also reduces activity of ascending sympathetic pathways. Again, there is major synergy with opioids, with much deeper sedation seen when combinations of the drugs are used together.

Dose-sparing effects

If alpha 2 agonists are used for premedication, they hugely reduce the required dose of subsequent anaesthetic agents, both induction and maintenance, by up to 80%. Premedication with an alpha 2 agonists provides a very stable background of analgesia and sedation intraop, and care must be taken to check data sheet recommendations of dose reductions of other agents to avoid relative overdosing. The onset of action of induction agents can also be prolonged due to the slowed heart rate and vasoconstriction seen after an alpha 2 agonist (it takes relatively longer for the induction agent to be pumped round the body and reach the brain), so again check data sheets timings and avoid the temptation to whack in another bolus before the first one has had a chance to work. Prior administration of an alpha 2 agonist can also prolong the duration of effect of other anaesthetics.

Temperature conservation

The peripheral vasoconstriction helps to conserve body temperature so although patients still need to be kept warm for 12 hours, body temperature will not drop as much as with other anaesthetic or sedative agents that cause vasodilatation.

Cardiovascular effects

Changes in heart rate and blood pressure

When an alpha 2 agonist is administered it binds to postsynaptic receptors in the walls of small end arterioles, which

Box 8.1 **Main effects of alpha 2 agonists**

- Analgesia – central effect
- Sedation
- Anxiolysis
- Muscle relaxation
- Dose-sparing of other anaesthetic agents
- Temperature conservation

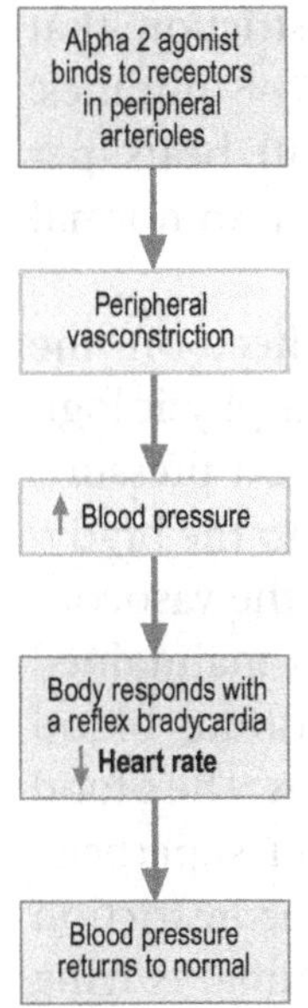

Figure 8.1
Summary of the cardiovascular changes seen after administration of an alpha 2 agonist.

causes a peripheral vasoconstriction. This will bump up systemic blood pressure as the same volume of blood is being pumped through relatively narrower tubes. Central arteries supplying the organs are unaffected. The body's pressure receptors, baroreceptors, detect this hypertension, and send a message up to the brain alerting it to the change. The brain sends a message back down to the heart, via the vagus nerve (increased parasympathetic tone) and slows down the heart rate, producing a reflex bradycardia. The bradycardia will bring the blood pressure back down to normal or just below normal. The initial hypertension only lasts about 7–8 minutes. After 15–20 minutes it's thought that the bradycardia is partly maintained by a central effect of the alpha 2 agonist reducing sympathetic tone. In dogs the heart rate is reduced to about 35–60 beats per minute, and about 60–80 beats per minutes in cats. Fig 8.1 summarises the cardiovascular changes produced by alpha 2 agonists.

Fig 8.2 plots the changes in both heart rate and blood pressure after an alpha 2 agonist was given to a group of dogs. Normal heart rate and blood pressures are shown at time 0, just before the dogs were given medetomidine.

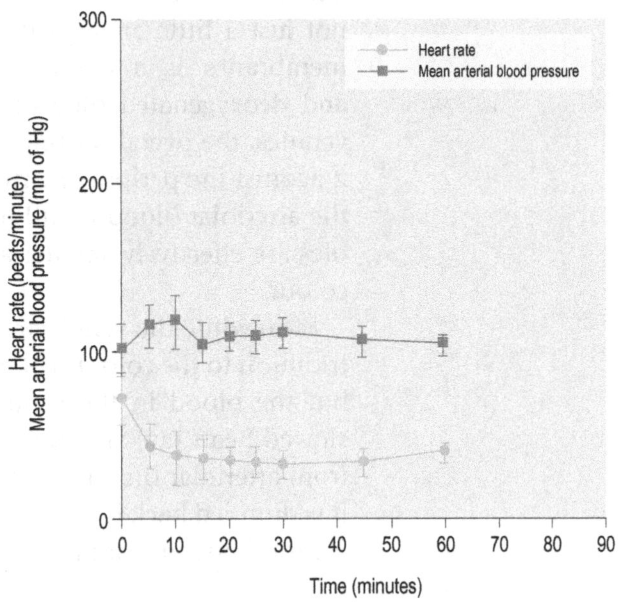

Figure 8.2
Changes in blood pressure and heart rate in dogs given medetomidine i.m. at 40µg/kg. Baseline values, pretreatment are shown at time 0 just before drug administration. (From Alibhai HIK, Clarke KW, Lee YH, et al. Cardiopulmonary effects of combinations of medetomidine hydrochloride and atropine sulphate in dogs. Vet Record 1996; 138:11–13, reproduced with permission.)

The medetomidine causes peripheral vasoconstriction that results in an initial hypertension for the first 7–8 minutes. At this time the heart rate slows to about 40 beats per minute and brings the blood pressure back down to normal values.

Alpha 2 agonists do not have a direct effect on the heart, the bradycardia associated with them is a physiological response by the body to an increase in blood pressure. There will be a reduction in cardiac output due to the bradycardia and increased peripheral resistance from the vasoconstriction, however, the blood supply to organs is maintained as the peripheral vasoconstriction will redistribute blood away from the periphery to the central vital organs. The blood flow to the peripheral tissues, i.e. the skin and superficial muscles, is reduced because of peripheral vasoconstriction and a reduced heart rate. However, when the animal is lying still under sedation or anaesthetised the O_2 demand by these tissues is very low anyway. More importantly the oxygen saturation of the arterial blood is maintained at normal levels.[1]

Mucous membrane colour

One of the things that clinicians find off-putting about alpha 2 agonists is the rather worrying shade of blue of the mucous membranes of patients. The immediate reaction is to think that there is a distinct lack of oxygen inside the patient and the anaesthetists become tachycardic, short of breath and not just a little anxious themselves. The colour of mucous membranes is a combination of oxygenated red blood and deoxygenated blue blood in peripheral arterioles and venules, the overall normal effect looks pink. After an alpha 2 agonist the peripheral arterioles vasoconstrict, so although the arteriolar blood is still nice and red, the narrowed arterioles are effectively smaller and contribute less to the overall colour.

Meanwhile the venules remain the same size so their contribution to the colour will be relatively greater. Not only that but the blood in the venules is bluer. This is because the slowed heart rate allows tissues more time to extract oxygen from arteriolar blood before it is pumped on, so by the time it is dumped back into the venules it is more desaturated and is more blue in colour. The combination of smaller red arterioles and bluer blood in the venules makes the mucous membranes look pale and blue, even though oxygen saturation in the blood supply to the tissues remains at normal levels.

Frequently pulse oximeters can give a false low reading with these drugs as they often rely on pulsatility to get a reading, and this is reduced in peripheral vessels that are constricted under an alpha 2 agonist. One way around this is to use a pulse oximeter that takes a reading more centrally, e.g. using a rectal probe, or one that is clipped onto the tongue. Gently massaging the tongue to increase local blood flow before taking a reading is a good idea.

Other side effects

Respiration Alpha 2 agonists can reduce respiratory rate and breaths may show a clustered pattern, but in their favour they increase the depth of respiration. The likeliest cause of profound respiratory depression is a relative overdose of other anaesthetic agents used concurrently.

GI tract A proportion of cats and dogs vomit shortly after being given alpha 2 agonists; giving it i.v. or in combination with an opioid can reduce the risk of this occurring. Binding of alpha 2 receptors present in the gut wall results in slowing down of gut motility.

Endocrine effects One of the central effects of these drugs is to inhibit the release of antidiuretic hormone (ADH) from the pituitary gland, leading to a slight increase in urine production. Apparently anecdotal reports from the human side indicate that coming round from an anaesthetic desperate for a wee is an extremely uncomfortable experience, so it seems prudent to gently empty the patient's bladder at the end of a long procedure. This also prevents them urinating on recovery and getting wet and cold in the kennel. Alpha 2 agonists acting on receptors in the pancreas can reduce secretion of insulin, resulting in a mild transient increase in blood glucose levels (still within the normal range and not exceeding the renal threshold).

Box 8.2 Side effects of alpha 2 agonists

Main side effects

- Cardiovascular
  - Peripheral vasoconstriction
  - Physiological bradycardia
  - Initial hypertension (7–8 min)
  - Normo- or mild hypotension thereafter
- Reduced respiratory rate
- Vomiting

Minor side effects

- Slowing of gut motility
- Mild increase blood glucose
- Mild increase urine production

Reversal

Atipamezole can be used to reverse alpha 2 agonists. However, if the alpha 2 agonist has a longer half-life than atipamezole, then it will hop back on the receptors once the atipamezole has been cleared out of the body and re-sedation will be seen. Atipamezole has a half-life of about 160 minutes in cats and dogs. Atipamezole will reverse both sedation and analgesia within minutes of administration, so if used intraop there will be a dramatic jump in the patient's plane of anaesthesia, which is not ideal.

Patient selection

Alpha 2 agonists are useful drugs in otherwise healthy animals; they provide predictable dose dependent effects that can easily be reversed. They are ideal as part of the multimodal approach to analgesia, having major synergistic effects with opioids. However, they do cause changes in the cardiovascular system, so the patient needs a normal cardiovascular reserve that can cope with the changes. They are not designed for use in compromised cases, such as the 22-year-old hyperthyroid cat with cardiomyopathy and half a kidney. Patient selection is important, and so is weighing the patient to ensure correct dosages are used (not all cats weigh 5 kg). Data sheet recommendations for the dose reductions of other anaesthetic agents need to be followed to avoid relative overdosing.

Metabolism

Alpha 2 agonists are metabolised by the liver and excreted mainly by the kidneys in urine.

Contraindications

Alpha 2 agonists should not be used in animals with cardiovascular or respiratory compromise, or those with hepatic or renal impairment. Extra care is needed in juveniles less than 4–6 months of age, as they do not cope with cardiovascular changes as well as mature animals. These drugs can induce vomiting so are not suitable where an increase in intraocular or oesophageal pressure is detrimental.

Drug interactions

It is not advisable to use atropine or other antimuscarinic drugs with alpha 2 agonists. Atropine is often used to raise the heart rate, but in the presence of a peripheral vasoconstriction this will cause a severe hypertension.

Individual drugs

Medetomidine

The half-life is 60–90 minutes in both cats and dogs so it will be nicely reversed by atipamezole (half life 160 minutes) without the risk of re-sedation. There is evidence medetomidine[4] (and dexmedetomidine[5]) can reduce the risk of adrenaline-induced cardiac arrhythmias. It is the most specific alpha 2 agonist licensed for small animals, and it is also licensed for use in combination with butorphanol in both dogs and cats, and with ketamine in cats. It has been shown to provide 60–90 minutes of good quality analgesia (without reversal) and can be used at microdoses as an infusion for analgesia and sedation.

Xylazine

This is an older alpha 2 agonist and has been used in veterinary practice since 1968. It is less specific for alpha 2 receptors than medetomidine, and there is great species variation in susceptibility to its effects. Horses, dogs and cats require 10 times the dose needed in cattle.

Romifidine The half-life is 120 minutes in dogs and 360 mins in cats, and re-sedation can be seen after reversal with atipamezole (particularly in cats). It is a partial agonist and less potent than medetomidine so greater volumes are needed to produce the equivalent effects. It is not specifically licensed as an analgesic used alone in small animals.

Future developments

As already mentioned, alpha 2 agonists are regaining popularity as analgesics used at very low doses as constant rate infusions or as repeated injections. The relatively tiny doses are well below data sheet recommendations but seem to provide impressive levels of analgesia as part of a multimodal approach, with minimal cardiovascular changes, and still a great deal of dose-sparing of other agents is seen. In the future this technique of administration may well become more popular.

Dexmedetomidine is an alpha 2 agonist currently licensed for use in humans, and rather surprisingly to the more veterinary minded, is used in intensive care patients at very low dose infusions to provide sedation and analgesia. Most surprisingly it is actually recommended for use in surgical patients with coronary vascular heart disease where the effects of alpha 2 agonists seem to be beneficial, i.e. decreased heart rate, increased peripheral resistance (due to the peripheral vasoconstriction), decreased stress response (due to central sympathetic inhibition), and reduced cardiac output. It is used preop and continued up to 72 hours postop in these patients and has been shown to reduce other anaesthetic drug requirements, reduce oxygen consumption and the stress response to surgery, steady heart rate and blood pressure intraop, and even reduce postop mortality and shivering.[6,7] Very few animals suffer from coronary vascular disease, probably because of lifestyle differences (not many pets have a penchant for smoking or access to cooked breakfasts) but there are other diseases where alpha 2 agonists are being investigated to see if their cardiovascular effects could be beneficial, such as periop use in cats with hypertrophic cardiomyopathy or dynamic left ventricular outflow tract obstruction.

Key summary points of alpha 2 agonists for analgesia

1. Alpha 2 agonists cause sedation, analgesia, muscle relaxation and anxiolysis.
2. They act on receptors in the sympathetic nervous system and pain pathway in the spinal cord and brain to provide short duration analgesia equivalent to a partial opioid. Degree of analgesia may vary between individual drugs.
3. They have major synergy with opioids; both drugs can be used together at lowered doses to produce enhanced sedation and analgesia. There is also synergy with ketamine.
4. Alpha 2 agonists are very dose-sparing of other anaesthetic agents and can prolong their onset and duration of action.
5. Alpha 2 agonists produce a peripheral vasoconstriction resulting in bradycardia and an initial hypertension followed by a return to normal blood pressure (or a mild hypotension).
6. Other side effects include respiratory depression, vomiting, slowed gut motility, and mild increases in blood glucose and urine production.
7. Used at microdoses intraop and postop, medetomidine can provide good background sedation and analgesia whilst minimising cardiovascular changes.
8. Alpha 2 agonists can be reversed with atipamezole, an alpha 2 antagonist.
9. Consideration must be given to patient selection; patients should ideally be otherwise healthy.

LOCAL ANAESTHETICS

Local anaesthetic molecules consist of a tertiary amine connected to an aromatic ring by an ester or an amide linkage and are therefore classed as either aminoesters (e.g. procaine) or aminoamides (e.g. lidocaine, bupivacaine). Local anaesthetics just act at their site of injection; they block the transmission of pain impulses along nociceptor fibres, providing complete analgesia in the area. Nociceptor impulse transmission is prevented because the local anaesthetics stop the flow of sodium ions through nerve membranes, which slows down depolarisation and prevents an action potential (electrical impulse) being generated. Rather conveniently Aδ fibres are the most susceptible to these drugs, followed by small unmyelinated C fibres, so pain is the first sensation to be lost. The duration of effect depends on how long the drug is in contact with the nerves, and this depends on various chemical properties of the drug and its rate of absorption from the tissue, which in turn depends on blood flow.

A vasoconstrictor, most commonly adrenaline, is often added in to local anaesthetics to reduce blood flow and prolong the duration of effect. Vasoconstrictors are not recommended in high-risk patients (they can increase the risk of cardiac arrhythmias) or for local blocks of appendages (distal extremities like paws) where blood flow should not be compromised. Local anaesthetics are ideal for pre-emptive use as they can potentially block all nociceptive impulses travelling to the spinal cord from the target tissue, and therefore prevent the development of central sensitisation. Preop use will reduce the anaesthetic requirements during surgery. Local and regional anaesthetic techniques are ideal for use with other analgesics as part of the multimodal approach. Local anaesthetics show synergy with opioids when used in combination for epidural analgesia.

Analgesic techniques using local anaesthetics

Local anaesthetics can be administered topically, or injected locally into tissue at a particular site to block a small area of tissue or a whole region. They can also be used to block specific nerve trunks or instilled into a body cavity. Epidural and spinal administration is also a widely used technique. These different techniques for local anaesthetic administration mean they are suitable for the relief of dermal and mucosal pain and somatic pain associated with trauma, inflammation and surgery.

Topical anaesthesia

Local anaesthetic sprays are available, e.g. lidocaine, 10% that produces anaesthesia of mucosa up to 2mm depth, 1–2 minutes after application, for a duration of 15–20 minutes. Lidocaine sprays are useful in sedated patients to desensitise oral, nasal and pharyngeal mucous membranes for minor invasive or diagnostic procedures such as foreign body removal, endoscopy, placement of nasal catheters for tube feeding or oxygen supplies. Sterile lidocaine jelly 2% will also vastly reduce the discomfort of urinary catheter placement in patients. Another use of these gels is to spread some on the rectum after rectal or perirectal surgery to provide analgesia and reduce postop straining (tenesmus).

EMLA cream is a human preparation containing both lidocaine and priocaine useful in veterinary patients. It is applied to the skin, a dressing is used to cover the area for at least

20 minutes and cutaneous anaesthesia will take effect after about 1 hour. If the skin is inflamed the duration of action is shortened as the local anaesthetics are absorbed more quickly. It is useful in the more fractious veterinary patient to facilitate intravenous injection or catheter placement. Care must be taken not to exceed the safe maximum dose with these topical preparations, as they are still very well absorbed systemically from mucous membranes. Other topical local anaesthetic preparations are commonly used on the eye to desensitise the cornea, usually to allow examination. Proparacaine (0.5%) is an example, but should not be used repeatedly as it can reduce the speed of healing of the cornea.

Local anaesthetics can be applied directly to exposed nerve trunks or tissue during surgery to provide excellent immediate postop analgesia. For example the brachial plexus can be bathed in local anaesthetic 2–3 minutes prior to transection during a forelimb amputation, to help reduce the huge barrage of nociceptive signals resulting from nerve damage. Topical use of local anaesthetic like this may possibly reduce the chance of phantom limb pain developing. Alternatively local anaesthetic can be injected into the perineurium of the nerves that are being cut.

Local tissue infiltration

Local infiltration involves injecting small blebs of local anaesthetic subcutaneously along a line or in a V shape. It can provide skin desensitisation for the suturing of lacerations or the removal of small skin tumours or biopsies. For larger tumours or subcutaneous ones the local needs to be placed deeper and in a rectangular or triangular pattern around the mass. The size of the lesion is the limiting factor in small dogs and cats because it's easier to exceed the total safe dose of local anaesthetic, which must be carefully calculated before use. Local infiltration can be done either before the incision is made, or at the end of surgery before wound closure and it does not delay healing. Possible complications include inadvertent intravenous injection of the local or excessive bleeding due to sympathetic blockade and resulting vasodilatation (this can be reduced by using a preparation containing adrenaline). Unfortunately the injection of local itself is known to sting; warming the local to body temperature beforehand can ease this.

Local tissue infiltration to block a region, 'ring blocks'

Local anaesthetic can be injected around the base of a digit or distal limb to provide a ring block of all the nerves supplying the region, prior to amputation or distal limb surgery. Preparations *without* a vasoconstrictor should be used, to avoid reducing local blood flow, which could result in tissue ischaemia and damage.

Intravenous regional anaesthesia

This technique is used to produce short-term (less than 2 hours) analgesia of distal extremities, e.g. paws in dogs. An Esmarch bandage is applied to the extremity to desanguinate it; the elastic bandaging material begins at the distal end of the limb and is wrapped in a proximal direction to push the blood out of the area. A tourniquet is then applied proximal to the bandage and the bandage removed. Lidocaine solution is then injected into a vein distal to the tourniquet (cephalic or saphenous vein). This will desensitise the paw within 10 minutes, and the tourniquet can be left on for up to 90 minutes. When the tourniquet is removed sensation returns within 15 minutes and analgesia persists up to another 30 minutes.[8] Complications may arise if the tourniquet is left on for too long and causes ischaemic limb damage, and systemic local anaesthetic toxicity could occur if the tourniquet isn't tight enough.

Specific nerve blocks

If the anatomy of an area is well known then local anaesthetic can be injected to block a specific nerve trunk carrying pain impulses from the surgical site to the spinal cord. Careful aseptic technique should be used and the syringe aspirated before injection to ensure the needle is not in a blood vessel. Ideally, local blocks should be done preop to make the most of a pre-emptive effect. Examples include infraorbital and mandibular nerve blocks before dental surgery to provide analgesia of the upper and lower teeth arcades respectively and intercostal nerve blocks before and after intercostal thoracotomy surgery for pain relief. Table 8.2 lists the indications and some commonly used nerve blocks that are possible. Further details on how to perform these blocks and the anatomical landmarks can be found in the references listed at the end of the chapter. Care must be taken to observe patients for signs of self-mutilation of the numb area on recovery after local blocks, and loss of sensation to the mouth

Table 8.2 Indications and areas of analgesia of specific nerve blocks[8,9]

Indication	Nerve block	Area of analgesia
Dental surgery of upper arcade	Infraorbital nerve	Maxillary teeth Soft and hard palates Muzzle
Dental surgery of lower arcade	Inferior alveolar nerve	Lower arcade teeth Chin
Total ear canal ablation Bulla osteotomy	Auriculotemporal nerve Great auricular nerve	External and middle ear
Elbow and distal limb surgery, forelimb amputation	Brachial plexus	Forelimb distal to elbow
Thoracotomy	Intercostal nerves	Adjacent area of chest wall
Distal forelimb and paw	Radial/ulnar/median nerves	Antebrachium and paw of forelimb

can make some animals quite anxious. Aseptic techniques are needed to avoid infection at injection sites.

Instillation into a cavity

Local anaesthetic can be instilled into the thoracic cavity for postop analgesia following thoracotomy in the sedated or anaesthetised patient. A thoracostomy tube needs to be surgically placed and local flushed into the thoracic cavity. The dog is then placed with the incision side down for 10–20 minutes to allow the local to pool near the incision site, where it diffuses across the pleura and blocks intercostal nerves adjacent to the site. Alternatively an over-the-needle catheter can be put aseptically into the pleural space for administration of local, however this can be painful in the conscious patient.[8] Potential complications include pneumothorax, accidental pulmonary trauma during catheter placement and infection.

Local anaesthetic can also be placed in the abdomen for the alleviation of upper abdominal pain such as acute pancreatitis. Again a strict aseptic technique is required and very careful dosing as the local will be readily absorbed across an inflamed peritoneum. A diluted volume of local is placed in the abdomen via abdominocentesis at the level of the umbilicus. Ideally the patient should be placed in dorsal recumbency for 10 minutes then ventral recumbency with the hindquarters slightly raised for another 10 minutes.

Intra-articular analgesia

Joints can be injected with local anaesthetic before or after surgery once the joint has been effectively sealed. This is most commonly employed for stifle and shoulder arthrotomy and seems to be a relatively simple, safe and effective way of providing postop analgesia (Fig 8.3). Aseptic precautions are very important for injecting into joints.

Epidural administration

Epidural anaesthesia can be used as an adjunct to general anaesthesia to provide profound intra- and postop analgesia for hind limb and caudal body surgery, and reduce requirements for anaesthetic inhalation agents. This is useful, as using lower doses of these latter agents will reduce cardiopulmonary depression of the patient. Epidural anaesthesia provides pre-emptive, intraop and excellent prolonged postop analgesia as well. Occasionally, epidural anaesthesia plus sedation (and oxygen supply) could be considered as an alternative to a full general anaesthesia in high-risk patients for certain surgical procedures caudal to the diaphragm. Epidural administration means the drug is injected into the

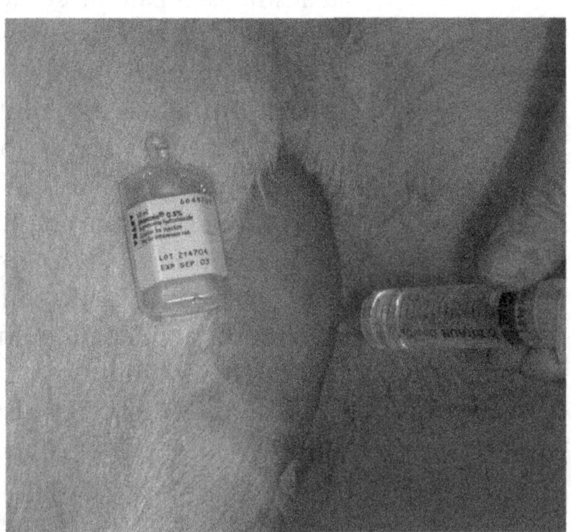

Figure 8.3
Intra-articular bupivacaine can provide excellent postop analgesia after stifle joint surgery.

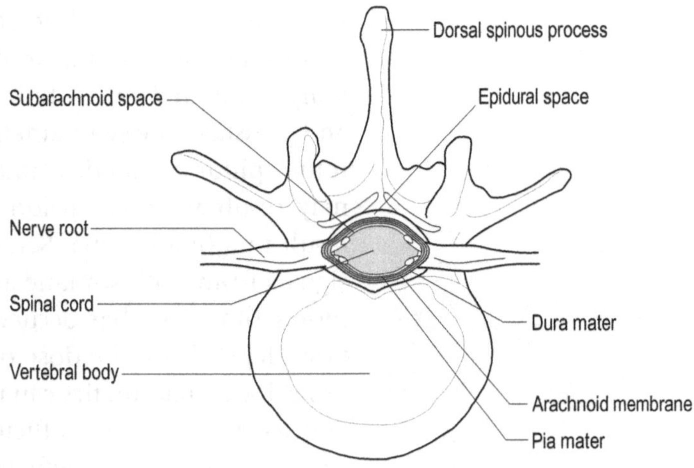

Figure 8.4
Cross-section diagram of the spine showing the coverings of the spinal cord; pia mater, arachnoid membrane and dura mater.

space between the dura mater (the outermost layer covering the spinal cord) and the periosteum of vertebrae. This space is referred to as the epidural space and contains fat, fluid and venous plexuses. The arachnoid membrane lies on the inside of the dura mater – this encloses the subarachnoid space that contains cerebrospinal fluid (CSF). Finally, the deepest layer is the pia mater that covers the spinal cord itself. Fig 8.4 is a simplified schematic diagram showing a cross section of the spinal column and the various layers. There are dorsal, dorsolateral and ventral spinal arteries associated with the pia mater, which need to be avoided when attempting epidural or spinal anaesthesia.

Local anaesthetics can be given epidurally, alone or in combination with opioids or alpha 2 adrenoreceptors agonists, preop to provide excellent analgesia for the caudal body, or even extending up to the forelimbs. When given into the epidural space there seem to be three mechanisms by which analgesia is produced. Local anaesthetics will diffuse through the dura mater into the subarachnoid space where it acts on nerve roots – this is thought to be the primary site of action. The drug will also cross the dura mater and act directly on the spinal cord. Finally, the local may diffuse into the paravertebral areas through the intervertebral foramina and block nerves distally, resulting in multiple paravertebral blocks.

As local anaesthetics penetrate a nerve trunk, sympathetic nerves are blocked first, followed by sensory nerves and then motor nerves. Of the different types of sensory nerves Aδ and C fibre nociceptors transmitting pain are blocked preferentially compared to Aβ fibres that are responsible for touch and pressure. The sympathetic blockade can be of significance if the epidural extends cranially because blocking of T5 to L3 may result in hypotension, and blocking of T2 to T4 can result in a bradycardia. Sensory blockade will interrupt pain signals from both somatic and visceral tissues. The degree of motor blockade that occurs, producing loss of motor function, depends on the dose of local used. At lower concentrations, local anaesthetics can produce analgesia without motor deficits, but it's very difficult to titrate this accurately and some proprioceptive deficits are probably inevitable. Sometimes higher doses are indicated to produce total sensory and motor blockade, resulting in absolute pain control and to allow physiotherapy postop of a very painful limb. In contrast, epidural morphine results in long-lasting analgesia with no motor effects at all. Bupivacaine and ropivacaine appear to provide the most differential block, interrupting sensory impulses whilst having the least effect on motor function.[3] Table 8.3 lists onset and duration times of epidural analgesia using each local anaesthetic in the dog. Note that timings can vary depending on the concentration of drug used. The addition of adrenaline can prolong effects but also increases the risk of systemic uptake and toxicity.

Local anaesthetics can be used in combination with opioids for epidural analgesia. There does seem to be a synergy between the two types of drug, and clinical use of morphine plus bupivacaine (the most popular combination) provides an increased degree and duration of analgesia

Table 8.3
Local anaesthetics for epidural analgesia in the dog

Local anaesthetic	Onset of action	Duration of action
Lidocaine 2%	5 min	45–90 min
Bupivacaine 0.5%	20 min	2–6 h
Ropivacaine 0.5%	15 min	1.5–7 h
Mepivacaine 2%	5 min	60–90 min

(From Torske KE, Dyson DH. Epidural analgesia and anaesthesia. Vet Clinics of North America: Small Animal Practice 2000; 30(4):859–874, reproduced with permission.)

compared with either drug used alone, and there are minimal cardiopulmonary changes. It allows lower doses of each drug to be used, therefore reducing the potential for their side effects. Since there is no significant evidence for any detrimental effects using a combination, it makes sense to use both drugs wherever possible.

Side effects

Most of the potential side effects of local anaesthetics are seen if they are overdosed and/or given intravenously by accident. Systemic toxicity of local anaesthetics primarily involves the heart and CNS – acute CNS toxicity occurs at much lower doses than those required to produce acute cardiac toxicity. Doses in small dogs and cats in particular should be carefully calculated. Muscle twitching and convulsions are usually the first signs of local anaesthetic toxicity in small animals. With large overdoses, such as inadvertent intravenous administration, convulsions can be followed by unconsciousness, coma and respiratory arrest. Convulsions can be controlled with a benzodiazepine such as diazepam or midazolam, and patients suffering respiratory depression may require ventilation.

Systemic absorption of high doses of local anaesthetic can reduce the excitability, conduction and force of contraction of cells in the myocardium (heart wall muscle). In fact lidocaine can be used therapeutically for these effects, to treat cardiac dysrhythmias in an emergency situation. However, local anaesthetics can themselves cause dysrhythmias (e.g. AV block) and hypotension (via arteriolar dilatation). If this occurs, intravenous fluids are needed to support the circulation and the heart should be monitored with an ECG. Further treatment may be indicated if a bradycardia or ventricular tachycardia or fibrillation develop. Bupivacaine should not be given i.v. as it is the one most likely to be cardiotoxic.

Very rarely, local anaesthetics can cause direct damage to tissues (particularly if vasoconstrictors are used), allergic reactions and methaemoglobinaemia have been seen.

Absorption and metabolism

Local anaesthetics with a fast rate of absorption have a fast onset of action but a shorter duration of action and a greater risk of side effects. Bupivacaine and ropivacaine are longer acting with a higher safety margin and therefore do not need to be given with a vasoconstrictor. Most local anaesthetics used in veterinary patients are metabolised in the liver, or are dependent on breakdown by enzymes produced by the liver; metabolites are excreted in urine. Care is therefore needed with their use in patients with severe hepatic disease.

Drug interactions

Local anaesthetics are highly protein-bound so their concurrent use with other highly protein bound drugs could in theory lead to their displacement and an increased risk of toxicity.

Contraindications

The two contraindications for any epidural anaesthesia (with local, opioid or alpha 2 agonist) are sepsis and coagulopathies (clotting disorders). If one of the numerous vessels in the epidural space is punctured by a needle and continues to bleed it will increase pressure in the spinal canal, and ultimately put pressure on the cord itself leading to paresis and paralysis. Sepsis or localised infection of the skin over the epidural injection site is the other contraindication because it increases the risk of introducing infection into the epidural space.

Individual local anaesthetics

Lidocaine Lidocaine 2% is available as an injection and topical spray licensed for veterinary use. A 2% gel is also made for human use. It is a very versatile local anaesthetic – it can be given topically, injected for regional and nerve blocks, intravenous regional anaesthesia and used epidurally. Solutions containing adrenaline must not be given i.v. As mentioned earlier it can be given for the treatment of certain ventricular arrhythmias. It has an onset of 10–15 minutes and duration of action of 45–60 minutes without adrenaline. This is extended to 1–2 hours when adrenaline is added.

Bupivacaine This has a slower onset of action of up to 20–30 minutes but longer duration than lidocaine, 4–6 hours. Bupivacaine is not as effective topically but is very useful for local infiltration and epidural analgesia. A 0.5% solution is available, and a preservative-free formulation can be used for epidurals. Low doses produce good sensory blockade whilst preserving most of the motor function. It is often the local anaesthetic of choice in small animals due to its effect and duration. However, it should not be used in patients with ventricular arrhythmias as it is the most cardiotoxic of the local anaesthetics and must not be given i.v.

Ropivacaine This local has recently been licensed in humans, it has a rapid onset of 5–10 minutes and a duration of 3–5 hours. It can be used for local infiltration and epidurals; a 0.5% solution is available. It produces selective blockade of sensory over motor nerves comparable to bupivacaine and its main advantage is that ropivacaine has only half the cardiotoxic potential.

Mepivacaine Mepivacaine is not effective topically but can be used for local and epidural administration. It has a rapid onset of 5–10 minutes but a short duration of 90–180 minutes. It causes less tissue irritation than lidocaine and has a higher therapeutic index; a 2% formulation is available.

Future developments

Recent studies have looked at the efficacy of low dose i.v. infusions of lidocaine for the treatment of hyperalgesia and neuropathic pain states in people. Experimental studies have found that sodium channel blockers like lidocaine can reduce the sensitivity and spontaneous firing of nociceptors in neuromas and the dorsal horn associated with neuropathic pain (e.g. phantom limb pain) at doses too low to block nerve conduction altogether (see chapter 10 for more details). Systemic lidocaine has also been shown to reduce pain caused by nerve damage in diabetic patients that suffered from peripheral neuropathies. Analgesia lasted as long as 3–21 days after an i.v. infusion of lidocaine and allodynia was also alleviated. Unfortunately, cancer-related pain was not alleviated by systemic lidocaine.[11,12]

Another area of research is looking at structural differences in sodium ion channels on peripheral nerves to try and develop local anaesthetics that only interrupt nociceptor fibres and leave other sensory and motor nerves unaffected.

Key summary points of local anaesthetics

1. Local anaesthetics interrupt the transmission of pain impulses along nociceptors, producing a unique absolute analgesia and preventing central sensitisation.
2. They can be administered topically, or by local infiltration to desensitise an area, injected to block specific nerves innervating a surgical site and by the epidural route. They can also be instilled into body cavities and joints.
3. They are ideal to use pre-emptively as part of a multimodal approach. They reduce anaesthetic requirements and provide prolonged postop analgesia.
4. Excellent synergistic analgesia for hind-limb and caudal body surgery can be provided by an epidural using both a local anaesthetic and an opioid, e.g. bupivacaine plus morphine
5. Local anaesthetics are relatively safe if given correctly but they can produce CNS and cardiac toxicity from systemic absorption or accidental intravenous administration. Total doses must be carefully calculated, especially in small dogs and cats.

KETAMINE

At higher doses ketamine is a dissociative anaesthetic agent, it dissociates the brain from the rest of the body, which characteristically produces profound analgesia combined with only superficial sleep. It is also classed as an NMDA antagonist – it antagonises or blocks NMDA receptors in the spinal cord that would normally be bound by the neurotransmitter glutamate. Both NMDA receptors and glutamate are very important in the development and maintenance of central sensitisation in the spinal cord. Ketamine can therefore help prevent the development of central sensitisation and may be useful for abolishing it once it is established. At low doses that avoid dissociative anaesthesia the duration of analgesia is about 30 minutes. Low dose infusions can be used for analgesia, and it can also be administered as a bolus, i.m., via the epidural route or even topically on burn injuries. Reports are mixed on its efficacy as an epidural analgesic (a preservative-free formulation is required).[3]

In humans it has been shown to be useful for the treatment of phantom limb pain, opioid resistant pain, severe burns pain and in subcutaneous infusions to control postop and trauma pain. For continuous analgesia, ketamine should be combined with an opioid, which produces a synergistic analgesic effect, or a sedative. Ketamine alone can cause CNS excitation, particularly in dogs, so it is preferable to use it in drug combinations to avoid this 'ketamine effect'. Unusually for an anaesthetic agent ketamine has a stimulatory effect on the cardiovascular system but can also depress respiration. It is currently licensed for use with medetomidine for sedation or full anaesthesia with or without butorphanol for feline anaesthesia.

NITROUS OXIDE

Nitrous oxide is the only inhalation agent to provide significant analgesia. Nitrous oxide is a gas delivered to patients alongside other anaesthetic inhalation agents and is routinely used in humans to provide good analgesia during surgery. It seems to have efficacy in small animals as well and needs to be administered at a concentration of at least 50% to provide analgesia. The analgesia is not long lasting – once administration of the nitrous is stopped the effects rapidly wane within 5 minutes as the gas is blown off. Its mechanism of action is unknown but part of the effect may be due to inducing the release of opioids or catecholamines. It is contraindicated where gas accumulation in a cavity or viscera would be detrimental, e.g. gastric dilatation.

FUTURE ANALGESIC DRUG DEVELOPMENTS

As described in Chapter 5, the pain pathway involves many different mechanisms, neurotransmitters and receptors, so there are a lot of potential therapeutic targets. Antagonists at the following receptors in the pain pathway may prove to be useful:

- NMDA receptors
- Neurokinin 1 receptors
- Vanillioid receptors
- Metabotropic glutamate receptors
- Calcitonin gene-related peptide CGRP receptors
- Cholecystokinin receptors.

Other current areas of interest in the development of new analgesics are:

- Modulation of key neurotransmitters involved in sensitisation and pain transmission, e.g. substance P, nerve growth factor (NGF).

- Nicotinic receptors agonists – these have been shown to be analgesic in lab studies, but with side effects.
- Tetrodotoxin resistant sodium channel blockers – these channels are over expressed in painful neuromas.
- Ca channel blockers – used to treat cardiovascular disorders, but have been found to reduce other analgesic drug requirements.
- Capsaicin and its receptors (VR-1) – (see Chapter 10); this topical compound is already available on the human side.
- Nerve growth factor (NGF) antagonists – NGF and its receptor trk-A play a key role in peripheral and central sensitisation.
- Cannabinoids – reported to have an analgesic effect in humans, particularly in chronic pain. There is growing evidence that some cannabinoids, e.g. delta 9-THC, may produce analgesia by several mechanisms:[13]
  - Suppression of trk-A expression (see last point)
  - Enhancing endogenous opioid mechanisms
  - A metabolite of delta 9-THC can inhibit COX
  - They seem to inhibit firing of second order wide dynamic range neurones in response to noxious stimuli in the dorsal horn of the spinal cord
  - Inhibiting release of some neurotransmitters involved in nociception in the spinal cord, e.g. glutamate
  - Local administration may inhibit sensitisation of neurones.

  Cannabinoids are not, strictly speaking, drugs of the future – the marijuana plant was used medicinally in the nineteenth century and apparently Queen Victoria was known to partake in a spot of cannabis consumption for migraine relief. The marijuana plant actually contains over 460 compounds, 62 of which have a cannabinoid structure, with differing properties and effects. Research is aimed at producing a cannabinoid with analgesic action but without the undesired side effects.
- Nitric oxide synthase inhibitors – nitric oxide is an inflammatory mediator involved in peripheral sensitisation.

There are other drugs that have weak or non-existent analgesic effects when administered alone but can enhance pain relief when they are given alongside conventional analgesics.

These are referred to as adjuvant analgesics and are discussed in detail in Chapter 10 where non-pharmacological methods of pain management are also looked at.

FUTURE ROUTES OF ADMINISTRATION

It is doubtful that we will discover any new orifices or vessels now (anatomy has been pretty well covered over the years) but new ways of delivering currently available analgesics are being developed. Ketamine and more local anaesthetics are being incorporated into topical gels, which avoids systemic side effects and may be useful for neuropathic and burns pain. NSAIDs are another group of analgesics that are already used topically in humans for acute and chronic pain. A nasal spray containing butorphanol is available for people in the USA and a subcutaneous implant containing hydromorphone has been licensed for human cancer patients, which provides 4 weeks continuous release of the opioid. Veterinary patients may benefit from some of these new products in the future.

REFERENCES

1. Ko JCH, et al. Cardiorespiratory responses and plasma cortisol concentrations in dogs treated with medetomidine before undergoing ovariohysterectomy. J Am Vet Med Assoc 2000; 217(4):509–514
2. Campoy L. Epidural and spinal anaesthesia in the dog. In Practice 2004; 26(5): 262–269
3. Dobromylskyj P, Flecknell, Lascelles BD, et al. Management of postoperative and other acute pain. In: Flecknell P, Waterman-Pearson A, eds. Pain management in animals. London: Saunders; 2000:81–145
4. Alibhai HI, Clarke KW, Lee YH, et al. Cardiopulmonary effects of combinations of medetomidine hydrochloride and atropine sulphate in dogs. Vet Record 1996; 138: 11–13
5. Hayashi Y, Sumikawa K, Maze M, et al. Dexmedetomidine prevents epinephrine-induced arrhythmias through stimulation of central alpha 2 adrenoceptors in halothane anaesthetised dogs. Anesthesiology 1991; 75(1):113–117
6. Pascoe PJ. Alpha 2 agonists and cardiovascular disease: an oxymoron? Proceedings of the Association of Veterinary Anaesthetists Spring Meeting 15–16 April 2004; London UK
7. Grounds M. Sedation and analgesia for patients requiring intensive care. Proceedings of the Association of Veterinary Anaesthetists Spring Meeting 15–16 April 2004; London UK
8. Lemke KA, Dawson SD. Local and regional anaesthesia. Vet Clin N Am: Small Animal Practice 2000; 30(4):839–857
9. Tranquilli WJ, Grimm KA, Lamont LA. Analgesic techniques. In: Pain management for the small animal practitioner. Jackson: Teton Newmedia; 2000: 32–72

10. Torske KE, Dyson DH. Epidural analgesia and anaesthesia. Vet Clin N Am: Small Animal Practice 2000; 30(4):859–874
11. Lamont LA, Tranquilli WJ, Mathews KA. Adjunctive analgesic therapy. Vet Clin N Am: Small Animal Practice 2000; 30(4):805–813
12. Boivie J. Central pain. In: Wall PD, Melzack R, eds. Textbook of pain, 4th edn. Edinburgh:Churchill Livingstone; 1999: 879–914
13. Neeleman M.P. Cannabinoids, magic mushrooms and pain: its place in human medicine. Proceedings of the Association of Veterinary Anaesthetists Spring meeting May 2003, Doorwerth, The Netherlands

CHAPTER 9 MANAGEMENT OF ACUTE PAIN

GENERAL PRINCIPLES

There are four important principles of pain management that should be applied to try and ensure optimal pain relief:

- timing of analgesia
- multimodal analgesia
- principle of analogy
- an individual approach.

Timing of analgesia

Pain should always be prevented in surgical patients, or treated as soon as possible in trauma and other cases. This approach will minimise the development of sensitisation and a heightened pain state (hyperalgesia and allodynia) making the pain easier to control. The prevention of pain entails administering analgesics preop, but also ensuring that doses are adequate and dosing intervals are not too long to avoid pain breakthrough intra- and postop. Every time the patient is exposed to a deluge of nociceptive signals a degree of sensitisation will occur and pain will become increasingly difficult to relieve. The greater the surgical stimulus or level of pain expected, the greater the amount of pre-emptive analgesia required. Another advantage of this approach is that the resultant intraop analgesia reduces the doses of other anaesthetic agents that are needed and hence their side effects such as cardiovascular depression are also minimised. Preop analgesia will also give a more stable plane of anaesthesia and a smoother recovery.

Multimodal analgesia

The second principle is based on the fact that nociception and pain perception involve many different cell mechanisms and neurotransmitters, so it is unlikely that one type of analgesic alone will completely alleviate pain. Using combinations of different classes of analgesic that act on different parts of the pain pathway produces the most effective analgesia; and this often results in a synergistic effect where the resulting analgesia is greater than the sum of the individual drugs used alone. It also allows drugs to be used at lower doses, which reduces their side effects. As the level of pain increases, interrupting the pain pathway at more and more points will give the best pain control, i.e. add in different classes of analgesic, rather than just increasing the dose of the one drug. The multimodal approach also helps prevent gaps in analgesia caused by drugs having a slow onset of action or short duration. For example, a preop NSAID may not have peak effect until near the end of surgery, but may last 24 hours. If an opioid is given preop as well, this may provide good intraop analgesia whilst the NSAID is starting to work, but wear off within a couple of hours when the NSAID has taken over.

Principle of analogy

The timely administration of analgesics is crucial for pain relief, but often there can be some debate as to whether an animal is actually in pain and, if so, how severe it is. As discussed in Chapter 3 the recognition and assessment of pain in animals is itself a monumental challenge in the practice environment. The solution is to use the Principle of Analogy, which states that if a stimulus is likely to cause pain in a human, assume it will be painful to animals as well and provide appropriate analgesia, i.e. give animals the benefit of the doubt – if you think a procedure or injury, etc. would be painful to you, assume it will be painful to your patient and provide analgesia. One of the best ways to diagnose pain is to give an analgesic and look for a change in the patient's demeanour. The dose of analgesic and duration of ongoing analgesia should match the anticipated level and duration of pain. All surgical procedures should include pain relief, as they would for humans.

An individual approach

It is vital to repeatedly assess patients to look for changes in behaviour that indicate whether an analgesic has worked, or if further medication is required, and to ensure dosing intervals are not too long. Patients need to be treated on an individual basis, for example some animals may need repeat doses of an opioid much earlier than another patient. Durations of action of analgesics are a guideline, and may vary between different individuals. However, care must be taken to avoid overdosing and toxicity, something that the multimodal approach helps prevent. Do not assume that one analgesic protocol will suit every case undergoing the same procedure, some patients may require more analgesia or just not respond as well to certain drugs, or even be more sensitive to the side effects of a particular drug.

Box 9.1 **General principles of acute pain management**

1. Timing of analgesia – minimise sensitisation
   - Pain should be prevented whenever possible by using preop analgesia. Where pain is already established, e.g. trauma patients, pain should be treated as early as possible.
   - Avoid pain breakthrough by using adequate doses of analgesics and dosing intervals that are not too long.
2. Multimodal analgesia – provides the most effective pain relief and avoids gaps
   - Use different classes of analgesic together to interrupt the pain pathway at multiple points. This gives a synergistic effect and a greater degree of analgesia.
   - As the level of pain increases, add in more types of analgesic.
3. Principle of analogy – treat pain even if its presence and severity are not obvious
   - If a stimulus would cause pain in a human assume it will also cause pain in an animal and provide analgesia. All surgical procedures should include pain management.
   - Match the dose and duration of analgesic treatment to the anticipated level and duration of pain.
   - Use the provision of analgesia as a tool to diagnose the presence of pain.
4. An individual approach – tailor pain relief to each patient
   - Individuals have varying analgesic needs and responses to drugs.
   - Reassess patients at regular intervals to ensure adequate pain relief is provided for long enough.

IMPLEMENTING AND DEVISING PAIN MANAGEMENT PROTOCOLS IN PRACTICE[3,4]

To implement a successful pain management programme in a practice it is important that all of the staff are bought into the idea and see it as a common goal. Emphasis needs to be put on the value of achieving optimal pain relief in all the patients, and then conveying this to the clients. As discussed in Chapter 2, unrelieved pain is detrimental to the recovery, healing, welfare and quality of life of patients. Some top tips for achieving a best practice approach to pain management are as follows:

- educate and include all professional and lay staff
- client education
- create an in-house 'pain team'
- establish pain management protocols
- ensure patient follow-up
- develop discharge protocols.

Educate and include all professional and lay staff

The alleviation of pain and patient comfort should be a common objective and priority of every member of the practice. All nursing staff and vets should have training on the recognition and assessment of pain and how to provide appropriate care. All lay staff should be trained to educate clients on the importance of pain management.

Client education

Use consent forms and itemised bills so the owners are made aware of the practice's commitment to effective pain management. Do not make analgesia an optional extra – it is as important as any other surgical procedure or medication. Surgery without analgesia is like offering surgery without instruments. When quoting a price for an operation, give the owner an idea of the real value, don't just state the sum. For example, a bitch spay may cost £*X.XX*, and this can be qualified by explaining that it includes all the pain relief medication necessary to ensure the pet is as comfortable as possible, during hospitalisation and after discharge at home. Suggested wording for consent forms can be along the lines of the following:[3]

'Our practice strongly believes in quality, compassionate medical care for all our patients. During your pet's stay, pain-relieving medication (analgesics) will be administered as necessary to ensure that your pet is as comfortable as possible. All surgical patients will receive analgesics during and after surgery and in addition, medication may be dispensed for use at home after discharge.'

Create an in-house 'pain team'

There may already be members of staff that colleagues will refer to who have specialist interests in areas such as orthopaedics or dermatology. The same expertise can be developed in pain management by having a group of nurses and vets who are responsible for establishing and developing analgesic protocols and overseeing their implementation.

Establish pain management protocols

Every patient examination should include pain assessment whatever the original reason for presentation, and ideally an in-house standardised pain scoring and recording system established for use in the patients notes. Protocols for preventing as well as treating pain in every patient should be written and posted around the practice so the information is readily accessible and used by everybody. Rescue protocols should also be developed for the recognition and treatment of pain in patients unresponsive to the standard protocols. Protocols should be continually monitored and revised on the basis of their success or shortcomings. All members of staff need to be kept up-to-date with any changes made to protocols. Written pain management protocols ought to contain the following information:

- Guidelines for pain assessment examinations, scoring and recording for every patient
- Guidelines on the training of new staff and ongoing training of experienced staff on pain management
- Listings of procedures, diseases or circumstances known to be associated with pain and their anticipated level of pain
- Methods of recognising the presence of pain, its severity and identifying the cause
- Methods of pre-emptive pain control, postop analgesia, and other acute and chronic pain management
- Methods for rescue analgesia in unresponsive cases

- A list of the available analgesic drugs, with their mechanism of action, doses, potential side effects, contraindications and drug interactions
- Adjunctive methods of pain management (drugs and non-pharmacological methods)
- How to educate clients on recognising pain, the importance of pain relief and home care techniques including advice on analgesics and signs of any adverse effects.

Ensure patient follow-up

Write guidelines for staff on the continuing reassessment of patients to ensure ongoing pain is treated after the immediate postop period. Regular pain assessments should be made whilst the patient is hospitalised and recorded in the medical notes. Pain assessment ought to be continued even after discharge, at postop checks and longer-term follow-up examinations. Owner input is crucial for assessing pain in outpatients.

Develop discharge protocols

When patients are discharged from the practice it is important they leave with sufficient analgesic medication. This will also require client education to explain how important the medication is in terms of facilitating recovery, how to administer it and to make them aware of any signs of potential side effects. Pain doesn't stop just because the animal has left the building. Clients should be taught to recognise signs of pain in their pet and asked to contact the practice if they feel their pet is in pain.

The above suggestions are an 'ideal model' and anyone who has been in general practice will be well aware that change takes time – after all it can take a good 3 years or more just to order a new pair of bandage scissors in some places. However, the value of pain management cannot be overemphasised and putting in place such protocols will be self-promoting as the results will hopefully speak for themselves, not least in terms of job satisfaction.

When devising specific pain management protocols, the practice needs to take into account:

- the drugs available
- the choice of analgesic techniques

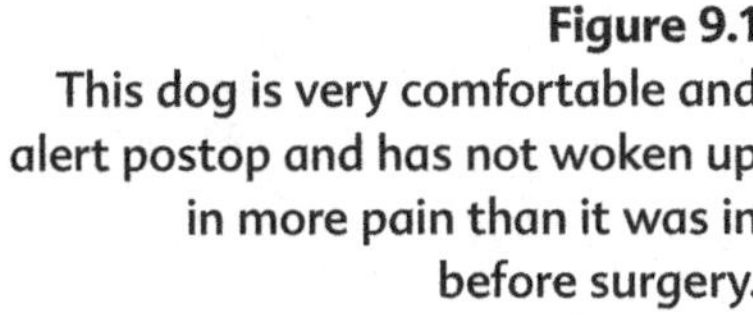

Figure 9.1
This dog is very comfortable and alert postop and has not woken up in more pain than it was in before surgery.

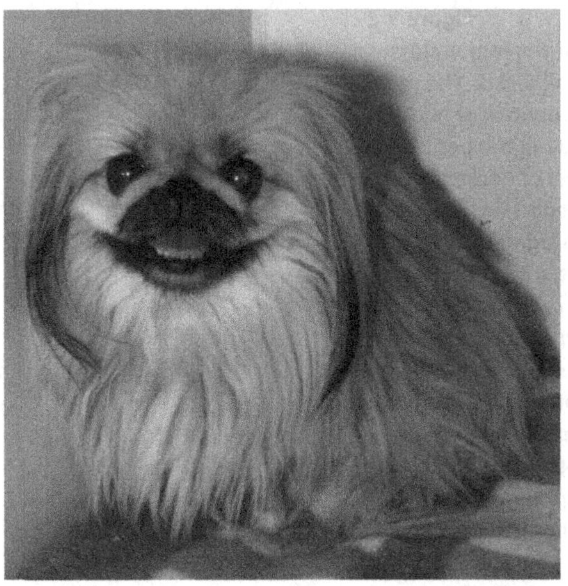

- the anticipated degree of pain in both surgical and non-surgical patients.

Ideally the protocols should ensure that surgical patients do not wake up in more pain than they were before the operation.

CLASSES OF ANALGESIC DRUGS

It is important to understand where along the pain pathway different analgesic drugs have their action, how they work and their potential side effects (see Chapters 6, 7 and 8 for more detail). This provides a basis for the rational choice of analgesic protocol for patients with varying intensities and types of pain and in some cases complicating concurrent problems. It also allows a multimodal approach to be taken which becomes increasingly valuable in cases of more severe pain. Common analgesic drugs used in companion animal practice for acute pain are:

- opiates and opioids
- non-steroidal anti-inflammatory drugs (NSAIDs)
- alpha 2 adrenoceptor agonists
- local anaesthetics
- ketamine
- nitrous oxide.

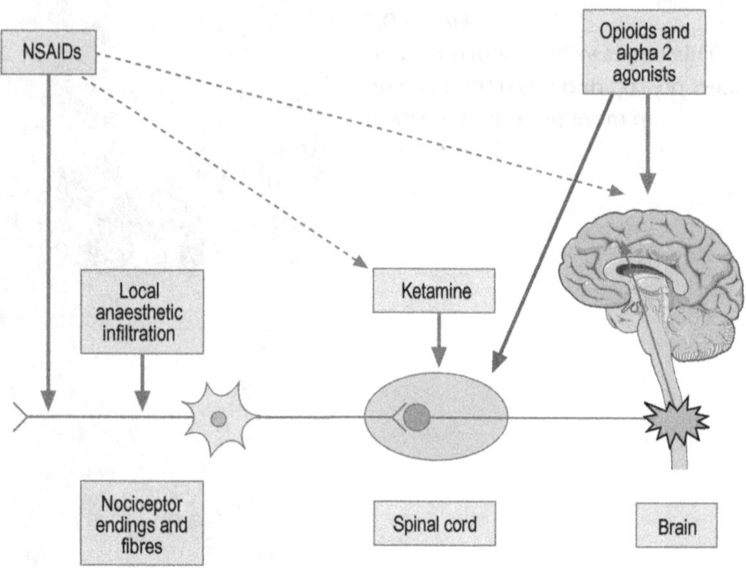

Figure 9.2
Sites of action of the major classes of analgesics. N.B. The main mechanism of actions of NSAIDs was thought to be in the periphery, at the level of nociceptors in damaged tissue. However, they also have a significant central effect, interrupting pain transmission in the CNS. Opioid receptors are expressed in the periphery associated with inflammation and therefore do have some peripheral analgesia. Local anaesthetics and opioids given via the epidural route block pain at the level of the spinal cord.

Fig 9.2 shows where each major class of analgesic works along the pain pathway, although the mechanism of action of nitrous oxide is still a bit of a mystery. Adjunctive therapies for analgesia and their proposed sites of action are detailed in Chapter 10, along with further non-pharmacological methods of pain management that can also have a very important role in acute pain management.

ANALGESIC TECHNIQUES

There is a wide range of analgesic therapies available for managing acute pain in hospitalised patients (listed below). General anaesthesia itself does not provide analgesia as the pain pathway will still be firing away during surgery. It just renders the patient unconscious so they don't perceive the pain, but it will still allow the development of peripheral and central sensitisation. This is why pre-emptive analgesia is so important (see Chapter 5).

Pharmacological analgesia techniques for acute pain

- opioids – injection of boluses, constant rate infusions (CRI), orally
- NSAIDs (only some are suitable for preop use) – injection, orally
- local anaesthetic nerve blocks

- local anaesthetic tissue infiltration
- epidural anaesthesia with local anaesthetic and/or opioid
- fentanyl transdermal skin patches
- intra-articular local anaesthetic and/or opioid
- alpha 2 agonists – as part of the premed or micro dose CRI
- ketamine – as part of the anaesthetic or low dose CRI
- nitrous oxide.

Some of these agents also double up as sedatives (opioids, alpha 2 agonists) or can be full anaesthetics themselves (ketamine, alpha 2 agonists). Other techniques that may be useful in acute pain are:

- topical local anaesthetic
- local anaesthetic instillation into a body cavity
- sedation in addition to analgesia.

In cases of severe unremitting pain, heavy sedation or full general anaesthesia may be indicated whilst the pain is controlled with analgesics. Sedation with analgesia is also indicated if patients are anxious. Sedatives help to calm the animal, but must always be used in conjunction with analgesics as they can also reduce an animal's ability to express pain – this can be mistaken for pain relief. General anaesthesia per se does not prevent firing of the pain pathway; analgesia must always be provided during surgery in addition to unconsciousness.

Other methods to help alleviate acute pain (see also Chapter 10)

Stress and anxiety will potentiate pain and make the whole experience much worse. In humans it is been demonstrated that anxiety leads to the release of serotonin, a neurotransmitter in the CNS. Serotonin seems to directly excite sensory neurones including those in the pain pathway, effectively leading to an increase in the amount of information processed as pain information (i.e. allodynia). Therefore an integral part of managing pain is to minimise stress and anxiety of patients by providing a pleasant as possible environment during their stay in the practice.

Hospitalised patients need ongoing close observation and compassionate care. Patients should have ample soft warm dry bedding, free from soiling from faeces and urine. Gentle

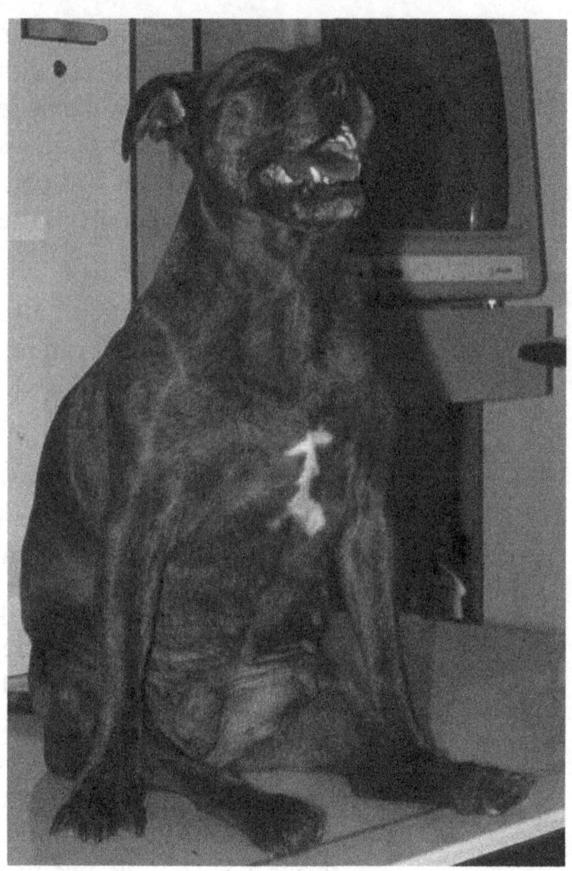

Figure 9.3
This dog with acute spinal pain is also very anxious and distressed due to the accompanying paresis and will benefit from sedation as well as analgesia.

grooming and cleaning of skin and teeth may be required. Cats need to be housed in a separate room from dogs, whilst well-socialised dogs benefit from being in a central area where they can watch and interact with people. Frequent petting and speaking softly will help reduce anxiety, especially when it comes to wound examinations and dressing changes. Not all individuals appreciate hands on TLC, smaller prey species may get more stressed by handling, and need to be housed well away from predators.

Just the odour of other species on nurses' clothing can be stressful for animals. It makes sense to handle 'small furries' before cats and dogs, and ensure kennels are cleaned thoroughly to remove traces of previous occupants. The temperature should be warm and constant, avoiding large fluctuations and draughts. Indwelling catheters can be placed in patients that need multiple blood sampling, to avoid repeated venepuncture. Where appropriate try and avoid painful i.m. and s.c. injections; use i.v. or oral administration. A full bladder is very uncomfortable and patients are often reluctant to pass urine in a kennel or strange surroundings, particularly if it involves a painful stance. In such circumstances it may be necessary to catheterise some patients to prevent discomfort or to relieve them.

Surgical technique can greatly influence the degree of postop pain. Gentle handling of tissues and minimising tissue trauma will reduce stimulation of the pain pathway and sensitisation. Avoiding too much tension on suture lines, the use of padded dressings to protect traumatised tissue and splinting to reduce movement at the site of injury will all aid postop pain management.

WHERE ACUTE PAIN MAY ARISE

Obviously any tissue damage or trauma will lead to stimulation of nociceptors and pain. It is also reasonable to assume that all surgical procedures, many diagnostic procedures, and injuries or diseases that would cause pain in humans will cause pain in animals. Any condition where tissue inflammation is present (and this isn't always associated with overt tissue damage), such as a cat bite abscess, impacted anal glands, cystitis, conjunctivitis, otitis externa and other infections can be extremely painful. Another source of significant pain is distension of tissues; this can be a result of a tumour or abscess formation, etc. Hepatitis, pancreatitis and other conditions leading to organ distension and stretching of organ capsules can be intensely painful. Stretching of the periosteum is one of the main sources of the severe pain associated with bone tumours.

Tissue ischaemia will produce acute pain; common examples include gastric dilatation/volvulus, intestinal obstruction, and aortic thromboembolism. Neuropathic pain (pain from direct injury to nerves) is particularly severe and difficult to treat and can cause acute pain as well as chronic pain syndromes, e.g. meningitis, nerve root compression secondary to intervertebral disc disease. Many serious conditions like pancreatitis and infections lead to the release of systemic inflammatory mediators that result in a fever and contribute to sensitisation, so the patient generally feels 'more sore' all over (a bit like the generalised aching accompanying a fever

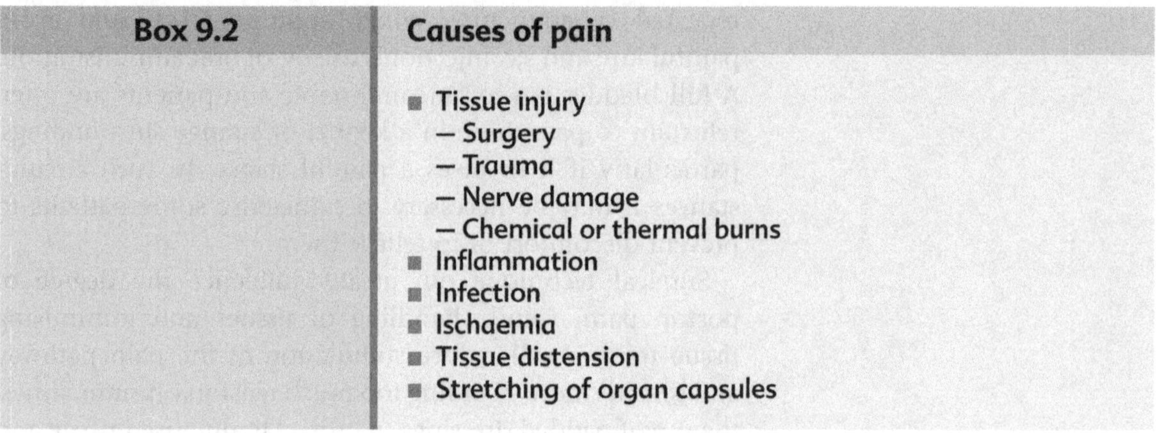

Box 9.2 Causes of pain

- Tissue injury
  - Surgery
  - Trauma
  - Nerve damage
  - Chemical or thermal burns
- Inflammation
- Infection
- Ischaemia
- Tissue distension
- Stretching of organ capsules

commonly reported in people). It is important to remember to treat the pain as well as the underlying cause.

Clinicians also need to be aware that they can inadvertently subject patients to further pain and intensify pain already present with diagnostic techniques or invasive treatments, e.g. positioning for radiography, thoracocentesis, abdominocentesis, arthrocentesis, catheter placement in veins or the bladder, drains, etc. These procedures can also induce a lot of stress and anxiety (that will potentiate pain) from the feeling of airway obstruction, sensation of foreign bodies in the airway or urethra, and just the physical restraint. Appropriate analgesia and sedation must be provided, along with gentle handling and good nursing care.

PERIOP PAIN MANAGEMENT

Once a suitable anaesthetic protocol has been decided upon, the analgesic requirements of the patient should be gauged and included in the premed. The exact choice of analgesics may vary depending on the anaesthetic agents, and doses of anaesthetics may need to be adjusted to take account of sedative effects of certain analgesics and any dose-sparing properties. Further intraop and postop requirements must also be anticipated and organised before surgery. The anticipated degrees of pain associated with common surgical procedures are listed below and are based on the expected amount of tissue trauma and invasiveness of surgery. The duration of surgery and tissue trauma or handling is another variable to take into account and depends on the attending surgeon and their experience and technique. This is just a rough guide – each patient must be judged on an individual basis. See Chapters 3 and 4 for further details on assessing pain in animals.

LEVELS OF PAIN ASSOCIATED WITH SURGERY

Mathews[1] has suggested a scheme for describing the levels of pain following various surgical procedures. (See Box 9.3.)

GENERAL APPROACH TO PERIOP PAIN MANAGEMENT

Every surgical procedure and many diagnostic procedures will cause a degree of pain. Pain is never beneficial to the patient; it leads to a prolonged recovery, increased morbidity, increased stress and suffering (see Chapter 2). Everything possible should be done to prevent and alleviate pain; this includes minimising the factors that potentiate painful experiences – anxiety, sleeplessness and stress. It may be better to admit surgical cases on the day of the procedure where it is feasible rather than the night before as this avoids the animal being in a novel, strange environment which will cause a great deal of anxiety and lack of sleep. The patients should always be handled kindly and gently, with a soft voice and kept in a comfortable environment (see above). These concerns are even more important in geriatric patients

a

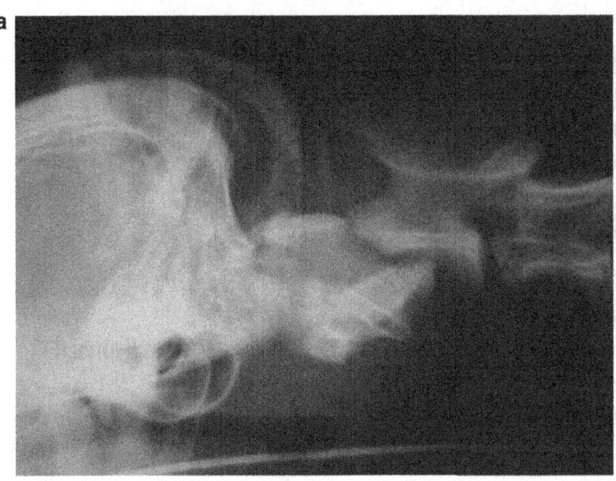

b

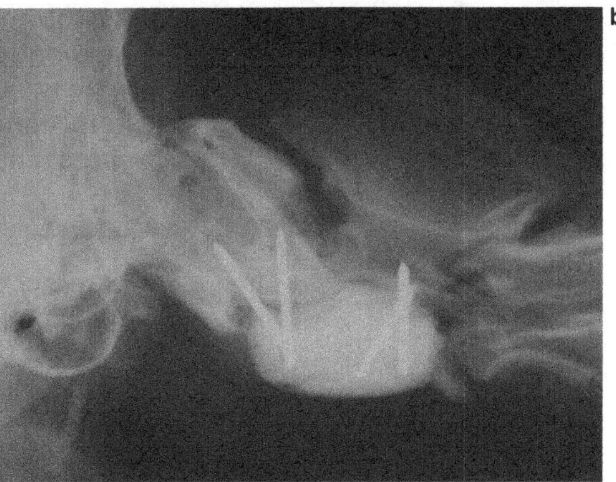

Figure 9.4
(a) Spinal surgery, such as repair of this C2 neck fracture, would be classed under severe to excruciating pain. (b) Postop repair of C2 neck fracture.

Box 9.3 **Anticipated levels of pain associated with surgical procedures**

Severe to excruciating pain

- multiple fracture repairs with extensive soft tissue injury (including intraop manipulation)
- major fracture repair
- some cranial cruciate repairs, e.g. tibia plateau levelling osteotomy
- major orthopaedic procedures, e.g. total hip replacement, osteotomy
- any surgery with extensive soft tissue injury or inflammation postop
- spinal surgery* or surgery involving direct nerve damage (neuropathic pain).

*Although loss of pain sensation can be a clinical sign of intervertebral disc disease, pain is often severe following surgery.

Severe and moderate-to-severe pain

- intra-articular surgery
- fracture repair
- limb amputation
- onychectomy (de-claw of cats; not done in UK)
- gastric torsion
- testicular torsion
- mesenteric and other torsions
- thoracotomy
- exploratory laparotomy
- intestinal foreign body
- splenectomy
- cystotomy
- traumatic diaphragmatic hernia repair (with organ and extensive tissue injury)
- total ear canal ablation
- mass removal with extensive tissue disruption.

Moderate pain

- external fixator orthopaedic repair
- tail amputation
- exploratory laparotomy of short duration with minimal manipulation and no inflammation
- inguinal hernia repair
- simple acute diaphragmatic hernia repair (no organ injury)
- mass removal
- ovariohysterectomy*
- castration*

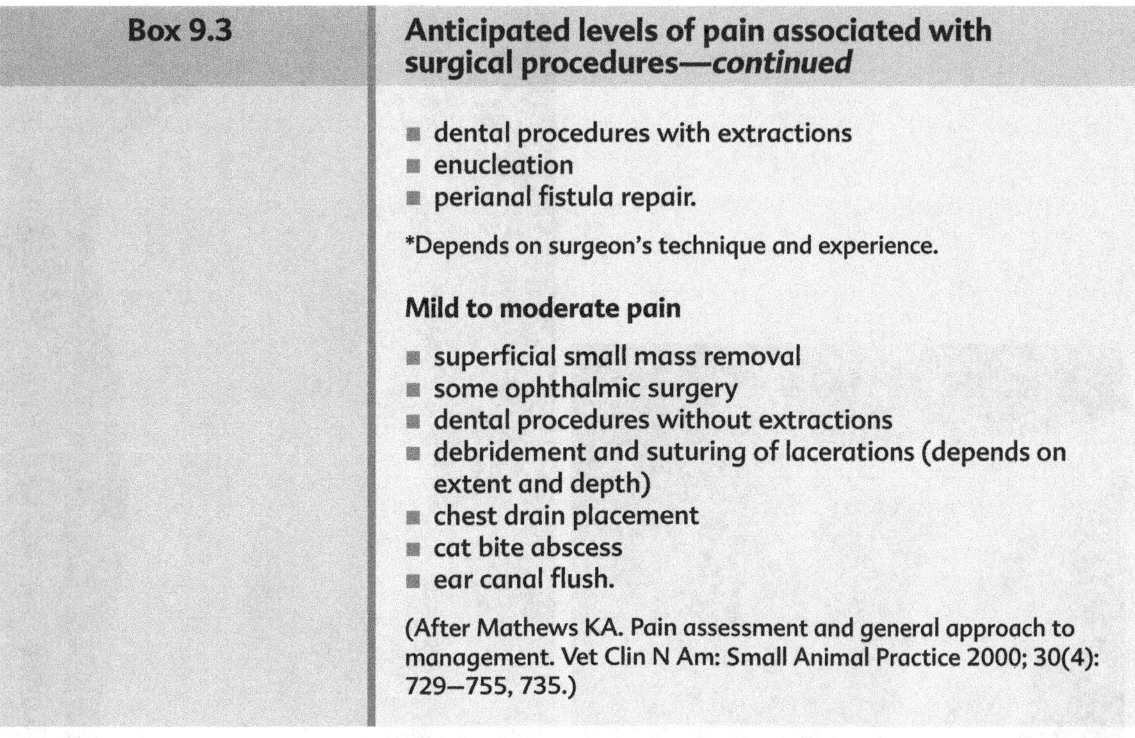
Box 9.3 **Anticipated levels of pain associated with surgical procedures—*continued***

- dental procedures with extractions
- enucleation
- perianal fistula repair.

*Depends on surgeon's technique and experience.

Mild to moderate pain

- superficial small mass removal
- some ophthalmic surgery
- dental procedures without extractions
- debridement and suturing of lacerations (depends on extent and depth)
- chest drain placement
- cat bite abscess
- ear canal flush.

(After Mathews KA. Pain assessment and general approach to management. Vet Clin N Am: Small Animal Practice 2000; 30(4): 729–755, 735.)

as ageing tends to reduce animals adaptability to new situations.

Premedication

The aim of premedication is to reduce anxiety, provide pre-emptive analgesia, reduce the dose of subsequent anaesthetic agents and counteract their side effects, and help smooth induction and recovery. Acepromazine is widely used and alpha 2 agonists are also useful as they provide sedation with analgesia, but patient selection is important due to their effects on the cardiovascular system. Acepromazine is not without side effects either; it causes peripheral vasodilatation and hypotension. In older patients, opioids seem to produce more sedation, so less sedative may be required. For severe and excruciating pain, high doses of opioid full mu agonists are indicated – morphine is still the gold standard analgesic. Fentanyl, methadone, hydromorphone and oxymorphone (available in the USA) are also useful. Pethidine (although very short-acting) and partial agonists such as buprenorphine are suitable for more moderate pain. Morphine tends to cause vomiting when given preop to non-painful dogs; this is less likely with methadone and oxymorphone. Intravenous morphine is best avoided as it can cause histamine release and

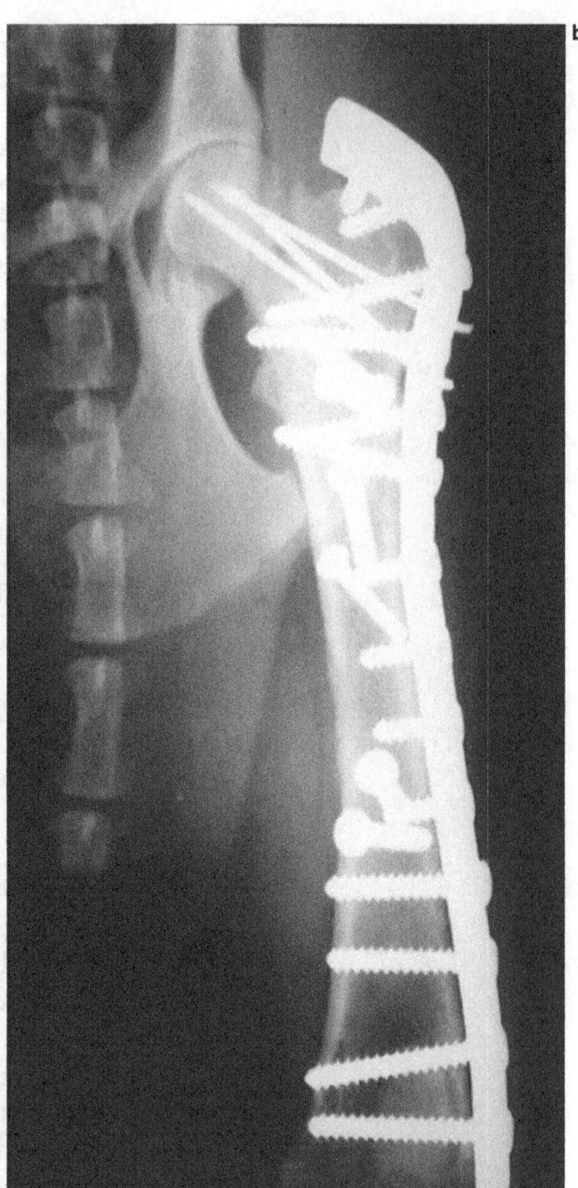

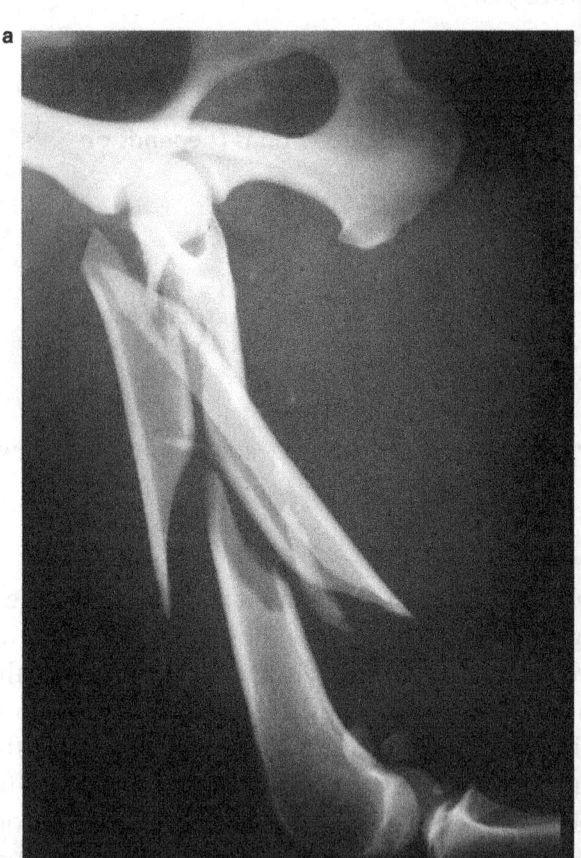

Figure 9.5
(a) This comminuted diaphyseal fracture repair may be classed as severe pain. (b) Postop repair of comminuted diaphyseal fracture.

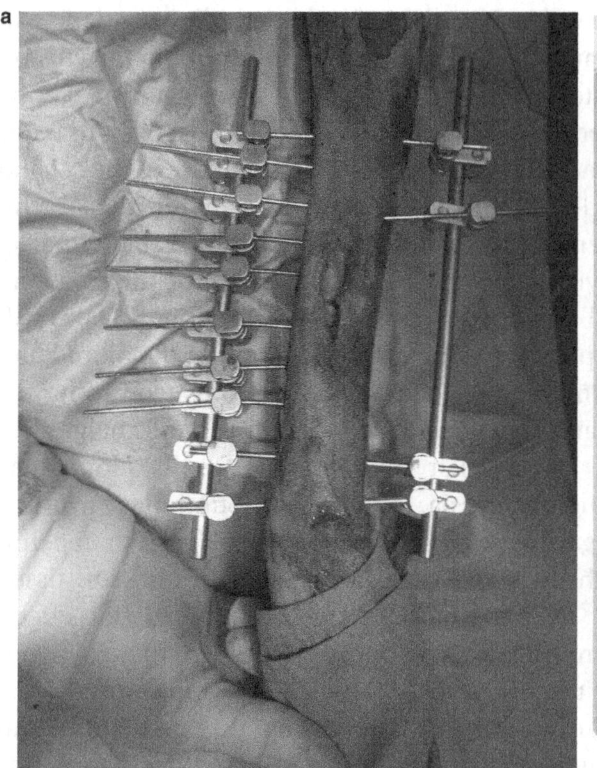

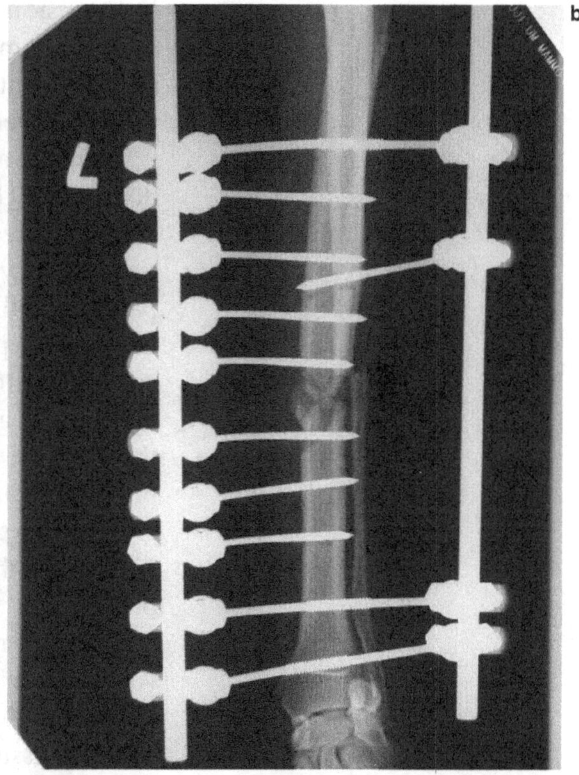

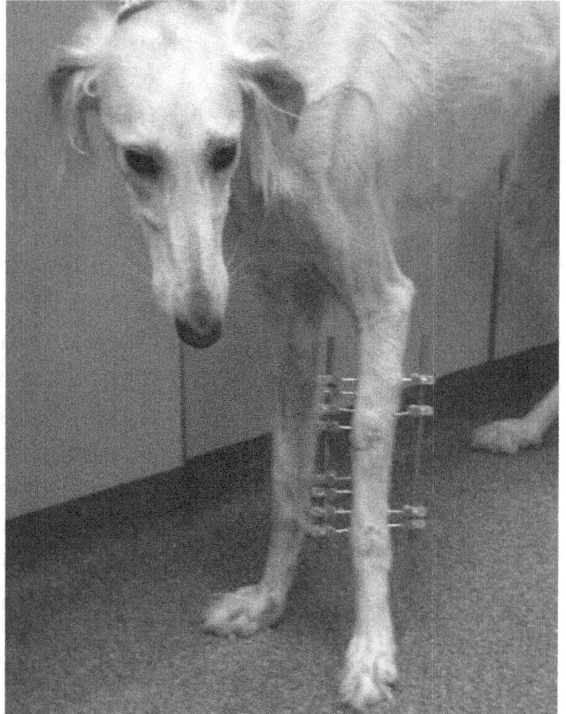

Figure 9.6
(a) An external fixator repair of this radius fracture may be classed as moderate to severe pain.
(b) Postop radiograph of radius fracture repair.
(c) Postop the dog is quite comfortable with its external fixator that has stabilised the fracture.

hypotension unless given very slowly. Pethidine similarly will cause histamine release i.v., and should only be given i.m. (the s.c. route is not very efficacious). Pure agonists can be used at lower doses for the management of less severe pain.

There are now NSAIDs licensed for preop use in the cat and dog in the UK – carprofen and meloxicam and their inclusion in a premed with opioids will provide excellent analgesia with a synergistic effect, suitable for moderate to severe pain. As well as reducing pain and sensitisation, NSAIDs will help reduce postop swelling. They will outlast the opioid and ensure continuing analgesia postop. Opioids tend to have a faster onset and so will provide more immediate analgesia at the start of surgery. For milder pain, NSAID alone may provide enough analgesia. Studies have found that carprofen given preop gave as good as, if not better analgesia than pethidine, in both dogs and cats for orthopaedic and soft tissue procedures.[6,7] NSAIDs have a range of potential side effects and should not be used preop in cases where there is hypovolaemia or the risk of haemorrhage or compromised renal perfusion during surgery. Supporting the circulation and blood pressure with i.v. fluids can reduce the risks of side effects. Giving NSAIDs postop is another option in higher risk situations as long as alternative preop analgesia is provided. In some cases they will be contraindicated altogether (see Chapter 7 for further details).

Preop administration of an NMDA antagonist such as ketamine will reduce pain and the development of central sensitisation. Studies in humans found preop and intraop ketamine decreased wound hyperalgesia for up to 7 days postop.[8] It has synergy with opioids and alpha 2 agonists. Dogs and cats should not receive ketamine at higher doses alone because it can produce convulsions and therefore it should be used in combinations with, for example, a benzodiazepine or an alpha 2 agonist.

Local anaesthetic nerve and regional blocks are often given before induction (or intraop); they are ideal for blocking nociceptive impulses from the surgical site. Specific ones are indicated for particular procedures (see Chapter 8).

Maintenance

Induction and maintenance agents like propofol, thiopentone, halothane and isoflurane do not provide any analgesia.

Therefore if a procedure is particularly invasive or involves extensive disruption of tissue, further intraoperative analgesia is indicated in addition to the preop analgesics. This will have the added benefit of reducing the dose of anaesthetic agents, and they all depress the cardiovascular system so it is a bonus if this effect is minimised. Nitrous oxide is a very good analgesic to use intraop where indicated, but it is rapidly blown off and provides no residual effect postop.

For moderate to excruciating pain, intraop boluses or infusions of opioids provide excellent analgesia. Opioids with a very short duration of action, e.g. fentanyl, alfentanil, are suitable for this. They are dose-sparing of inhalant anaesthetics; however, respiratory depression can be significant and the patients usually need ventilating. Intra-articular morphine and/or bupivacaine are now being used at the end of joint surgery after the joint has been sealed, to provide very good postop analgesia. They could also be injected into the joint before surgery for a pre-emptive effect.[2,8]

Epidural anaesthesia with local anaesthetic, e.g. bupivacaine and/or morphine, using preservative-free formulations, is indicated for moderate to severe pain from surgery involving caudal body parts and hind limbs. They are often administered after induction but before surgery starts. Care must be taken to closely monitor patients that have epidurals with local anaesthetic as they can get significant motor blockade, which can cause problems on recovery. They can develop hypotension intraop if sympathetic lumbar or thoracic blockade occurs. Some patients may try to mutilate a numb area on recovery or become very anxious at the loss of sensation after epidurals or local anaesthetic blocks.

Constant rate infusions (CRI) of low doses of ketamine or micro-doses of alpha 2 agonists such as medetomidine can be used to provide excellent intraop analgesia; infusions can also be continued postop for analgesia in very painful circumstances. Medetomidine used this way provides a very steady plane of background analgesia and sedation intraop and is very dose-sparing. It is also known to reduce the stress response to surgery and its cardiovascular side effects are reduced at micro-doses. Ketamine or medetomidine infusions can be given alongside an opioid infusion for a synergistic effect. Low dose ketamine infusions have a lovely pre-emptive effect and have been shown to reduce the requirements for opioids after major surgery in dogs. The big advantage of using infusions (opioids, ketamine or alpha 2 agonists) is that analgesia is continuous, there is no drop-off between repeat doses and it minimises the risk of pain breakthrough.

Postop

The use of preop and intraop analgesics with a sedative effect will tend to prolong the recovery period, especially opioids that suppress the cough reflex and therefore allow animals to tolerate the endotracheal tube for longer. A slower recovery can be beneficial to avoid excitation or anxiousness. Animals should recover with ample fully effective analgesia already on board, but they still need to be continually assessed on recovery to check analgesia is maintained. Individual requirements for analgesia can vary greatly, so do not assume a set pain management protocol will be enough for every patient. If severe intractable pain is apparent on recovery, the patient can always be re-anaesthetised to stop it experiencing the pain, whilst more effective analgesia is administered.

Dogs often show a short period of excitation on recovery that usually passes with some comforting and care but pain can be a contributing factor. One way to diagnose the presence of pain in this situation is to give a short-acting opioid with a fast onset of action i.v., e.g. fentanyl or alfentanil. If the dog is still showing excitation despite further analgesia then it probably is very anxious so try giving a tranquilliser, e.g. low dose i.v. acepromazine or medetomidine. Once the patient is calmer, carefully examine the painful body part, to see if the patient is sensitive to manipulation, which would indicate the need for further analgesia. If the animal continues to be agitated this may be due to opioid excitation – this can be confirmed by giving more fentanyl or alfentanil i.v. If the agitation gets even worse then an opioid antagonist is indicated. Nalbuphine is a mixed antagonist/agonist that will reverse mu agonist effects but leave some analgesia from kappa agonism. Alternatively naloxone (a full antagonist) can be titrated slowly to effect. If, however, the extra opioid actually improves matters then the animal is probably in pain and a longer-acting opioid can

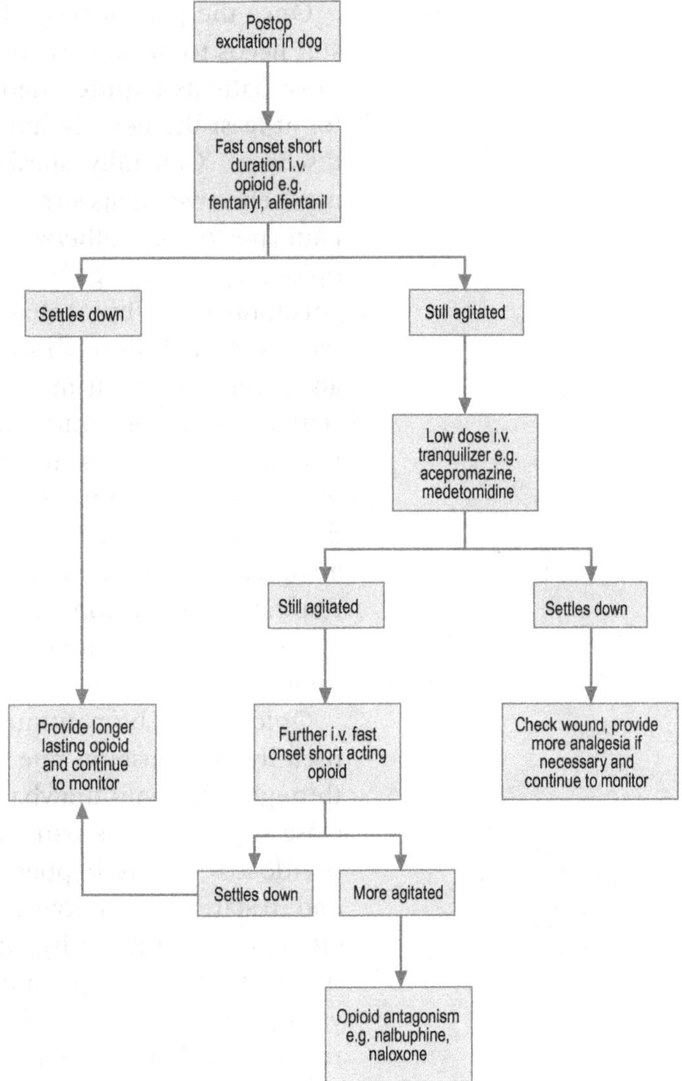

Figure 9.7
Decision making tree for postop excitation in dogs.

be used to continue the analgesia. Fig 9.7 summarises the approach to postop excitation.[8]

A similar approach can be taken with cats, bearing in mind they are more susceptible to opioid excitation than dogs. Cats in unrelieved pain may start to throw themselves violently around the recovery cage, and medetomidine is a useful sedative/analgesic in some of these cases (acepromazine can be a bit unpredictable in cats), particularly as it can be reversed with atipamezole if necessary.

Once the patient has fully recovered from anaesthesia, it still needs to be reassessed and monitored for signs of pain. Most patients require ongoing analgesia after major surgery for at least the next 24 hours and then for several days after discharge. Generally speaking, opioids are the safest and most effective analgesics available for the treatment of acute pain (postop and otherwise). As discussed before, the partial opioid agonists, e.g. buprenorphine, and mixed agonists/ antagonists, e.g. butorphanol, have a ceiling effect whereby increasing their dose above a certain point may not increase analgesia – in fact it may start to be reversed. It is better to start using a pure mu agonist, e.g. morphine or oxymorphone, if analgesia is still inadequate after a partial agonist,[9] or consider an epidural, local anaesthetic block, or microdose medetomidine CRI, etc. There is no upper limit to the analgesia from pure mu agonists, the main limiting factor is respiratory depression – although this is rare in dogs and cats – so increasing increments can be carefully used to bring pain under control.

Opioids can be continued postop by injection, or more usefully in constant rate infusions to avoid pain breakthrough. The only drawback of opioid CRI is the need for close supervision as patients can become heavily sedated if overdosed. If this happens, temporarily stop the infusion and restart it at a lower dose. The other potential side effects of opioids are hypotension and bradycardia; the use of i.v. fluids will help support the circulation. The problem with waiting for signs of pain to appear before doses are repeated is that a degree of sensitisation will develop each time the analgesic wears off and pain becomes increasingly harder to control. If opioid infusions are not possible then use their average durations and patient response as a guide to dosing intervals (as well as referring to data sheets). Fentanyl patches can also be applied postop to continue analgesia, although there is a 12–24 hour delay before onset of analgesia and they do not always work in every patient. As mentioned earlier, very painful patients may benefit from ongoing CRI of ketamine or medetomidine, and even continuing epidural analgesia via placement of an epidural catheter.

NSAIDs will usually provide 24 hours of analgesia; they have synergy with opioids and they may be given preop in some animals. In higher-risk patients it may be preferable to wait until after anaesthesia before giving a NSAID and oral preparations can then be dispensed for longer-term follow-up at home. NSAIDs have little dose flexibility, unlike the opioids, and are usually restricted to a single dose over a 24-hour period, and cannot be titrated to effect. They can provide very effective analgesia, especially in combination with opioids, but there are many more restrictions on their use compared with other types of analgesic. See Chapter 7 for more details on their use. NSAIDs would not be indicated for particular surgical conditions such as gastric dilatation where the blood supply to the gastric mucosa has been compromised. Signs of NSAID intolerance include vomiting, diarrhoea with or without blood and general depression, whereupon the NSAID should be withdrawn and the patient investigated and treated appropriately. It is advisable to make owners aware of the signs of side effects of any medication that is dispensed for use at home.

Severe unremitting postop pain

If a patient shows unexpectedly severe pain after surgery with allodynia and causalgia (where light touch elicits great pain) the possibility of nerve entrapment by a ligature or implant should be considered. Treatment entails re-operating to free the nerve; meantime the pain needs to be controlled. A loading dose of opioid is indicated followed by a CRI and maybe a NSAID added in. In situations of excruciating pain (postop or otherwise), where the priority is immediate intense analgesia, morphine can be diluted in saline and given very slowly i.v. over 5–10 minutes (to try and avoid histamine release). This can be followed by a morphine CRI, with the dose tailored to the animal's response. For other opioids the normal dose over a given period can be divided up and given as an infusion. Ketamine can also be administered, as can a local block or epidural, and as mentioned earlier the patient can be re-anaesthetised whilst the cause of the pain is investigated.

Table 9.1 gives very general guidelines for periop analgesic protocols for various levels of anticipated pain. It basically demonstrates the multimodal technique of interrupting the pain pathway at an increasing number of points to provide more analgesia. One question that gets asked is

Table 9.1
General approach to preop pain management protocols

Level of anticipated postop pain	Suggested preop analgesia	Further postop analgesia
Mild pain	Opioid full/partial agonist Or NSAID	Provide further postop analgesia as needed: NSAID Or opioid full/ partial agonist
Mild to moderate	Opioid full agonist + NSAID ± Alpha 2 agonist ± Epidural analgesia or local anaesthetic infiltration/block	One or more of these if necessary: NSAID Micro dose alpha 2 agonist infusion Opioid full/partial agonist
Moderate to severe	Opioid full agonist preop, consider further doses intraop + NSAID + Epidural analgesia with bupivacaine and/or morphine + Local anaesthetic nerve or regional blocks ± Ketamine or micro dose alpha 2 agonist infusion intraop	Opioid agonist If necessary also: Higher dose of opioid or increased frequency Additional epidural drugs Additional local anaesthesia, e.g. into body cavity Ketamine or micro dose alpha 2 agonist infusion Adjunctive analgesia

NB If a patient shows signs of anxiety on recovery, consider using a sedative such as acepromazine or diazepam, or low doses of alpha 2 agonist

whether or not it is possible to provide too much analgesia. The answer is probably not, but the potential for side effects needs to be taken into account and balanced against a reasonable assessment of the requirement for analgesia. There is a radical and somewhat controversial argument for giving every patient as much analgesia as possible regardless of the level of anticipated pain, to ensure no patient ever suffers unnecessarily.

SPECIFIC EXAMPLES OF PAIN MANAGEMENT PROTOCOLS FOR SURGICAL CASES

Table 9.2 gives some ideas for suggested protocols for specific procedures in dogs. It just gives some suggestions, and Table 9.3 lists examples of analgesics, and durations of action. When using these tables and those for cats (Tables 9.4, 9.5) it is important to note:

1. For all drugs check the individual data sheets for appropriate doses, contraindications and warnings.
2. Doses of sedatives and other anaesthetic agents may need adjusting according to dose-sparing effects of any analgesics given preop. It is strongly advised that clinicians check all individual drugs for data sheet recommendations.
3. Always refer to the licensing cascade in the UK and choose analgesics not contraindicated by the patient's condition or disease.
4. Only use NSAIDs that are specifically licensed for preop use: carprofen (Rimadyl®) and meloxicam (Metacam®) in the UK.
5. Medetomidine (Domitor®) is not licensed for use with opioids other than butorphanol in the UK.
6. Some drugs are not licensed (particularly the opioids) for veterinary use.
7. Further information on dose rates can be found by contacting manufacturers and in the references cited in 'Further Reading'.
8. More comprehensive lists of analgesics and constant rate infusions (CRI) can be found in the references in 'Further Reading'.
9. The approximate durations of actions of analgesics in dogs and cats can be used as a rough guideline for dosing intervals but opioids in particular have a lot of individual variation, and animals should be treated on an individual basis.
10. Postop oral NSAIDs, e.g. carprofen and meloxicam, should be started 24 hours after their preop injection in dogs.
11. Acepromazine is not an analgesic; it is included as an example of a sedative that can be used in the premed. Other sedatives that are useful in combination with opioids are diazepam and midazolam.

Table 9.2
Example protocols for surgical pain in dogs

Canine procedure	Anticipated degree of pain	Examples of preop analgesia	Examples of intraop analgesia	Examples of postop analgesia
Severe abdominal pain, e.g. pancreatic tumour removal or pelvic split	Severe to excruciating	Acepromazine + morphine + NSAID	Epidural morphine + bupivacaine ± fentanyl CRI* ± microdose medetomidine/ ketamine CRI	Continue epidural + medetomidine CRI if necessary + morphine + NSAID
Hind-limb fracture repair, cruciate repair, orthopaedic surgery (or amputation)	Moderate to severe or excruciating	Protocol 1 Acepromazine + morphine + NSAID	Protocol 1 Epidural morphine + bupivacaine	Protocol 1 Morphine after epidural worn off + NSAID for 7–10 days
		Protocol 2 Sedative + opioid agonist + NSAID + fentanyl patch 12–24 h before surgery	Protocol 2 Intra-articular bupivacaine (or bupivacaine into nerves before resection for amputations)	Protocol 2 May need repeat opioid – depends on timing of application offentanyl patch + NSAID 7–10 days postop
Forelimb fracture or orthopaedic surgery (or amputation)	Moderate to severe or excruciating	Acepromazine + morphine + NSAID	Brachial plexus block with bupivacaine ± fentanyl CRI	Morphine + NSAID for 7–10 days postop
Exploratory laporotomy, splenectomy, intestinal foreign body	Moderate to severe	Protocol 1 Acepromazine + morphine	Protocol 1 Incisional local anaesthetic block + fentanyl CRI	Protocol 1 Morphine after CRI + NSAID for 7–10 days postop if appropriate
		Protocol 2 Sedative + Morphine + Fentanyl patch 12–24 h before surgery		Protocol 2 May need more morphine – depends on timing of fentanyl patch application Leave patch on 3–5 days

Table 9.2
Example protocols for surgical pain in dogs—*cont'd*

Canine procedure	Anticipated degree of pain	Examples of preop analgesia	Examples of intraop analgesia	Examples of postop analgesia
Thoracotomy	Moderate to severe	Sedative + morphine + NSAID	Intercostal nerve blocks ± epidural morphine Consider opioid CRI	Morphine + Intrapleural local anaesthetic if chest drain in place + NSAID
Total ear canal ablation	Moderate to severe	Sedative + morphine+ NSAID	Auriculotemporal and great auricular nerve block	Morphine + NSAID
Caesarean section	Moderate	Acepromazine + pethidine + NSAID	Consider nitrous oxide	Repeat pethidine then buprenorphine
Ovariohysterectomy and castration	Moderate	Acepromazine + buprenorphine + NSAID	Incisional local anaesthetic block	Repeat buprenorphine + NSAID 3–5 days postop
Perianal fistula repair	Moderate	Sedative + morphine + NSAID	Epidural morphine and bupivacaine	Epidural bupivacaine + NSAID
Dental with extractions	Moderate to severe	Acepromazine + buprenorphine + NSAID	Infraorbital ± mandibular ± maxillary nerve blocks	If whole mouth or multiple molar extractions, may need more morphine NSAID for 3–7 days postop

NB Only use NSAIDs that are specifically licensed pre-op and continue the same one postop as per data sheet
*CRI = constant rate infusion

Table 9.3
Some examples of analgesics for use in dogs

Drug	Route	Approx time to onset of analgesia	Approx duration
Opioids for moderate to severe pain			
Morphine	i.m., s.c.	15 min	2–4 h
Oxymorphone	s.c., i.m., i.v.	15 min 1 min	3–5 h
Methadone	s.c., i.m.	15 min	2–4 h
Fentanyl patches	Transdermal	12–24 h	72+ h
Fentanyl injection	i.v. (low dose)	1 min	20–30 min
Opioids for mild to moderate pain			
Pethidine	s.c., i.m.	15 min	1–2 h
Buprenorphine	s.c., i.m.	45 min	6–8 h
Butorphanol	s.c, i.m., i.v.	20 min 1 min	15–60 min
NSAIDs			
Carprofen	s.c., i.v., p.o.		24 h
Meloxicam	s.c., i.v., p.o.		24 h
Local anaesthetic nerve blocks, infiltration			
Bupivacaine		20–30 min	4–6 h
Lidocaine		10–15 min	45–60 min (longer with adrenaline)
Epidural analgesia (use preservative-free drugs)			
Bupivacaine	epidural	10–15 min	2–6 h
Lidocaine	epidural	5–10 min	1–1.5 h
Morphine	epidural	20–60 min	16–24 h
Sedatives (not analgesics)			
Acepromazine	s.c., i.m., i.v.	30–45 min 20 min	2–6+ h
Diazepam	i.v.	Within minutes	Up to 6 h
Midazolam	i.v., i.m.	Within minutes	Up to 6 h

EXTRA NOTES ON PERIOP PAIN MANAGEMENT IN CATS[9,11,12]

The use of EMLA local anaesthetic cream may be indicated more often in cats to facilitate placement of an intravenous catheter preop. Apply the cream to the shaved area and cover it for at least 20 minutes before venepuncture.

As in dogs, opioid pure mu agonists are the analgesics of choice for severe pain. Morphine and methadone are both very useful in cats as are oxymorphone and hydromorphone (widely used in the USA). Morphine may be less effective in cats than dogs, as cats produce very few metabolites of morphine that would normally contribute to the analgesia, as seen in other species.[2] Pethidine also works well in cats but is relatively short-acting – only 1–2 hours. Buprenorphine is a highly effective analgesic in cats and relatively long-acting, rarely causing dysphoria or vomiting. It can be given preop and recent work has found it to be very effective given via transmucosal absorption through the oral mucous membrane. This buccal administration is a very patient- and owner-friendly technique for ongoing pain relief.[12] Butorphanol is a mild short-acting analgesic in both cats and dogs and rarely the first choice for surgical pain.

Fentanyl skin patches are particularly useful for cats as they are so 'hands off' (always a bonus when dealing with the vast majority of tortoise-shells). The onset of analgesia may be quicker than dogs; studies have found steady state plasma concentrations achieved in 6–12 hours in cats compared with 18–24 hours in dogs. However, the plasma concentrations of fentanyl can vary widely between individual cats, probably due to differences in weights, body temperature and skin permeability. It is important not to rely entirely on these patches and to evaluate each patient carefully to see if further analgesia is needed. Fentanyl and alfentanil have been used successfully in cats as intraop intermittent boluses or CRI.

Opioids cause marked dilation of the pupils in cats (mydriasis), bear this in mind – avoid bright lighting in their environment and startling them on approach. There have also been reports of opioids causing hyperthermia in cats, and open mouth breathing was seen as a result.[12] This was treated using active cooling with fans and cool water or reversing the opioid with naloxone. Epidural analgesia can be used in cats although it is technically more difficult. Morphine provides very effective analgesia (with few systemic side effects) up to the level of the forelimb and can be used for forelimb, abdominal, hindlimb and thoracic surgery. Analgesia is nicely enhanced by the inclusion of bupivacaine. Epidural local anaesthetics can also be used for hindlimb and abdominal surgery but the larger volumes needed for more cranial analgesia cannot be used because they cause respiratory and cardiac depression. Epidurals are normally administered after induction and before surgery, as this technique is a bit tricky to perform in the average conscious cat.

Cats are particularly susceptible to the toxic effects of NSAIDs because as is often the case with this species they do not metabolise the drugs as well as dogs due to deficiencies in the glucuronidation pathways in the feline liver. Cats must be dosed very accurately with NSAIDs as there is a narrower safety margin than in dogs, and great care must be taken when repeating doses to leave a long enough dosing interval to avoid an accumulation of the NSAID. Data from other species on NSAIDs cannot be simply extrapolated to cats – they are not 'small dogs' in the world of pharmacology. Carprofen is licensed for preop use in cats and a single injection may provide from 48 up to 72 hours analgesia. Meloxicam is also licensed preop in cats and gives similar levels of analgesia. Ketoprofen and tolfenamic acid are both good analgesics in cats, giving at least 18 hours of analgesia comparable to carprofen and meloxicam, but they should only be given postop (neither are licensed preop). Similar warnings and contraindications apply to cats and dogs regarding the use of NSAIDs.

Ketamine is usually used as a dissociative anaesthetic agent in cats, rather than at low doses for analgesia. However, anaesthetic protocols incorporating ketamine do result in less postop pain, as do those including medetomidine. Transmucosal absorption of medetomidine via oral administration has been described as efficacious in cats and is a very useful technique in the less cooperative cat. Local anaesthetic blocks in cats are just as good for analgesia as in dogs, and of similar duration, but great care is needed to check the total dose does not exceed safe levels.

Table 9.4 gives some ideas for suggested analgesic protocols for a range of surgical procedures in cats. Table 9.5 gives further examples of some analgesic drugs that can be used in cats.

Table 9.4
Example protocols for surgical pain in cats

Feline surgical procedure	Anticipated level of pain	Examples of preop analgesia	Examples of intraop analgesia	Examples of postop analgesia
Hind-limb fracture repair, orthopaedic surgery (or amputation)	Moderate to severe to excruciating	Protocol 1 Acepromazine + morphine + NSAID Protocol 2 Sedative + morphine + fentanyl patch 8–12 h before surgery	Protocol 1 Consider epidural morphine Protocol 2 Consider ketamine CRI	Protocol 1 Buprenorphine (buccal admin) Protocol 2 Repeat morphine depending on timing of fentanyl patch application Consider continuing ketamine CRI
Forelimb fracture or orthopaedic surgery (or amputation)	Moderate to severe to excruciating	Protocol 1 Acepromazine + morphine + NSAID Protocol 2 Sedative + morphine + fentanyl patch 8–12 h before surgery	Protocol 1 Brachial plexus block with bupivacaine Protocol 2 Consider ketamine CRI	Protocol 1 & 2 Buprenorphine (buccal admin) Repeat opioid depending on timing of fentanyl patch application
Exploratory laporotomy, splenectomy, intestinal foreign body	Moderate to severe	Protocol 1 Sedative + morphine Protocol 2 Acepromazine + morphine + fentanyl patch 6–12 h before surgery	Protocol 1 Incisional block with bupivacaine + opioid, e.g. fentanyl or morphine CRI or ketamine CRI	Protocol 1 Buprenorphine buccal admin once clear of CRI Protocol 2 Repeat opioid depending on fentanyl patch Remove patch after 3–5 days
Ovariohysterectomy	Moderate	Acepromazine + buprenorphine + NSAID	Incisional block with bupivacaine	Repeat opioid, consider buccal buprenorphine 2–4 days

Table 9.4
Example protocols for surgical pain in cats—*cont'd*

Feline surgical procedure	Anticipated level of pain	Examples of preop analgesia	Examples of intraop analgesia	Examples of postop analgesia
Castration	Mild to moderate	Acepromazine + buprenorphine ± NSAID		NSAID if not had it preop. Repeat opioid
Dental with extractions	Moderate to severe	Protocol 1 Acepromazine + opioid agonist Protocol 2 Medetomidine + ketamine + butorphanol + NSAID	Protocols 1 & 2 Infraorbital ± mandibular nerve block with bupivacaine	Protocol 1 Repeat opioid NSAID if not given preop Protocol 2 Repeat opioid, consider buccal buprenorphine 2–4 days
Dental without extractions	Mild to moderate	Protocol 1 Acepromazine + opioid agonist Protocol 2 Medetomidine + ketamine + butorphanol + NSAID		Protocol 1 NSAID if not given preop if significant gingivitis present Protocol 2 Repeat opioid, and consider buprenorphine buccal admin for 2–4 days if significant gingivitis

GERIATRIC PATIENTS

Elderly humans are reported as needing lower doses of opioids and of being more susceptible to the ulcerogenic effects of NSAIDs. Although not proven in cats and dogs it would be prudent to bear this in mind for veterinary patients. Elderly patients are more likely to be suffering from concurrent disease that may mean NSAIDs are contraindicated or should be reserved for postop use only, or they may be receiving other medications with the potential to interact with analgesics. Animals on corticosteroids should not receive concurrent NSAIDs. Another serious drug interaction

Table 9.5
Some examples of analgesics in cats

Drug	Route of admin	Approx onset of analgesia	Approx duration of action
Opioids for moderate to severe pain			
Morphine	i.m., s.c.	15+min	2–6h
Oxymorphone	i.m., s.c.	15min	2–6h
	i.v.	1min	
Fentanyl patches	Transdermal	12–24h	72+h
Fentanyl injection	i.v. bolus	1min	20min
Opioids for mild to moderate pain			
Buprenorphine	s.c., i.m. buccal	45min	6–8h
Pethidine	i.m.	15min	1–2h or less
Butorphanol	s.c., i.m., i.v.	20min	2h
NSAIDs			
Carprofen	s.c, i.v.		48–72h
Meloxicam	s.c.		24+h

reported in humans is between selegiline (used for senility and Cushings) and some of the opioids (see Chapter 6). Local anaesthetic blocks may be an alternative form of pain management in some cases. Ketamine combined with a benzodiazepine is considered a good premed in geriatric or unstable cats.

Geriatric patients often suffer from osteoarthritis, which can make them very stiff and painful if they lie in an awkward position whilst under general anaesthesia. A high heart rate and raised blood pressure, often in response to changes in body position, during an operation unrelated to surgical stimulation may well be due to musculoskeletal pain. The patient's limbs and back need to be supported to try and minimise eliciting joint pain, and even patients undergoing non-invasive procedures such as radiography may require analgesia.

NEONATES

Neonates are usually more reactive to a pain stimulus than adults. There is some evidence suggesting they do actually have a lower threshold for pain.[8] Recent studies have found that puppies may require lower doses of opioids to achieve analgesia. They also seem to be more sensitive to the respiratory depressant effects of morphine, whilst fentanyl may have a greater safety margin in canine neonates. Generally it is advisable to use lower than average doses of opioids in neonates initially then give additional doses slowly to titrate to effect. NSAIDs also need to be used with greater care, and preferably at the low end of the dose range. Local anaesthetics seem to work well, but care is needed to avoid overdosing. Ketamine seems to be less effective in neonates compared to adults, probably due to differences in neurotransmitters in the pain pathway.

PREGNANT AND LACTATING PATIENTS

Opioids are known to be detrimental to the fetus in humans taking opioids through pregnancy, but animals rarely have such long courses of opioids and there is no data available looking at their effects in pregnant cats and dogs. A very small amount of opioid will pass into the milk of dams but in humans it is only 1% of the maternal dose. Opioids and NSAIDs are widely used in the very short term for perioperative pain management of caesareans in dogs and cats without noticeable side effects. High doses of opioids given preop can result in respiratory depression in the pups or kittens. If this occurs then respiration can be stimulated with doxapram, or the opioid reversed with naloxone.

NSAIDs may increase the length of gestation and have side effects on the fetus if used for long periods during pregnancy (see Chapter 7 for further details). NSAIDs are also excreted at very low levels in milk. NSAIDs with better safety profiles (the more COX 2 selective ones) are expected to have fewer detrimental effects on the offspring as well as the dam. The risks need to be carefully weighed up against the necessity for analgesia in each pregnant or lactating patient. If a NSAID is used, choose one with minimal side effects in normal animals – use it at the lowest dose and for the shortest time possible.

NON-SURGICAL ACUTE PAIN MANAGEMENT

Illness and trauma are some of the other causes of acute pain. Examples of non-surgical pain and the anticipated level of severity are shown in Box 9.4:[1,2]

Box 9.4 Anticipated levels of pain associated with non-surgical causes

Severe to excruciating pain

- neuropathic pain
  - meningitis
  - peripheral nerve entrapment, inflammation
  - intervertebral disc herniation
- peritonitis
- fasciitis (streptococcal)
- cellulitis
- necrotising pancreatitis
- necrotising cholecystitis
- pathologic fractures
- bone cancer
- burns (depends on severity).

Moderate to severe pain

- osteoarthritis
- acute polyarthritis
- peritonitis — bacterial, urine, bile, pancreatic
- capsular pain from organomegaly — hepatitis, pyelonephritis, splenitis, splenic torsion
- hollow organ distension — gastric dilatation
- torsion — mesenteric, gastric, testicular
- obstruction — urethral, ureteral, biliary
- pleuritis
- acute pancreatitis
- trauma — orthopaedic, extensive soft tissue injury, head trauma
- degloving injury with ligament and bone involvement
- rewarming after hypothermia
- frostbite
- cancer pain
- mucositis after radiation therapy
- thrombosis or ischaemia — aortic thrombosis
- hypertrophic osteodystrophy
- panosteitis
- corneal ulceration or abrasion
- acute conjunctivitis, distichiasis, keratitis
- glaucoma
- uveitis
- parturition
- dermatitis (depends on extent of inflammation and severity)
- mastitis
- early or resolving stages of surgical procedures classed as moderate to excruciating

Box 9.4 Anticipated levels of pain associated with non-surgical causes—*continued*

- early or resolving stages of illness and trauma described above.

Moderate pain

- early or resolving pancreatitis
- less severe soft tissue injuries
- early or resolving stages of surgical procedures classed as moderate to severe.

Mild to moderate

- cystitis
- otitis
- early or resolving surgical procedures classed as mild to moderate pain.

Mild

- early or resolving stages of some of the above surgical procedures and illnesses.

(After Mathews KA. Pain assessment and general approach to management. Vet Clinic N Am: Small Animal Practice 2000; 30(4):729–755, 735.)

SPECIFIC EXAMPLES OF NON-SURGICAL ACUTE PAIN

All the analgesic drugs and techniques discussed above for perioperative pain management can also be applied to other forms of acute pain. An added consideration is getting a rapid onset of analgesia – this often indicates intravenous drug

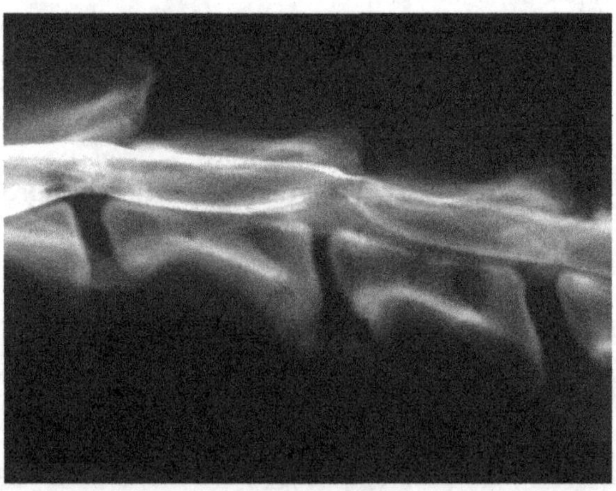

Figure 9.8
Intervertebral disc herniation as seen on this myelogram can be a cause of severe to excruciating pain.

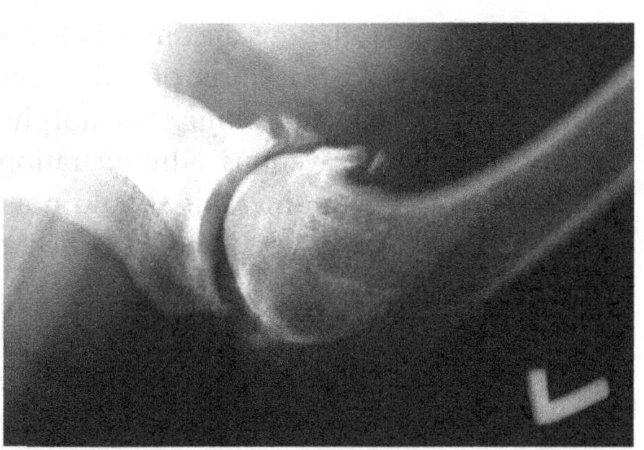

Figure 9.9
Osteoarthritis can be classed as causing moderate to severe pain depending on it stage. Evidence of new bone characteristic of osteoarthritis can be seen in this shoulder joint.

administration, and great care is needed with morphine using this route because of the risk of histamine release and hypotension. It can be diluted and a bolus given very slowly over 5–10 minutes.[11] Methadone and oxymorphone are less likely to cause histamine release. Opioids can be titrated to effect and continued as CRI if indicated. Obviously the underlying cause of pain also needs to be treated. There may also be more contraindications in non-surgical patients due to concurrent injuries and underlying disease, and certain classes of drugs like NSAIDs may need to be avoided initially.

TRAUMA PATIENTS

On first presentation the trauma patient needs a rapid and thorough physical examination. Special attention should be given to the cardiovascular and respiratory systems and a neurological examination should be included. The patient must be stabilised appropriately, using the ABC adage (airway, breathing, circulation). Details of stabilisation are beyond the realms of this book and can be found in the appropriate emergency medicine texts. A large bore venous catheter should be put in place, and i.v. fluids provided once haemorrhage has been controlled to adequately support the circulation and major organ perfusion. It can be very difficult to determine the presence and severity of pain in these patients, but they must be given the benefit of the doubt and provided with appropriate analgesia as soon as they have been assessed and as the circulation is being restored. Analgesia will often aid examination as animals usually fiercely guard painful body parts. The best analgesics to use in such situations are almost always mu agonist opioids as they have a quick onset of action and are the most potent analgesics, e.g. morphine, oxymorphone, fentanyl, alfentanil. Careful intravenous administration of a mu agonist is ideal (not pethidine, this should not be given i.v.) and the opioid can be slowly titrated to effect to minimise the risk of histamine release.

Otherwise healthy animals tolerate i.v. opioids better than animals with concurrent cardiovascular instability that are more susceptible to opioid side effects because of altered drug pharmacokinetics. This means even greater care is needed with the i.v. route of administration of opioids in trauma patients and in the presence of hypovolaemic shock. There is some evidence suggesting that animals in endotoxic or septic shock should not receive mu agonists, as they may reduce survival rates.[13] Morphine usually produces a useful degree of sedation, but if more sedation is indicated to reduce the patient's anxiety and stress, then consider adding in a tranquilliser such as acepromazine or low-dose medetomidine (ensure the circulation and respiratory system function have been restored). Medetomidine has the added advantage of being an analgesic itself and will contribute to a multimodal approach. Occasionally dogs can show signs of opioid dysphoria, with disorientation, anxiety and agitation, often with incessant vocalisation. There are several options if this situation arises:

1. Give higher doses of the same opioid to push the patient into sedation; if dysphoria gets worse then administer a sedative (see option 2) or partially reverse the opioid (see option 4)
2. Give acepromazine or medetomidine for sedation to retain the opioid analgesia
3. Do both options 1 and 2
4. Partially reverse the opioid with a partial or full antagonist.

The same principles can be applied to cats, but they are less tolerant of higher doses of opioids. Take care to administer small i.v. doses every 3–5 minutes to effect or until the pupils dilate, which usually indicates an analgesic dose has been reached.[14]

Once the patient has been stabilised and pain has been relieved, ongoing pain management needs to be organised.

Some patients with minor trauma may not require any more after the first doses of opioids. Those with more severe injuries will need ongoing opioids – a CRI or fentanyl patch can provide good quality background analgesia that can be topped up with further analgesics if necessary, e.g. ketamine, alpha 2 agonists, further opioids. Fentanyl patches need applying as soon as possible; they take up to 24 hours to reach effective plasma levels in dogs, but probably a bit sooner in cats at nearer 12 hours.

All patients will therefore need supplemental analgesia for at least the first 24 hours after the patch is applied to cover the gap, and there is a great deal of individual variation in the final blood levels reached – do not assume adequate analgesia will always be provided. Local anaesthetic analgesia can be added in, and if the circulation and blood pressure are well supported NSAIDs can be administered for ongoing pain relief. If the patient is likely to undergo surgery in the near future use a NSAID that has a preop licence initially, so the same one can be continued. Trauma patients with haemorrhage, recent blood loss or coagulopathies are probably more susceptible to the side effects of NSAIDs. Alpha 2 agonists are also unsuitable in the presence of haemorrhage as they cause vasoconstriction and hypertension that would make matters worse.

Animals with serious injuries to the abdomen, pelvis or hind limbs are candidates for epidural anaesthesia. An epidural catheter can be placed for the administration of local anaesthetic and/or opioids. The pain from fractured ribs can be alleviated by interpleural administration of bupivacaine via a chest drain. Care must be taken not to inadvertently overdose smaller patients with local anaesthetic. Patients with a marginal respiratory reserve are at higher risk of respiratory failure as the bupivacaine can induce diaphragmatic paralysis.

Patients with extensive soft tissue injuries will need regular dressing changes, which can be a source of a lot more pain and discomfort during hospitalisation. In addition to the constant levels of analgesia, this extra handling and movement needs further pain relief and sedation. Small i.v. doses of medetomidine are very useful in patients that have a stable cardiovascular system, or low doses of propofol titrated to effect can be used.

HEAD TRAUMA

Patients with head trauma and suspected increased intracranial pressure (ICP) are particularly tricky to treat with analgesics. Firstly, assessment of pain is even more difficult because of depressed mental state and abnormal behaviour, and the choice of systemic analgesic is more restricted. A thorough physical and neurological examination should be performed before any pharmacological intervention alters CNS activity. Vital signs and neurological function need close monitoring, and appropriate supportive treatment must be put in place. ICP depends on brain tissue volume, CSF fluid volume and the volume of blood in the cranium. Cerebral blood flow is related to arterial carbon dioxide levels, $PaCO_2$ – anything that depresses ventilation will increase $PaCO_2$ resulting in an increase in cerebral blood flow and ICP. Pain itself can increase ICP, as can opioids via respiratory depression. Low doses of opioids should not depress respiration in normal cats and dogs, but those with CNS depression (such as head trauma cases), are more susceptible to this effect. Therefore opioids must be used very carefully in head trauma patients with normal or slightly depressed mentation but avoided in those with more severe signs or comatose. It is prudent to monitor blood gases for signs of hypercapnea as a good indicator of respiratory depression, and there is always the option of intubating and ventilating patients.

Where analgesia is needed for more than a few hours, consider using NSAIDs in head trauma cases rather than systemic opioids. Ensure the circulation isn't compromised and there are no bleeding problems. Low-dose ketamine in combination with low-dose opioids (synergy allows dose reduction) or with propofol sedation may be an option in a head injured patient for pain relief. Other more local methods of pain relief are very useful alternatives in these patients and should be considered for any accessible areas. If there is hindlimb or caudal body pain, use an epidural – morphine administered via this route and at epidural doses is very unlikely to cause respiratory depression, and any systemic effects can be reversed with naloxone without touching the epidural analgesia. Mandibular and maxillary nerve blocks may be useful for fractures of the mandible or maxilla. Head trauma patients are at risk from developing seizures, so any drugs that precipitate fits are contraindicated, e.g. acepromazine.

BURNS

Burns pain is considered one of the most severe forms of acute pain in humans, and has two main components – resting pain that is constantly present and procedural pain of great intensity when wounds are debrided and dressing changes are carried out. The depth of the burn and area of tissue involved will determine the severity of pain, but later on it is thought that neuropathic pain and hyperalgesia can become significant contributors. Animals with partial-thickness burns over extensive areas will need ongoing analgesia such as a fentanyl patch or opioid CRI to control pain. For some animals this analgesia may still be inadequate and recent reports have suggested additional low doses of ketamine orally or by infusion may be efficacious for severe burns pain.[13] Low-dose infusions of lidocaine have been used successfully in human burns patients for analgesia.[15]

These patients will also need regular dressing changes that can be very painful. Heavy sedation or anaesthesia can be induced with ketamine and benzodiazepine (e.g. diazepam) combinations to facilitate treatment. Care is needed with drug doses in burns patients as they can lose a significant amount of protein through their wounds, and may be hypoproteineamic as a result. Therefore any highly protein-bound drug can have exaggerated effects, as there is more free drug circulating in the animal. This would be a reason to take even greater care with NSAIDs but these drugs tend not to be used early on in treatment anyway as burns patients are high risk for gastric and duodenal ulceration associated with stress (and bleeding problems from changes in platelet function).[13] NSAIDs are more useful later on during the healing and physiotherapy stages to provide enough pain relief to allow the patient to move affected skin and joints. Epidural and local anaesthetic techniques are very limited because there is such a high risk of infection associated with burns. Topical water-soluble lidocaine lubricant can be used on very painful burns, but duration of therapy should be short as there is significant potential for systemic absorption and toxicity, especially in cats. Wound healing does not seem to be affected by topical EMLA cream (lidocaine and prilocaine).[14]

NEUROPATHIC PAIN

Neuropathic pain (see Chapter 5 for more details) results from direct damage, injury or inflammation of neural tissue and results in sensory deficits combined with allodynia, hyperalgesia and referred pain syndromes. Chronic neuropathic pain is discussed further in Chapter 11. For short-term relief, opioids can be quite ineffective and animal studies suggest that patients may respond better to NMDA antagonists like ketamine and alpha 2 agonists. The combination of ketamine plus an opioid may give the best analgesia. Ketamine can be given as a low-dose CRI, repeat injections or orally. It should be used in a combination to avoid the risk of adverse effects. There are successful reports of ketamine being made up into a paste and applied topically and a human case where epidural ketamine proved effective for neuropathic pain.[13] Other less conventional treatments being looked at are gabapentin (primarily an anticonvulsant) and topical capsaicin (a drug that depletes cells of substance P, a neurotransmitter involved in nociception; see Chapter 10).

ACUTE PANCREATITIS AND PERITONITIS

The pain from these two conditions can be excruciating and even contribute to mortality. Treatment of the underlying causes must be instigated along with aggressive supportive measures to support the cardiovascular system, control vomiting and relieve pain. Pethidine is cited as a useful opioid in pancreatitis, but in severe cases an epidural is required as well. The epidural catheter can be placed with the end of the catheter at around T13–L2. A combination of bupivacaine and morphine can be very effective and epidural morphine is unlikely to affect abdominal sphincter pressures. There is an argument for using NSAIDs as well because a component of the pain is inflammatory, but there is a concern that there could be an increased risk of GI ulceration in a lot of these cases.

FURTHER INFORMATION For more details on drug doses, local anaesthetic nerve blocks, epidural techniques and epidural catheter placement please refer to the texts listed under 'Further reading' below.

REFERENCES

1. Mathews KA. Pain assessment and general approach to management. Vet Clin N Am: Small Animal Practice 2000; 30(4):729–755
2. Tranquilli WJ, Grimm KA, Lamont LA. Pain management for specific conditions and procedures. In: Pain management for the small animal practitioner. Jackson: Teton Newmedia; 2000:74–103
3. Gaynor JS, Short C, Tranquilli W, et al. Practical approach for improved pain management in animals. A pain management handbook. Companion Animal Pain Consortium supported by Pfizer Animal Health.
4. American Animal Hospital Association Pain Management Standards 2003.
5. Hellyer PW, Gaynor JS. How I treat acute surgical pain in dogs and cats. Compend Contin Educ 1998; 20:140
6. Lascelles BDX, Butterworth SJ, Waterman AE. Postoperative analgesic and sedative effects of carprofen and pethidine in dogs. Vet Record 1994; 134:187–191
7. Balmer TV, Irvine D, Jones RS, et al. Comparison of carprofen and pethidine as postoperative analgesics in the cat. J Small Animal Pract 1998; 39:158–164
8. Pascoe PJ. Perioperative pain management. Vet Clin N Am: Small Animal Practice 2000; 30(4):917–932
9. Dobromylskyj P, Flecknell B, Lascelles BD, et al. Management of postoperative and other acute pain. In: Flecknell P, Waterman-Pearson A, eds. Pain management in animals. London: Saunders; 2000:81–145
10. Hellebrekers LJ. Practical analgesic treatment in canine patients. In: Hellebrekers LJ, ed. Animal pain. The Netherlands: Van Der Wees; 2000:117–130
11. Mathews KA. Management of pain in cats. In: Hellebrekers LJ, ed. Animal pain. The Netherlands: Van Der Wees; 2000:131–144
12. Robertson SA, Taylor PM. Pain management in cats – past, present and future. Part 2. Treatment of pain-clinical pharmacology. J Feline Med Surg 2004; 6:321–333
13. Pacoe PJ. Problems of pain management. In: Flecknell P, Waterman-Pearson A, eds. Pain management in animals. London: Saunders; 2000:161–177
14. Hansen B. Acute pain management. Vet Clin N Am: Small Animal Practice 2000; 30(4): 899–916
15. Pal SK, Cortiella J, Herndon D. Adjunctive methods of pain control in burns. Burns 1997; 23(5):404–412

FURTHER READING

Flecknell P, Waterman-Pearson A, eds. Pain management in animals. London: Saunders; 2000

Mathews K.A. Ed. Vet Clin N Am: Small Animal Practice 2000; 30(4)

Tranquilli W.J, Grimm K.A, Lamont L.A. Pain management for the small animal practitioner. Jackson: Teton Newmedia; 2000

CHAPTER 10 ADJUNCTIVE METHODS OF PAIN MANAGEMENT

DEFINITION OF ADJUNCTIVE ANALGESIA

There are both pharmacological and non-pharmacological adjunctive methods for helping to alleviate pain that can be added in to pain management protocols. They tend to be particularly useful in the management of chronic pain, although they can have a role in acute pain as well. Adjunctive analgesics are drugs that have a weak or non-existent analgesic effect when used on their own and usually have other primary indications, but they can enhance the effect of conventional analgesics when used in combination. Non-pharmacological adjunctive methods include physical and behavioural therapies that are known to help relieve pain and improve quality of life of patients, especially those with non-curable progressive painful conditions. A lot of the information on these types of therapies is extrapolated from the human side; some remain unproven in veterinary patients. None-the-less, it's reasonable to consider adding in techniques that are known to be helpful in human pain management, considering the very close similarities in the anatomy and physiology of the pain pathways in both groups of patients.

THE COMPLEXITY OF THE PAIN EXPERIENCE[1]

The pain that a human experiences as a result of a stimulus, or as is often the case in chronic pain states as a result of peripheral and central sensitisation, seems to be influenced by factors in addition to the sensory input from nociceptors. A few of these factors include previous experience, anxiety, stress and visual information. In the case of phantom limb pain, the pain seems to arise when there is a total lack of sensory input coming in, as the painful limb is no longer present. It's also known that widespread areas of the brain are involved in pain – there is not just one discrete area that sorts it all out. This has led to a new theory of pain called the neuromatrix theory, which suggests that the body's perception of itself is inherent in the brain as a set of neural networks or patterns that exist independently of any sensory inputs from mechanoreceptors or nociceptors, etc.

Sensory input may trigger these resting patterns to stimulate behaviour, movement and emotional changes, but they are not responsible for generating the patterns in the first place. The idea is that these neural patterns are genetically determined but they are also modified by a wide variety of influences from elsewhere in the brain, e.g. information from the environment, previous experiences, stress, etc. These inherent patterns, or neurosignatures, are a product of a complex network of neurones and synapses in the brain called the neuromatrix that is also modified by sensory inputs over time. Sensory inputs are processed by the neuromatrix, and it adjusts the constant output of its neurosignatures accordingly – these characteristic patterns are then projected onto the rest of the brain and give us our stream of awareness, actions, movements, emotions and learning. This means the information from nociceptors is only one of many influences that determine any pain experiences the patient has. In summary, the neuromatrix, which is genetically determined and modified by sensory experience, is the primary mechanism that generates the neural pattern that produces pain. Its output pattern is determined by multiple influences that converge on the neuromatrix, of which the nociceptive input is only one part (Fig 10.1).

The neuromatrix theory not only explains chronic pain states that exist even without obvious pathology, or poorly correlated to pathology, but it also explains why a lot of the adjunctive analgesics and techniques can be effective for relieving pain, because they are modifying inputs other than the nociceptive pathway that contribute to the overall pain experience. The huge complexity of nociception as a discrete pathway – with its multitude of transmitters, receptors, plasticity and interactions with other body systems – implies that a wide range of drugs may affect it via mechanisms that are not yet fully elucidated. Therefore it makes sense that drugs other than the conventional analgesics may have the potential to facilitate pain relief.

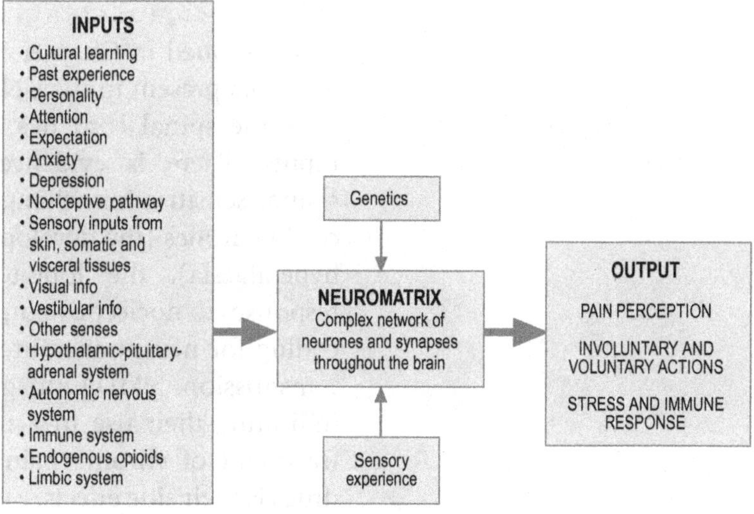

Figure 10.1 The neuromatrix theory of pain proposes there are many different influences on the final pain experience as well as the nociceptive pathway input into the brain. (From Melzack R. Pain and the neuromatrix in the brain. J Dent Educ 2001; 65(12):1378–1382, reproduced with permission.)

PHARMACOLOGIC ADJUNCTIVE ANALGESICS

A range of medications has been found to be a useful adjunct in pain management protocols:

- NMDA receptor antagonists
- corticosteroids
- antidepressants
- benzodiazepines
- phenothiazines
- sodium channel blockers
- anticonvulsants
- capsaicin
- St Johns wort
- nutraceuticals and other drugs used in osteoarthritis
- topical treatments
- biphosphonates.

Several of these drugs are not licensed at all in animals and details regarding their use in animals are purely anecdotal – effective dose rates and safety profiles have not always been established. If such drugs are to be used it's important to discuss this with owners. Further information can be found in the listed references and by contacting referral centres (e.g. university veterinary hospitals) to discuss case selection and protocols with clinicians who have first hand experience of their use.

NMDA receptor antagonists

As mentioned in Chapter 5, NMDA (N-methyl-D-aspartate) receptors present in the CNS pain pathway become activated once the spinal cord has received a deluge of nociceptive inputs. There is evidence these receptors contribute to central sensitisation: changes in the receptive field of spinal cord neurones (the development of allodynia and secondary hyperalgesia), the long-term enhancement of neuronal responses to nociceptive inputs and the switching on of genes coding for neurotransmitter and receptors involved in pain transmission. NMDA antagonists can attenuate these effects, indicating their use in acute pain and the prevention and treatment of chronic pain states. The problem with these drugs is their side effects, e.g. ketamine needs to be given with an opioid or sedative to avoid convulsions, excitation and dysphoria. Ketamine has been shown to be a useful analgesic administered as a low-dose infusion, i.v. bolus, i.m., s.c. infusion, epidurally or even applied topically to burns, in addition to being a dissociative anaesthetic agent (see Chapter 8).

Dextromethorphan is another NMDA antagonist that is actually available as a cough remedy, and there are clinical trials in humans reporting that its long-term administration resulted in an 80% reduction in pain associated with diabetic neuropathy (comparable to the analgesic efficacy of tricyclic antidepressants). It has also been used successfully preop, followed by postop administration, for the management of postop pain in adults undergoing tonsillectomy, mastectomy and hysterectomy. Side effects included dizziness, fatigue, and confusion.[2,3] Amantadine and memantine are other NMDA antagonists currently being studied for potential analgesic effects on the human side.

Corticosteroids

Corticosteroids are primarily indicated as anti-inflammatory agents, by inhibiting the synthesis of inflammatory mediators including both the prostanoids and leukotrienes. They act on intracellular receptors to induce and also switch off protein production. One of these induced proteins inhibits phospholipase A2 at the start of the arachidonic acid cascade (see Chapter 7) and they have other anti-inflammatory effects such as stabilising cell membranes and inhibiting COX and iNOS (inducible nitric oxide synthase). They have a vast array of potential side effects and should not be given alongside NSAIDs. However, in some conditions they can be used to alleviate pain associated with inflammation at the site of tissue injury. They also appear to be useful via their membrane-stabilising properties, to reduce aberrant firing of damaged nerves and may be useful for chronic neuropathic and some cancer-related pain.[3] In terminally ill patients and those with progressive conditions of chronic pain the risk of side effects from corticosteroids are often out-weighed by the benefits to the patient of analgesia and an improved quality of life.

Antidepressants

Antidepressants are commonly used in humans as an adjunct for the treatment of chronic pain. Although a substantial minority of people with chronic pain are also clinically depressed, the use of antidepressants is known to alleviate both disorders. There is evidence to suggest that antidepressants have an analgesic action not mediated by an antidepressant effect. The analgesia is produced at doses much lower than those needed to treat clinical depression and the onset of analgesia is often more rapid than the onset of the antidepressant effect. Analgesia is also reported without an antidepressive response and is demonstrated in patients without any detectable depression to start with. Some of the various types of antidepressants useful for analgesia in humans are:

- Tricyclic antidepressants – These drugs block the re-uptake of two neurotransmitters in the CNS, serotonin and noradrenaline, allowing them to act for longer. Serotonin is involved in controlling mood and levels of consciousness.
- Monoamine oxidase inhibitors (MAOIs) – These drugs block the enzyme monoamine oxidase that breaks down noradrenaline and serotonin, therefore raising their levels in the CNS.
- Selective serotonin re-uptake inhibitors (SSRIs) – This subgroup selectively block the re-uptake of just serotonin, allowing it to act for longer.

Their effects on central neurotransmitters may produce an analgesic effect as well as an antidepressant one. Evidence suggests that serotonin and noradrenaline can inhibit pain transmission in the thalamus, brain stem and spinal cord. They are also involved in descending inhibition of the pain pathway and may interact with endogenous opioid mechanisms. Other possible minor effects of these drugs that may contribute to analgesia are mild sedation, reduced anxiety, muscle relaxation, restored sleep cycles and even a mild anti-inflammatory effect. In addition, TCAs have been shown to block neuronal sodium channels (see later) – this may account for some of their analgesic action.[4]

Tricyclic antidepressants (TCAs, e.g. amitriptyline, imipramine)

There is less evidence for the use of these drugs for acute pain than for chronic pain. Studies have found TCAs to be effective analgesics for migraines, tension headache, back pain, arthritis, rheumatoid arthritis, fibromyalgia and different types of neuropathic pain.[4] This subgroup of antidepressants is currently considered the first choice antidepressant for adjunctive treatment of pain in humans. A few human trials have reported that combinations of TCAs and an anticonvulsant or a neuroleptic (e.g. a phenothiazine) may produce even better analgesia. TCAs are now recommended as adjunctive treatment of cancer-related pain in veterinary patients.[3] Adverse effects in humans are related to the autonomic nervous system (via noradrenaline) and are often transient and mild, e.g. dry mouth, palpitations, but can be occasionally a bit more serious with postural hypotension and even lack of consciousness and impotence. They must be used with care in patients with cardiac problems. Some CNS signs are reported such as tremors, sedation, and seizures.

Monoamine oxidase inhibitors (MAOIs, e.g. phenelzine)

Phenelzine has been found to be an effective analgesic for people with chronic pain derived from migraine, chronic fatigue syndrome, facial pain and pain of a psychological origin. However, there is very little published data available at the moment. MAOI side effects are rare and include CNS signs, hypertension and a hepatotoxicity. There are several drug interactions known in people, such as with pethidine and some anaesthetics.

Selective serotonin re-uptake inhibitors (SSRIs, e.g. fluoxetine – Prozac®)

Generally speaking it appears the SSRI subgroup is less efficacious for analgesia in humans than TCAs but is better tolerated. A limited number of trials have investigated their usefulness in arthritis, headaches, neuropathic pain, fibromyalgia and low back pain. Only half of these trials found the SSRIs to be significantly better than a placebo. Although not entirely confirmed as useful adjuncts for analgesia these drugs may be an option for patients intolerant of TCAs. There are several potential drug interactions to avoid with SSRIs including anticonvulsants, antiarrhythmic and other psychotropic drugs.

Benzodiazepines

Benzodiazepines, e.g. diazepam and midazolam, are primarily used as sedatives but are also known to reduce anxiety, muscle tension and insomnia, all of which can contribute to pain. They are considered useful in cases of acute pain associated with an element of muscle spasm, e.g. intervertebral disc problems with skeletal muscle spasm, and in the presence of high patient anxiety. The use of benzodiazepines for chronic pain is very controversial because not only can they worsen depression in people, they can also cause dependency.

Phenothiazines

The phenothiazines are a type of neuroleptic or tranquiliser. Acepromazine is the commonest one used in veterinary medicine. They have no inherent analgesic properties used alone, but can be used in conjunction with traditional analgesics to reduce patient anxiety, agitation and stress that would otherwise enhance the pain experience. They are useful in patients with opioid-induced excitement, as they treat the side effect without having to resort to reversing the opioid analgesia.

Sodium channel blockers

The local anaesthetics work by preventing nerve impulse conduction by blocking the sodium channels that are needed for the generation of a nerve impulse (action potential). One of the main components of neuropathic pain is the generation of ectopic impulses by damaged dysfunctional sensory neurones and their axons out in the periphery. Sodium channels play a key role in this impulse generation, and there are an increased number of these channels on damaged nerves, which seem far more sensitive to drug blockade than normal nerves. Therefore systemic sodium channel blockers such as local anaesthetics and other drugs can be used at low dose to treat this type of pain whilst avoiding interruption of normal nerve impulses.

Recent work has found that low-dose infusions of lidocaine can relieve pain, particularly neuropathic pain, and human studies have also found it useful in burns pain. However, results have been mixed for more acute postop pain. It seems that systemic lidocaine is able to stop the spontaneous firing of neuromas and dorsal horn neurones, and reduce their sensitivity at drug concentrations below those required to block nerve conduction altogether. The findings of various studies to date suggest that systemic lidocaine has the following actions. At low doses it suppresses ectopic impulses generated by chronically damaged peripheral nerves. Higher levels suppress central sensitisation, and central neuronal hyperexcitability. High levels have general analgesic effects and very high levels are associated with cardiac and CNS toxicity. Extremely high systemic doses will be lethal, as they will block all neuronal conduction.

Mexiletine is a sodium channel blocker normally prescribed as an antiarrhythmic. Human studies have found oral administration to be beneficial for neuropathic pain including multiple sclerosis and phantom limb pain.[5] Side effects include worsening of arrhythmias, GI upset and lightheadedness. Flecainide is another member of this class of drugs and is mentioned in human texts as an alternative for neuropathic pain where mexiletine side effects preclude its use.

Other sodium channel blockers may prove to have similar analgesic effects. This may be one mechanism by which the anticonvulsants phenytoin and carbamazepine and TCAs have an analgesic effect.

Anticonvulsants

Carbamazepine, phenytoin, and lamotrigine are all used as anticonvulsants, but they all have the ability to suppress the generation of ectopic impulses from sites of peripheral nerve injury and the associated dorsal root ganglia (large discrete collections of neurone cell bodies) up in the spinal cord by blocking sodium channels. By suppressing abnormal peripheral nociceptive inputs, there is a reduction in the release of excitatory neurotransmitters in the CNS, glutamate and aspartate. Another anticonvulsant, gabapentin, is known to be a very good analgesic but it does not block sodium channels. At the moment, gabapentin seems to be the anticonvulsant of most interest as an adjunctive analgesic for veterinary use.

Carbamazepine Carbamazepine is now the first-line analgesic for trigeminal neuralgia in people in the USA and it has been licensed as an analgesic for neuropathic pain as well as an anticonvulsant. Its primary mechanism of action is sodium channel blockade. The main drawback of this drug is adverse effects, particularly sedation and ataxia. People are started on very low doses and these are carefully increased to effect or until intolerance develops. The other disadvantage is that patients need regular monitoring of blood cells, as a rare side effect is an irreversible aplastic anaemia. Carbamazepine also affects the blood levels of other drugs, so concurrent use with other anticonvulsants and antidepressants needs careful monitoring.

Phenytoin This was the first anticonvulsant to be used as an analgesic, but is rarely used now. It is effective for neuropathic pain, and has been used to successfully control bouts of acute shooting pain that can occur with this condition. An intravenous form is available and has been used to give immediate relief from severe attacks of trigeminal neuralgia in people. Phenytoin can easily cause toxicity (nystagmus, vomiting, sedation) and interfere with the metabolism of other drugs.

Lamotrigine Lamotrigine, like phenytoin and carbamazepine, blocks sodium channels. Animal studies have found this anticonvulsant can reduce postop pain and analgesic requirements. From the small amount of published data available, it seems this drug has efficacy for central and peripheral forms of neuropathic pain. It has significant interactions with other anticonvulsants, increasing the risk of drug toxicity. Side effects include a rash, dizziness, ataxia and vomiting.

Gabapentin Gabapentin does not seem to reduce acute pain, but it does seem to be effective for chronic pain and reduces central sensitisation and hyperalgesia. Its mechanism of action is still pretty foggy – it may inhibit the release of excitatory neurotransmitters by sensitised neurones in the CNS, or block calcium channels (which may be important in nociceptor transmitter release and hyperexcitability of spinal cord neurones), or it may augment the descending inhibition of the pain pathway. Gabapentin has been used in people to treat neuropathic pain (arising from neuropathies, cancer, etc.), migraine and a wide variety of chronic pain states. In the USA, gabapentin is the anticonvulsant drug used most often for chronic pain because of its anecdotal evidence of good efficacy, ease of use, relative lack of drug interactions and relatively good safety profile. In some pain centres in the USA it is being used first-line as a treatment for all types of chronic pain in humans. Side effects are related to CNS depression, such as dizziness, ataxia and sleepiness.[5]

There are a few anecdotal reports emerging on the use of gabapentin in veterinary patients both as an adjunct and as a first-line analgesic.[3] A cat suffering from a malunion of a lumbar fracture with presumed neuropathic pain responded very well to gabapentin therapy alone, and the dose was titrated long-term to effect. Another cat with neuropathic pain and hind limb paresis from a low spinal fracture was unresponsive to a fentanyl patch, but did show a great improvement in the degree of allodynia within 48 hours of initiating gabapentin therapy. So far, case reports have started on lower doses and titrated upwards to effect, and reduced again once pain relief is achieved. Patients should be slowly weaned off gabapentin as sudden withdrawal of the drug can lead to rebound pain. Gabapentin is excreted unchanged in urine, so dose adjustments are indicated in patients with renal compromise. Signs of overdose in animals are reported to be reduced activity and sleepiness progressing to depression.

Capsaicin

Capsaicin is an extract of chili peppers used in topically applied preparations for local analgesia in humans. The proposed mechanism of action of capsaicin is that it binds to nociceptors in the skin and selectively stimulates the release of the neurotransmitter substance P from peripheral nociceptors until it becomes depleted – this produces pain relief in certain chronic pain states. There is an initial period of enhanced sensitivity, perceived as itching, pricking or burning with reddening of the skin when the substance P is released. This is followed by a refractory period with reduced sensitivity and after repeated applications, persistent desensitisation results as the nociceptors run out of substance P.[6] There is a small amount of evidence from an experimental study looking at the application of capsaicin in animals before a polyarthritis was induced that found it reduced subsequent joint swelling, implying an anti-inflammatory effect.[7] It has been used successfully to help reduce pain in people arising from arthritis, rheumatoid arthritis, diabetic neuropathy and psoriasis. The reduction in pain may not be huge but every little helps, especially in chronic pain. Reports of adverse effects at the site of application are not unusual.

There is a published experimental study looking at the effect of a topical analgesic balm containing capsaicin plus methyl salicylates applied over muscles of cats.[8] The balm attenuated the activity of afferent Aδ and C fibre nociceptors in the underlying muscle at 40 minutes after application. Another study on mice found that capsaicin alone attenuated sensory nerve activity at 20 minutes after application.[8] In a more clinically relevant study report, capsaicin ointment applied to the distal palmar digital nerves caused significant improvements in lameness score for up to 4 hours in horses with experimentally induced foot lameness.[8]

St Johns wort

The active ingredient of this compound is hypericin, and it has a similar mechanism of action as TCAs, raising levels of serotonin and noradrenaline – thought to enhance descending inhibition of the pain pathway and inhibiting nociception in higher parts of the brain. St Johns wort may be useful as an adjunctive analgesic for arthritis or neuropathic pain.

Nutraceuticals and other agents used in arthritis

The nutraceuticals are a group of orally administered agents that are not drugs, but substances that provide compounds required for normal body structure and function. They are produced in a purified or extracted form and aim to improve the health and wellbeing of patients.[9] They are commonly used as an adjunctive treatment for osteoarthritis as they may possibly have a chondroprotective effect (improving the structure of cartilage and reducing its breakdown in arthritis). As well as aiming to have a structure modifying effect they may have a symptom modifying effect, i.e. they may be analgesic and anti-inflammatory. Good quality published scientific evidence from veterinary trials to prove any of their effects is lacking, but anecdotally they are a popular treatment for canine arthritis alongside NSAIDs. Hyaluronic acid and pentosan polysulphate are two injectable potentially structure modifying drugs for use in arthritis that may also have an analgesic action. These are POM drugs (prescription-only medicines) and will have to have undergone a lot more scrutiny for efficacy and safety to gain a licence compared to a nutraceutical. The following discussion just focuses on the evidence for using these compounds as adjunctive analgesics in arthritis, rather than their potential structure modifying effect on cartilage.

Glucosamine

Glucosamine is thought to stimulate cartilage cells (chondrocytes) to synthesise more glycosaminoglycans (GAGs), a major component of cartilage matrix and joint fluid. Glucosamine itself is a precursor to GAG and is used by synovial cells to synthesise hyaluronic acid. In humans it is well absorbed from the GI tract and eventually incorporated into cartilage matrix. In arthritis, cartilage is broken down and its GAG content is reduced – this is closely related to the loss of biomechanical properties of cartilage. Laboratory studies have found that glucosamine may reduce inducible nitric oxide synthase (iNOS) during inflammation and have a weak anti-inflammatory action (independent of COX).

A recent paper in *The Lancet* followed the progression of knee arthritis in 212 human patients given either glucosamine sulphate for 3 years or a placebo.[10] After 3 years the group receiving glucosamine had significant improvements in their pain (and physical function) scores compared with the placebo group. The glucosamine group also rather interestingly showed significantly less narrowing of the joint space (reflecting less thinning of cartilage) than the placebo group, but rather oddly the change in joint space did not correlate well to symptoms, i.e. patients with severe joint narrowing could still have improved pain and function scores. Thus analgesia may not be directly dependent on any structure modifying effect on cartilage by glucosamine. A couple of other human studies have also found glucosamine to produce significantly better analgesia than placebo, and to be comparable to the NSAID ibuprofen in knee arthritis (but slower in onset).[11]

Overall, studies in humans suggest that glucosamine may help to control the clinical signs of osteoarthritis including pain. Glucosamine is considered relatively safe, however it is possible that it may raise blood glucose levels and therefore may be contraindicated in animals with type II diabetes or those obese animals at risk of developing it.

Chondroitin sulphate

Chondroitin sulphate is one of the main GAGs found in normal cartilage and is often manufactured from sharks' cartilage and bovine trachea. Oral doses are well absorbed from the GI tracts of humans and dogs. Some products contain both glucosamine and chondroitin, based on the theory there may be some synergism between the two substances in maintaining healthy cartilage structure. In experimental in-vitro studies, chondroitin sulphate has been found to have a mild anti-inflammatory action, although it's not clear this would translate to analgesia in a patient's joint. Studies in people with knee and hip arthritis found it did significantly reduce pain scores compared to placebo,[12] suggesting it does have a positive effect in humans.

Green lipped mussel

Green lipped mussel, rich in GAG, is prepared from the New Zealand shellfish *Perna canaliculus* and is available as a food supplement included in some complete dried diets for dogs. As with other members of this group of supplements, there is very limited peer reviewed published data available on the efficacy of this nutraceutical. One report did find that after 6 weeks of supplementing arthritic dogs' diets with green-lipped mussel supplementation there was a reduction in joint pain (plus swelling and crepitus; pain scoring was subjective).[13] The mechanism of analgesic action is speculated to be due to an anti-inflammatory effect by an omega-3 fatty acid in the preparation that may inhibit both arachidonic acid and COX, thereby reducing inflammatory pain. This, however, is not proven and is still a theory.[11]

Pentosan polysulphate (PPS, Cartrophen®)

This drug is a semi-synthetic GAG prepared from beech wood shavings and is structurally similar to heparin. It is administered as a course of weekly injections for 4 weeks subcutaneously. Apart from aiming to improve cartilage structure, there is conjecture that this compound has several analgesic actions. It seems that PPS may have antithrombotic and antifibrinolytic properties similar to heparin. One theory that remains unproven is that some of the pain in osteoarthritis originates from micro-thrombi (tiny blood clots) in the vasculature of synovial tissues (membrane enclosing the joint) and subchondral bone that sits beneath the cartilage pads at the end of long bones. If this is the case, then PPS could help breakdown the micro-thrombi and relieve pain. PPS may also inhibit pro-inflammatory mediators. One published study looked at the efficacy of a 4-week course of PPS in arthritic dogs compared to a 4-week course of a NSAID.[14] PPS dogs did have significant improvements in subjective pain score (plus lameness and orthopaedic score) compared to baseline values at each weekly assessment. Another study looked at varying doses of PPS over a 4-week treatment period in 40 arthritic dogs.[15] There were improvements in pain scores on joint manipulation from baseline values from week 3 onwards in the PPS group (at data sheet dose rate), whereas no change was seen in the placebo group.

Anecdotally, clinicians often say that they may not see a response in the patient until the third or fourth injection, but the effect seems to last for some time afterwards and that the best response is seen in cases of moderate to severe chronic arthritis.[15] PPS should not be given with NSAIDs or corticosteroids, because of the increased risk of reduced blood clotting. Generally, PPS seems to have a low incidence of side effects that are often mild and transitory, such as depression and inappetence for a few days after administration.[16]

Hyaluronan[17]

Intra-articular hyaluronan (IAHA) administration has been used for years for the treatment of osteoarthritis in horses, and has also been advocated in humans. Hyaluronan naturally occurs in joints; it is an important contributor to the compressive stiffness of cartilage, and is also responsible for providing the viscoelastic and lubricating properties of joint fluid. The synovial fluid of osteoarthritic joints contains decreased concentrations of hyaluronan and is of abnormally low molecular weight. This probably contributes to pain (and loss of joint function) as normal high molecular weight hyaluronan decreases the firing rate of joint nociceptors and may act as a filter, reducing the transmission of pain inducing mechanical stimuli, such as stretch and pressure to the sensitised joint nociceptor endings. IAHA may also reduce the production of inflammatory prostaglandins involved in pain. By injecting hyaluronan into joints the aim is to try and restore some of their physiological function. As yet there is little information available on its use in dogs, but it may turn out to be beneficial as an adjunctive treatment in the future.

Polysulphated glycosaminoglycans (PGAGs, e.g. Adequan®)

This is another product licensed for intra-articular or intramuscular injection in horses (and dogs in the USA). PGAGs inhibit enzymes that break down cartilage in osteoarthritis and stimulate chondrocyte and synovial cell metabolism. It is primarily used as a potential structure modifying drug but it can stimulate the synthesis of hyaluronan amongst other important molecules, and may reduce inflammatory prostaglandins, suggesting a direct analgesic effect.

Topical treatments

Topically applied NSAIDs are widely used in humans – dimethyl sulfoxide (DMSO) has been used as a topical anti-inflammatory analgesic in veterinary medicine for a long time. Topical medications are applied directly to the painful area and act locally on damaged tissue and peripheral nerves. The main advantage of these treatments is the minimal risk of systemic side effects but they also reduce the risk of drug interactions and can have a rapid onset of action. In inflammatory conditions they can reduce peripheral inflammation and concurrent sensitisation of local nociceptors. For neuropathic pain the aim is to target the abnormal firing of nerves and any ongoing neuronal inflammation. The main limitation in animals is the presence of fur and patients consuming the carefully applied treatment before it gets a chance to be absorbed.

Topical NSAIDs

Diclofenac and ketoprofen are just two NSAIDs widely used in humans in topical formulations for acute musculoskeletal pain (strains, sprains, bruising), postop pain, ophthalmic pain and for more chronic conditions like arthritis and rheumatoid arthritis. They constitute a vast market in human medicine, worth in the region of $150 million.[8] The exact vehicle formulation, active ingredient and application form, such as gel, cream, etc., can make a big difference to the efficacy and adverse effects of the preparation. Human studies looking at their use for acute soft tissue injuries show good responses to topical NSAIDs (diclofenac, ibuprofen and ketoprofen) after 7–14 days of use. One study found that preop application of topical piroxicam reduced postop pain in patients undergoing inguinal hernia repair.[7] Another study has found significant pain reduction with topical diclofenac for treatment of postop pain associated with corneal surgery.[7]

DMSO

Dimethyl sulfoxide has been used topically and parenterally as an anti-inflammatory for a long time in veterinary patients. It is licensed for the treatment of acute swelling caused by trauma in horses and inflammation associated with otitis externa in dogs, and is used for musculoskeletal pain in people. It penetrates mucous membranes and skin within 5 minutes of application and distributes into tissues in 20 minutes. It is thought to provide analgesia by blocking C fibre nociceptor conduction. It can cause irritation and inflammation at the site of application in some patients, which could unfortunately make matters worse.[3]

Menthol balm

A recent experimental study has reported that a menthol based balm used in humans for topical analgesia blunted Aδ and C fibre sensory afferents (muscle nociceptors) when applied over muscles in cats.[8] This was a model similar to the one used to study topical capsaicin and methyl salicylates discussed above. Menthol seemed to have a dramatic effect on the sensory afferent fibres 20 minutes after application. The mechanism of action of menthol balm is not clear but it is widely used in human preparations. It may work in a similar way to capsaicin, as a 'counter-irritant'. It often causes a feeling of coolness on skin, detected by receptors that include Aδ and C fibres, so it may be possible they become depleted of neurotransmitters, leading to analgesia after initial stimulation.

Biphosphonates

Biphosphonates are a group of drugs used in human patients to help relieve pain associated with bone cancer. These drugs are analogues of naturally occurring pyrophosphate compounds, which stick tightly to the surface of hydroxyapatite crystals in bone, and prevent their growth or breakdown. Their primary mechanism of action is to inhibit osteoclast activity (cells responsible for the breakdown and absorption of bone), they also inhibit cancer cell proliferation, induce programmed cell death apoptosis (often lacking in cancer cells), inhibit new blood vessel growth, and reduce the production of pro-inflammatory cytokines.[18] As well as relieving bone cancer pain they are also used as an adjunct in cancer therapy to treat hypercalcaemia associated with malignancy and inhibit bone metastases and pathological fractures.

Pamidronate is one of the most widely used biphosphonates in people, and there are newer ones arriving on the scene (ibandronate and zoledronate). Recommended regimes in humans for pamidronate are to give it i.v. initially – about 50% of patients are reported to respond in 7–14 days. It is then repeated every month or so for as long as the benefit is maintained.[19] Both i.v. and oral ibandronate have been shown to relieve moderate to severe metastatic bone pain in humans and the effect was sustained for over 2 years, significantly improving patients' quality of life and function.[20] These drugs are metabolically inert in the body but adverse effects can occur, e.g. pyrexia, oesophagitis, gastritis, and suppression of bone repair. Further research is needed into the role of biphosphonates as adjuncts to analgesia and the treatment of cancer in veterinary patients to fully establish their safety and efficacy, but they are already starting to be used for bone pain.

NONPHARMACOLOGICAL TECHNIQUES FOR ADJUNCTIVE ANALGESIA

As with many of the pharmacological adjuncts for analgesia, a lot of information for physical methods to aid pain relief is extrapolated from people, and may well not have been proven in either human or veterinary medicine yet. However, these methods may be of particular interest in patients unable to tolerate multiple medications and as a means to try and improve quality of life. They are not a replacement for proven analgesic techniques such as opioids, NSAIDs, etc. (nor are the pharmacological adjuncts), but sometimes adding in extra therapies may significantly enhance pain management.

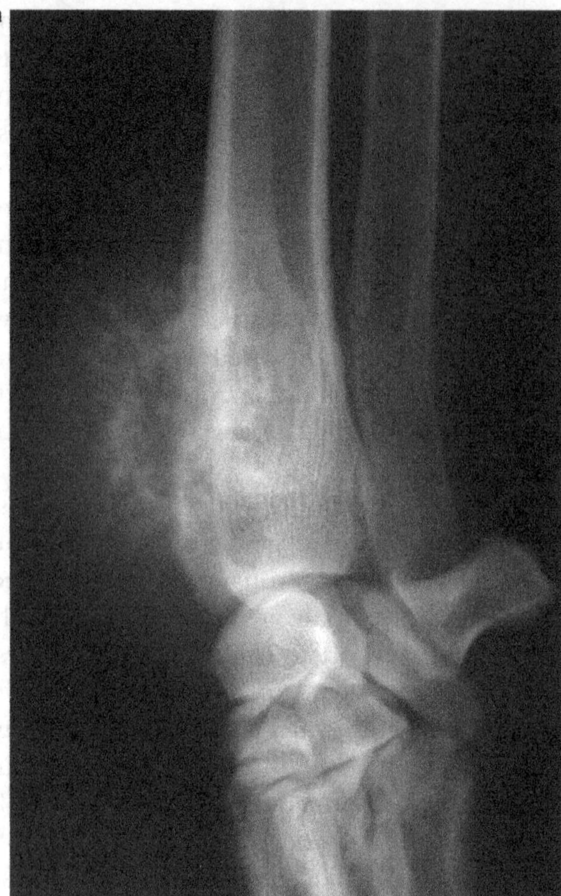

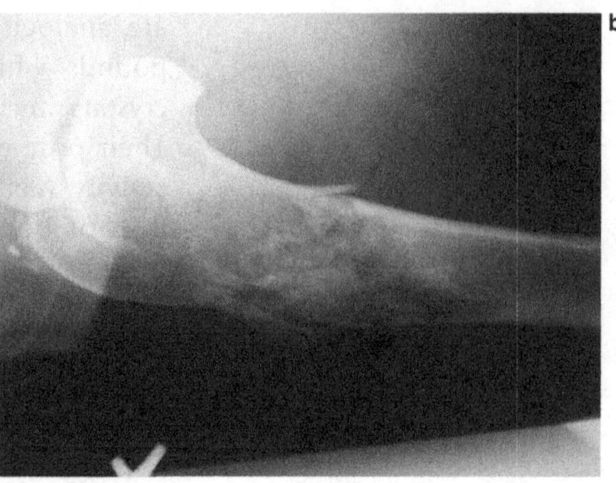

Figure 10.2
(a) Biphosphonates are starting to be used for the alleviation of bone pain associated with primary or secondary bone tumours such as these osteosarcomas of the radius and humerus. (b) Osteosarcoma of the humerus.

They can also provide the owner with opportunities to be more involved with their pet's pain management. Physical therapies for pain relief usually require special training on the part of the clinician and there are an increasing number of veterinary acupuncturists and physiotherapists who offer referral services and can be valuable contributors to pain management programmes. The following techniques are described below:

- acupuncture
- TENS
- massage
- heat
- environmental enrichment
- nursing care.

Acupuncture

Acupuncture is an ancient technique of traditional Chinese medicine; it is the stimulating of specific anatomical points, acupoints, just beneath the surface of the body to produce therapeutic or analgesic effects. Acupuncture is usually performed with a fine-gauge needle to puncture the skin, although heat and pressure may also be used. It was first described around 200 BC in one of the first manuals of Chinese medicine and has since become increasingly accepted in Western medicine as a valid form of treatment for many conditions. The literature refers to three main types of acupuncture therapies:

1. Classic acupuncture
2. Electrical stimulation (electroacupuncture)
3. Trigger point therapy.

There are other variations that aim to prolong effects by injecting physiologic saline or vitamin B12, or implanting gold beads into the acupoints.

Classic acupuncture is the best-known form and is based on the principles of ancient Chinese medicine. Health was believed to depend on the tension between two opposing forces in nature, yin (dark, female) and yang (light, male). Medical intervention aimed to balance these forces when they were considered out of harmony. Another important concept was that vital life energy 'chi' (or Qi) flowed through a set of interconnected channels called meridians. One of the internal organs was thought to be associated with each meridian, and the meridian would be named after this organ. Pain and diseases were classified according to the meridians involved and according to whether they had a yin (cold, hypofunctional) or yang (hot, hyperfunctional) nature. Excesses or deficiencies in flow of chi were said to cause pain or dysfunction. Invasion by exterior pathogens, interior cold or heat, stagnation of chi or blood, obstruction by phlegm and food retention, are examples of excess conditions leading to pain. Deficiencies in blood or chi, and consumption of body fluids from yin deficiency, could also cause pain, along with stagnation of chi distending the channels.

By inserting needles strategically along the meridians the balanced flow of chi throughout the body was restored. There are numerous variations on the classic approach, but generally, particular sets of meridian points are used to treat each type of pain problem. Electroacupuncture only differs from TENS (see below) by virtue of the fact that needles are used instead of broad electrodes. Basically, electrical stimulation using varying frequencies and intensity is applied to the acupuncture needles to aid pain relief. Apparently, electrical stimulation is nothing new; the Greeks and Romans used electric eels for pain relief in patients (which gave the leeches a bit of a rest anyway). Trigger point therapy uses the placement of acupuncture needles to relieve pain caused by trigger points in muscle. Trigger points are thought to be abnormal areas of skeletal muscle that can be felt as tender ropey strands or points associated with coldness, mild oedema, pain on palpation and fatigue (see Chapter 11).

The placement of acupuncture needles is now thought to relieve pain through several mechanisms involving the nervous system, endogenous opioids and humoral (blood-borne) factors. Meridians tend to follow the main nerves, vessels and fascial planes whilst acupoints (points used for needle placement) are closely related to the nerve branches – each of them has a specific location and function. Acupoints are characterised morphologically as a point or locus just beneath the skin comprising of a neurovascular and lymphatic bundle with a connective tissue sleeve that climbs up through the dermis towards the body surface. Both acupoints and meridians seem to be areas of decreased electrical resistance and increased conductance.

The various pieces of evidence that provide an explanation for the analgesic effects of acupuncture are as follows. Acupuncture analgesia fails to develop after local anaesthetic infiltration, or local block of the nerves innervating the acupoint, or sectioning of nerves proximal to the acupoint.[21] This implies that analgesia involves afferent input from peripheral nerves. MRI (magnetic resonance imaging) scanning has revealed that stimulation of acupoints causes measurable changes in specific areas of the human brain. There is activation of structures involved in the descending pathways that inhibit nociception (e.g. hypothalamus) and deactivation of brain structures involved in pain perception (e.g. limbic areas).[22] Thus acupuncture can lead to analgesia by modulating descending inhibition of the pain pathway and pain perception in the brain. Part of the analgesia is likely to be mediated through the release of endogenous opioids in the brain and spinal cord. Substances that antagonise opioids, e.g. naloxone, decrease acupuncture analgesia, and substances that block opioid breakdown can prolong acupuncture analgesia.

At a lower level down in the spinal cord, electroacupuncture has been shown to increase levels of endorphins and dynorphins in the spinal fluid of humans and rabbits. These endogenous opioids are involved in activating descending inhibition of the pain pathway in the spinal cord. Changing the frequency of electrostimulation activates different brain neuropeptides; correct needle placement and low frequency electrostimulation induce the release of central endorphins and enkephalins. This usually produces analgesia in 10–20 minutes and is considered to be cumulative, i.e. subsequent treatments produce better and better analgesia. High frequency stimulation induces the release of serotonin, adrenaline and noradrenaline and produces a non-cumulative analgesia. Low frequency stimulation is thought to have the best efficacy for most types of pain.[23] All these observations suggest that stimulation of acupoints induces the release of neurotransmitters and endogenous opioids, which can reduce the transmission and perception of pain impulses at several levels.

Acupuncture analgesia also fits rather well with the 'Gate Theory'. The propagation of pain impulses within the spinal cord can be inhibited by afferents from Aβ mechanoreceptors transmitting touch and pressure that are stimulated by needle insertion (see Chapter 5). A humoral mechanism may also be involved with the analgesia produced by acupuncture. Analgesia can be induced in animals that have not received needling, but have been cross-perfused with blood or CSF from animals that have undergone acupuncture.[24] Acupuncture also activates the local and central autonomic nervous system. At the point of needle placement redness and heat develop, with a feeling of warmth. An increase in skin temperature is also seen on the other side of the body to the acupoint. It is thought that stimulation of local autonomic nerves results in local vasodilatation and a centrally mediated effect to reduce sympathetic tone and increase parasympathetic tone.[22] In summary, acupuncture-induced analgesia seems to result from stimulating peripheral receptors and sensory nerves. This triggers the release of endogenous opioids, serotonin and noradrenaline in the CNS that act to inhibit nociception and pain perception.

There are several techniques of needle insertion but classically they are inserted into the skin and underlying tissue. Some therapists use a twisting motion on insertion and needle guide tubes are sometimes used. Needles should be sterilised or disposable ones used to avoid infections, and the skin wiped with an antiseptic prior to insertion. There are different principles of location of needle placement for the treatment of pain. The empirical approach is to place needles at points within the affected area, or for limb pain use the contralateral or opposite limb. This latter principle is useful if a dressing covers the affected limb, or the pain is associated with cancer because acupuncture is relatively contraindicated at the site of a tumour as it may increase local blood flow.[23] The other way is to use empirical points that have been shown to provide analgesia in one or more areas. A developing technique is to place needles at points proximal and distal to the painful area, or apply all of these principles simultaneously. For good analgesia using electroacupuncture, low frequency electrical stimulation should be applied for a minimum of 18–20 minutes. Details of suggested points to use are detailed in the references at the end of the chapter.

For the treatment of chronic pain, e.g. osteoarthritis, the patient would initially need frequent acupuncture sessions, e.g. three times a week, reducing to twice, then once a week, followed by intermittent sessions long-term to maintain analgesia. If chronic pain has been established for some time, the patient may require more frequent sessions at the start of treatment. It is important to discuss owner expectations before acupuncture is undertaken, so that clients are aware that chronically painful conditions can take six or more sessions to noticeably respond. Acupuncture and electroacupuncture can be used as an adjunctive treatment for acute pain as well as chronic conditions. It can be used preoperatively to reduce anaesthetic requirements and contribute to pain relief, or postop before recovery. Acupuncture is considered relatively safe, but as with any procedure there is always a risk, and there are reports of wayward needle insertion causing pneumothorax and even spinal cord or cardiac damage in the very occasional (and very unlucky) human recipient. Infections from dirty needles, and needle-breakage, where a piece of needle is left in the patient, are other possible complications to be aware of. Despite a lack of conclusive evidence in the scientific literature, acupuncture is now widely regarded in human and veterinary medicine as a valuable tool for adjunctive chronic pain management and can have a role in acute pain. It is something well worth considering offering to owners, either as an in-house option from a trained vet or by referral.

TENS (transcutaneous electrical nerve stimulation)

TENS uses a small battery-powered device to deliver an electrical current to one pair of pad electrodes applied to the skin of the painful area, or two pairs of electrodes (dual output) to stimulate Aβ mechanoreceptor fibres. By stimulating these fibres their input into the spinal cord will inhibit input from nociceptors converging at the same dorsal horn neurones, effectively closing the gate on the nociceptor (see Chapter 5 'Gate Theory'). With conventional TENS the electrodes are placed in the painful area and the intensity of electrical stimulation is increased to get an effect. Acupuncture-like TENS uses bursts of impulses and may be placed at a different location from the pain. There is a suggestion (unproven) that this latter form of TENS may involve the release of endogenous opioids as well as gating.

Both types of TENS are usually applied for at least 30–45 minutes, and it may relieve pain for up to several hours afterwards – although there may be no ongoing analgesia after TENS is stopped. There are successful reports of TENS helping to relive postop pain, e.g. after orthopaedic surgery (where it was also shown to enhance rehabilitation), early labour pains in women and after trauma (e.g. fractured ribs). Chronic pain studies with TENS in humans have mixed results. Good responses are reported in some reviews, for example one review found about 50% of patients derived a short-term benefit from TENS for various chronic pain states, and 25% of patients will use it for many years.[25] Several studies have found long-term TENS helps reduce the consumption of other analgesic medications by patients.[25] TENS is widely used in human medicine for chronic pain relief – it is simple to use and has few side effects – but again there is a lack of rigorous scientific evidence to support its use as an effective analgesic. The analgesia is often only experienced during treatment and is moderate in nature, making it useful only as an adjunctive therapy rather than a sole analgesic. Some patients get no benefit and it can make pain worse in some cases of neuropathic pain where normal touch evokes pain. Otherwise it is considered free from side effects and is only contraindicated in patients with pacemakers, over the neck, or over the pregnant uterus. Its use in veterinary medicine is uncommon at present.

Massage

Massage is defined as the application of touch or force to soft tissues (muscles, tendons, ligaments), without causing movement or change in the position of a joint. Massage encompasses stroking, kneading and deep massage techniques that are applied to tissues of increasing depth. Despite a lack of controlled studies, it is widely acknowledged in humans that rubbing or massaging sore muscles and joints produces a soothing feeling and pain relief. The mechanism of this action is unclear – it may be to do with gating in the spinal cord, or even the release of neurotransmitters centrally that enhance descending inhibition of nociception. Passive movement, stretching, and manipulation along with other physiotherapies are also used to increase muscle and joint function usually associated with specific orthopaedic conditions, which in turn helps relieve pain. For pets that appreciate grooming and stroking, like most family dogs and a lot of cats, these gentle actions may well reduce anxiety and aid relaxation – both effects are beneficial to pain relief.

Relaxation techniques are used in people with chronic pain and are thought to decrease central arousal and muscle tension, and improve patient symptoms. It also allows owners to have direct involvement with their pet's pain management and that is often beneficial for them as well. Massage may be something that can be incorporated into the long-term management of osteoarthritis – the owner may find it a useful technique before walking their dog or in the mornings to relieve joint stiffness. Patients where more specific physiotherapy is indicated should be referred to the appropriate expert.

Heat application

Heat can be applied via several techniques to raise the temperature of superficial and deep tissues to help relieve pain. There are four main effects of heating tissues:

- increasing local blood flow in an attempt to speed healing of non-acute soft tissue injuries
- muscle relaxation and facilitation of stretching
- reduction of joint stiffness
- pain relief.

The mechanism for an analgesic effect is not clear, but theories include the release of endorphins, general relaxation and vasodilatation reducing pain from ischaemia.[26] Heat application must be used with tremendous care in patients unable to communicate how hot they are getting, to avoid accidental overheating and even burns. Heat may be useful by itself but also as an adjunct to massage and prior to passive physiotherapy. Heat is contraindicated in acute musculoskeletal injury and acute inflammation of joints as it can increase haemorrhage and oedema. The general consensus is to avoid tumours as well, to avoid increasing their blood flow.

Modalities available for superficial heat application include heat pads and hot packs. Heat can be applied to deeper tissues using ultrasound waves, shortwave and microwave diathermy and low-frequency lasers. Evidence for the efficacy of ultrasound and lasers as analgesic adjuncts in human texts is still scant. Shortwave diathermy has produced significant analgesia in patients with soft tissue injuries. However, if they seem to give some relief for individuals then it is valid to use them as part of an overall pain management protocol. Care must be taken to use heat application techniques that are safe in the smaller than human veterinary patient, and it is advised that potential cases are referred to veterinary experts (e.g. veterinary physiotherapists) with experience in such novel techniques.

Environmental enrichment

Arrays of psychological therapies are utilised in chronic pain management protocols in people to try and minimise some of the factors that may potentiate pain states, i.e. tension, anxiety, stress, negative thoughts and immobility. These factors are thought to effectively oppose descending inhibition of pain afferents, opening the gate for nociceptive afferents in the spinal cord. Education and counselling are used to ensure patients understand their condition and help them adapt better. If a patient mistakenly believes the pain reflects a worsening of underlying pathology it results in an even greater loss of function. Relaxation techniques and stress management are used and this often improves symptoms. People are often given 'operant behavioural therapy' that involves setting goals in a step-like fashion that reinforces positive behaviour.

Another extremely important area of chronic pain management in humans is cognitive behaviour therapy. The basis is that the behavioural and emotional response to pain is primarily influenced by thoughts, i.e. personal beliefs and expectations, rather than the disease process itself. The aim is to change these thoughts and consequently the response to pain. Obviously these strategies are extremely limited in veterinary patients, but one technique that could sensibly be applied is that of diversion therapy. Diversion techniques decrease the perception of pain by switching patients' attention to other stimuli and this distraction can activate descending inhibition of the pain pathway. This therapy is utilising the mechanism underlying the situation where a dog only pulls up lame after the rabbit it was chasing has cleared off, even though it sustained the injury earlier on.

An assessment of what motivates the patient can be used to help identify environmental factors that may provide a pleasurable focus of attention. If appropriate (depending on underlying problems) it may involve more play activities, choosing different routes for walks, making use of food-stuffed toys, or hiding food to engage the dog in sniff-and-search activities. This sort of adjunctive therapy requires a highly motivated and dedicated owner who is bought into the idea, and the input of experienced pet behaviourists, who can play an extremely important role in chronic pain management protocols. There is further discussion on the role of environmental enrichment and overall quality of life in the next chapter, regarding chronic pain management.

Nursing care

As discussed in the previous chapter on acute pain management, good nursing care cannot be underestimated as an

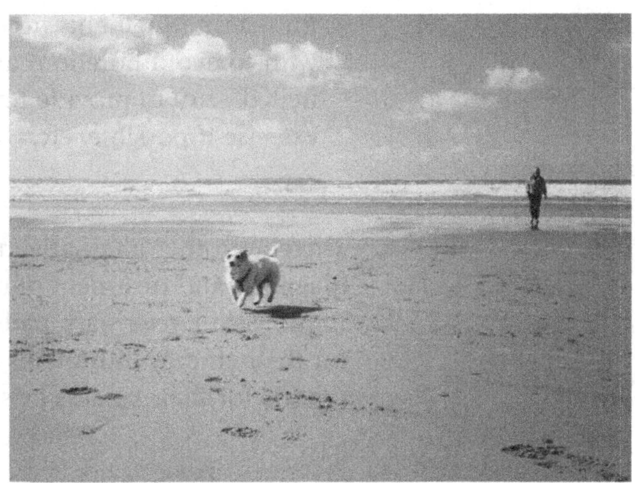

Figure 10.3
Environmental enrichment such as choosing novel routes for walks and outings to new places such as the beach can provide great pleasure and distraction from chronic pain for patients.

aid to minimising pain and discomfort. This involves providing:

- clean dry soft bedding
- ambient stable temperature
- keeping different species in different rooms (i.e. cats separate from dogs, and apart from prey animals such as rabbits) – if this isn't feasible, ensure cats have a covered bed so they can hide and feel safe
- the presence of a familiar toy or blanket can be reassuring for patients
- access to fresh food and water as soon as appropriate
- quiet surroundings to allow animals opportunity to sleep
- access to human interaction and company for socialised patients
- petting, stroking and grooming for amenable in-patients
- cleaning to avoid faecal and urine soiling ± teeth cleaning
- supportive dressings, where appropriate, that are regularly checked; cats may not tolerate dressings, particularly on hind limbs, so they may not always be as beneficial in this species
- splinting to immobilise painful body parts where appropriate
- oral and i.v. drug administration where possible to avoid painful i.m. injections
- ample opportunity to allow in-patients to defecate and urinate; many house-trained animals will hold on until they have access to the outside

- long-term in-patients need to be stimulated and interacted with to avoid boredom and frustration, whilst being kennelled – try to provide toys and access to a larger area for exercise if possible, etc.

FURTHER ALTERNATIVE METHODS

There are other alternative therapies used in people for the diagnosis and treatment of medical problems that are tempting to try in veterinary patients. There is a lack of evidence for their efficacy in humans as well as animals but anecdotal reports for their success exist.

Homeopathy

Homeopathy is a system of medicine started over 150 years ago by Samuel Hahnemann, who observed that substances that cause certain symptoms could be used to treat those same symptoms, i.e. using like to treat like. Hahnemann developed remedies with very low concentrations of the substance that could stimulate the body to eliminate symptoms produced by the same substance given at high concentrations. Remedies are described according to their concentration, and the more dilute the preparation the more potent they are considered by homeopaths. The main problem that advocates of Western medicine have with homeopathy is that the higher dilutions may well not contain any molecules of the original substance, but the idea is that the properties of the substance are preserved during serial dilutions. There are extremely few published studies on the use of homeopathy for pain relief in people, and it is not yet established as an adjunctive form of analgesia in humans (or animals, where there is even less information available). Homeopathic remedies are probably relatively safe as they contain so little of the original ingredient. The most likely adverse reaction would be an exacerbation of the clinical signs, although the homeopath may regard this as a good thing because the body is reacting to cure itself.

Herbal and plant medicine

Several analgesic drugs are derived from plants and herbs, e.g. opioids from poppies, salicylates from willow bark. Herbalists believe that the therapeutic benefit of the herb is due to the unique combination of ingredients provided by that specific plant, and that extraction of active ingredients may decrease the healing power. The whole plant is considered natural and therefore less likely to be toxic, whereas purified extracts can lead to more side effects. However, it is known that herbal and plant medicines can have serious side effects and negative interactions with pharmaceuticals.[27] The other safety issue regarding these medicines is their lack of regulation; the quality and concentration of active ingredients can vary widely and potentially dangerous contaminants can be present.[27] If clinicians consider using herbal remedies it is important they obtain them from a very reliable and rigorously controlled high standard source and that the exact content is known. The clinician must also be aware of any possible interactions with conventional drugs. There are a few human reports of some remedies being better than placebo in rheumatoid arthritis. The effect may have been due to the presence of salicylates and omega fatty acids and other ingredients that would affect inflammatory mediators.[27]

Chiropractic and veterinary manipulative therapy

Chiropractic is based on manual manipulation of the spine and the belief that many diseases are brought about by dysfunction of the spinal column. For example, problems with an abdominal organ could be due to the nerves controlling the function of the organ being compressed as they leave the spine. Although scantily used in small animals at present, chiropractic may be a future area of adjunctive pain relief to be researched.

Magnetic field therapy

Magnetism can be used therapeutically by applying static magnets to affected body parts wrapped in a dressing, or by using an electromagnet that requires a battery or electrical supply. Electromagnets can provide more powerful magnetic fields than static magnets and they can also be switched on and off to deliver pulsed electromagnetic fields (PEMF). PEMF has been used in people for various problems such as fracture non-unions, osteochondritis dissecans, chronic skin ulcers and osteoarthritis. One study did find an improvement in pain scores in 25 people with arthritis using PEMF compared to a placebo.[27] It is possible there may be some benefit in this rather unorthodox method as an adjunct to pain management. There are no serious side effects associated with this therapy, although there is the potential for an electric shock from a faulty PEMF device.

Key summary points of adjunctive analgesia

1. Pharmacological and physical methods of adjunctive analgesia can be useful tools to add to acute and chronic pain management protocols alongside conventional analgesics. When it comes to pain relief 'every little bit can help'.
2. Adjunctive therapies are not designed to replace conventional analgesia but to supplement them.
3. Many pharmacological adjuncts are unlicensed in animals and there is limited data available on their efficacy and safety. More information should be sought and owners made aware of the situation before they are used.
4. Non-pharmacological adjuncts are particularly useful for chronic pain and for patients who are less tolerant of drugs
5. Veterinary acupuncturists, pet behaviourists and veterinary physiotherapists can be extremely important in devising and providing long-term pain management protocols.

REFERENCES

1. Melzack R. Pain and the neuromatrix in the brain. J Dent Educ 2001; 65(12): 1378–1382
2. Max MB, Gilron IH. Antidepressants, muscle relaxants and NMDA receptor antagonists. In: Loeser JD, ed. Bonica's management of pain, 3rd edn. Philadelphia, USA: Lippincott Williams & Wilkins; 2001:1710–1726
3. Lamont LA, Tranquilli WJ, Mathews KA. Adjunctive analgesic therapy. Vet Clin N Am Small Animal Practice 2000; 30(4): 805–813
4. Monks R, Merskey H. Psychotropic drugs. In: Wall PD, Melzack R, eds. Textbook of pain, 4th edn. Edinburgh: Churchill Livingstone; 1999:1155–1186
5. Rowbotham MC, Petersen KL. Anticonvulsants and local anaesthetic drugs. In: Loeser JD, ed. Bonica's management of pain, 3rd edn. Philadelphia, USA: Lippincott Williams & Wilkins; 2000:1727–1736
6. Mason L, Moore A, Derry S, et al. Systematic review of topical capsaicin for the treatment of chronic pain. Br Med J 2004; 328:991–994
7. Galer BS. Topical medications. In: Loeser JD, ed. Bonica's management of pain, 3rd edn. Philadelphia, USA: Lippincott Williams & Wilkins; 2000:1736–1741
8. Ragan BG, Nelson AJ, Foreman J, et al. Effects of a menthol-based analgesic balm on pressor responses evoked from muscle afferents in cats. J Am Vet Med Assoc 2004; 65(9):1204–1210
9. Bauer JE. Evaluation of nutraceuticals, dietary supplements and functional food ingredients for companion animals. J Am Vet Med Assoc 2001; 218(11):1755–1760
10. Reginster JY, Deroisy R, Rovati LC, et al. Long term effects of glucosamine sulphate on osteoarthritis progression: a randomized, placebo controlled clinical trial. The Lancet 2001; 357:251–256

11. Creamer P. Osteoarthritis. In: Wall PD, Melzack R, eds. Textbook of pain, 4th edn. Edinburgh: Churchill Livingstone; 1999:493–504
12. McLaughlin R. Management of chronic osteoarthritic pain. Vet Clin N Am Small Animal Practice 2000; 30(4):933–949
13. Bierer TL, Bui LM. Improvement of arthritic signs in dogs fed green-lipped mussel (*Perna canaliculus*). Am Soc Nutr Sci J Nutr 2002; 132:1634s–1636s
14. Smith JG, Hannon RL, Brunnberg L, et al. A randomised, double blind, comparator clinical study of the efficacy of sodium pentosan polysulfate injection and carprofen capsules in arthritic dogs. Osteoarthritis Cartilage 2001; 9(Suppl B):S21–S22
15. Read RA, Cullis-Hill D, Jones MP. Systemic use of pentosan polysulphate in the treatment of osteoarthritis. JSAP 1996; 37: 108–114
16. Hannon RL, Smith JG, Cullis-Hill D, et al. Safety review of Cartophen Vet in the dog: review of adverse reaction reports in the UK. JSAP 2003; 44:202–208
17. Kuroki K, Cook JL, Kreeger JM. Mechanisms of action and potential uses of hyaluronan in dogs with osteoarthritis. J Am Vet Med Assoc 2002; 221(7):944–950
18. Milner RJ, Farese J, Henry CJ, et al. Biphosphonates and cancer. J Vet Intern Med 2004; 18(5):597–604
19. Twycross R, Wilcock A, Charlesworth S, et al. Palliative care formulary, 2nd edn. Oxon:Radcliffe Medical Press; 2002: 215–239
20. Heidenreich A, Ohlmann C, Body JJ. Ibandronate in metastatic bone pain. Semin Oncol 2004; 31(5 Suppl 10):67–72
21. Rogers PAM, White SS, Ottaway CW. Stimulation of the acupuncture points in relation to therapy of analgesia and clinical disorders in animals. Vet Annual 1977; 17: 258–277
22. Mittleman E, Gaynor JS. A brief overview of the analgesic and immunologic effects of acupuncture in domestic animals. J Am Vet Med Assoc 2000; 217(8):1201–1205
23. Gaynor JS. Acupuncture for management of pain. Vet Clin N A Small Animal Practice 2000; 30(4):875–884
24. Kho HG, Robertson EN. The mechanisms of acupuncture analgesia: Review and update. Am J Acup 1997; 25:261–281
25. Chabal C. Transcutaneous electrical nerve stimulation. In: Loeser JD, ed. Bonica's management of pain, 3rd edn. Philadelphia, USA: Lippincott Williams & Wilkins; 2000:1842–1847
26. Lehmann JF, Lateur BJ. Ultrasound, short wave, microwave, laser, superficial heat and cold in the treatment of pain. In: Wall PD, Melzack R, eds. Textbook of pain, 4th edn. Edinburgh: Churchill Livingstone; 1383–1397
27. Pascoe PJ. Alternative methods for the control of pain. J Am Vet Med Assoc 2002; 221(2): 222–229

FURTHER READING

Mathews KA, ed. Veterinary Clinics of North America Small Animal Practice 2000; 30(4)

CHAPTER 11 CHRONIC PAIN MANAGEMENT AND QUALITY OF LIFE

DEFINITION OF CHRONIC PAIN

Chronic pain of is often described as pain having duration of more than 3–6 months. Chronic pain can arise from a sustained noxious stimulus such as ongoing inflammation, but chronic pain can also persist even in the absence of the original noxious stimulus or beyond the expected time after an initial injury. Chronic pain can be constant or intermittent and vary in intensity and nature over time. It can manifest spontaneously or be provoked by external stimuli. This type of pain is sometimes referred to as pathologic pain, it has no useful purpose as it does not help the healing process or serve any protective function outside a clinical setting. In fact chronic pain often becomes the disease itself.

Chronic pain can result from changes in the pain pathway, i.e. sensitisation (detailed in Chapter 5), whereby a specific stimulus elicits much greater neuronal activity than it would in normal animals, with an exaggerated amplitude and duration. The result is hyperalgesia, an increased response to a stimulus that is normally painful, and allodynia, pain due to a stimulus that does not normally provoke pain. This creates a real problem when it comes to treatment because analgesic drugs will often be less effective when the patient has an altered pain pathway and patients will require higher, more frequent doses of increasingly potent analgesics to control their pain.

ASSESSING CHRONIC PAIN

Chapter 3 discusses the difficulties of assessing pain in animals and chronic pain is particularly challenging as associated behaviour changes can often be subtle, insidious in

Box 11.1	Chronic pain
	Pain lasting more than 3–6 months that can persist beyond, or in the absence of, the original painful stimulus

onset and go unnoticed by the owner, or mistakenly be put down to normal ageing. Another problem is that owners tend to be more concerned and aware of pain associated with an obvious external injury or surgical procedure rather than pain arising from less visible sources such as osteoarthritis and cancer. This is very likely to result in an underestimation of the pet's pain and discomfort. Generally speaking animals show similar signs of chronic pain to humans (see Chapter 4):

- sleep disturbances
- appetite depression
- irritability and aggression
- reduced activity levels
- social withdrawal
- lack of enthusiasm for activity
- depression
- lowered pain threshold.

Other major indicators of chronic pain reported in humans are constipation and abnormal illness behaviour, as well as the signs listed above.

Clinicians are more reliant on owner information to diagnose chronic pain, as the signs are often only apparent in the home setting, rather than on a short visit to the vets. Chronic pain is very debilitating for the sufferer; it has a widespread impact on many aspects of life and severely compromises quality of life (see below for further discussion on quality of life in veterinary patients). For this reason, quality of life is becoming increasingly used as a tool to measure the effectiveness of chronic pain treatment in people. It allows an assessment of treatment success when the underlying pathology may not be curable, focuses attention on what really matters to the patients and can highlight the true impact of any drug side effects in relation to their overall benefit. In humans, they specifically look at the elements of quality of life that are affected by poor health, called 'health-related quality of life' (HRQoL), and this is considered an even more reliable measure of human chronic pain than direct pain measures themselves.

An ability to assess HRQoL in veterinary patients would have all the advantages listed above for people with the addition of enabling clinicians and owners to more confidently decide when further treatment would not be in the best interest of the patient and euthanasia is the kindest option. A group at Glasgow University Veterinary School has started to develop a questionnaire for owners to evaluate HRQoL in their dogs suffering from chronic pain.[1] Preliminary work has involved interviewing pet owners to establish areas or domains of behaviour that are relevant to chronic pain assessment and identification of descriptive words (descriptors) for these behaviours that owners use to convey the degree and nature of their pets' pain. The researchers have then used the domains and descriptors to create a questionnaire that has undergone preliminary validation and will be tested out further in the field in due course.

Table 11.1 lists the domains and descriptors found to be relevant to assessing chronic pain in dogs. Interestingly, these preliminary findings are very similar to the range of domains used in long-established human HRQoL questionnaires. This information, although representing the results of early research, provides a very useful framework for clinicians when dealing with patients in chronic pain. By careful questioning of owners at the outset before treatment, and at follow-up consultations after treatment, the relative success of chronic pain management protocols can be assessed and adjusted accordingly. It also helps focus everybody's attention on quality of life[2,3] rather than the nuances of underlying pathology, which is often progressive and irreversible – although obviously treatment of the underlying disease must always be paramount. Redirecting owners to what really matters to the patients is also a valuable approach when it comes to managing owner expectations. The clinician needs to be aware that in some individual patients behaviour alterations may be due to physical impairment associated with the underlying disease, as well as pain.

Table 11.1
The qualities and quantities of behavioural domains relevant to assess dogs with chronic pain, and the descriptive terms used by owners to describe those domains

Domains of behaviour	Negative descriptors	Positive descriptors
Activity	Apathetic, apprehensive, lacklustre, lethargic, listless, reluctant, sleepy, slowed, sluggish, tired, weary	Active, boisterous, bouncy, energetic, lively, playful, tireless
Comfort	Complaining, groaning, moaning, pained, sore, stoic, uncomfortable	Comfortable, stretching
Appetite	Off food, picky	Enthusiastic about food, greedy, interested in food, thirsty
Extroversion–introversion	Detached, quiet, subdued, unresponsive, unsociable, withdrawn	Affectionate, bold, curious, eager, excitable, friendly, fun loving, nosy, outgoing, sociable
Aggression	Aggressive, grumpy, irritable, territorial or protective	Good-natured, even-tempered, placid
Anxiety	Anxious, cautious, distressed, frightened, nervous, panicky, strained, uneasy, upset	Accepting, easygoing, laid-back
Alertness	Depressed, dull, confused, uninterested	Alert, bright, inquisitive, interested, keen, obedient
Dependence	Attention seeking, clingy, comfort seeking, pathetic, pitiful	Confident, independent
Contentment	Miserable, sad, sorrowful, resigned, unhappy	Contented, happy
Consistency	Inconsistent	Consistent
Agitation	Agitated, crying, disturbed, panting, restless, unsettled, whining	Calm, at ease
Posture-mobility	Awkward, limping, stiff	Athletic, fit, relaxed
Compulsion	Compulsive	No terms

(From Wiseman-Orr ML, Nolan AM, Reid J, et al. Development of a questionnaire to measure the effects of chronic pain on health-related quality of life in dogs. Am J Vet Res 2004; 65(8):1077–1084, reproduced with permission.)

Box 11.2 **Chronic pain management**

The ultimate goal of chronic pain management should be to maximise quality of life, not necessarily quantity of life

ANALGESIA FOR CHRONIC PAIN MANAGEMENT

There are several problems with the provision of long-term analgesia to outpatients; it is not just the obvious issue of potential side effects of administering drugs long-term that can create difficulties. Firstly the route and frequency of analgesic drug administration has to be one that the owner can cope with and that avoids causing too much discomfort to the patient, and the drug should not be dangerous for the owner to handle or store. It is important to warn owners of the potential side effects of the drugs they are giving to their pets – make them aware of the risks and benefits, and if they are informed of the early signs of a problem the drug can be withdrawn and treatment adjusted to minimise the risk of any serious consequences. Unfortunately a lot of analgesics are only available for animals in an injectable form, are short-acting, or are controlled drugs that require careful dispensing to owners.

Owner compliance, once an analgesic has been dispensed, can be unbelievably poor when it comes to actually getting medication into the pet. A recent study looked at owner compliance with a mere 10-day course of antibiotics for common acute bacterial infections in dogs, ranging from wound infections and gastrointestinal upsets to pyometra and tooth infections.[4] Only 44% of the 95 owners included in the study gave the full course of antibiotics to their dogs. The study also found that compliance was significantly higher amongst owners who felt the vet had spent enough time on the consultation, presumably explaining their pet's condition and treatment. Compliance was significantly higher for owners of dogs with gastrointestinal disorders as well, possibly because cleaning up after the pets was more than enough motivation to get some tablets down them. An earlier veterinary study indicated that owners were failing to give tablets during the day because they were out at work, but this was not a significant factor in the later study.

On the human side it is worth noting that a doctor presented with an apparent treatment failure in a child is encouraged to consider lack of parent compliance first of all, something that vets may not always think of straight away in their patients. When dispensing long-term medication for pets it is wise to discuss potential compliance problems with owners and look at using easy to administer formulations,

Box 11.3	Practicalities of long-term medication
	■ Choose a route of administration that is owner friendly ■ Ensure the drug itself is safe to store and handle at home ■ Check that drug administration does not cause unacceptable patient discomfort or stress ■ The owner needs to be made aware of the early signs of potential side effects of the medication ■ Choose a formulation appropriate for both the owner and pet to maximise compliance ■ Monitor owner compliance and consider this in the event of apparent treatment failure ■ Consider having a practice nurse phone up owners to offer advice and help on medicating pets

preferably once or twice daily where possible. Merrily waving off an arthritic 90-year-old Rottweiler owner from the practice, clutching a bottle of torpedo-sized capsules for four times a day administration is not good practice. Similarly, seeing an owner nursing multiple lacerations bring back a cat with bits of tablet stuck all over its head is an indication that compliance may not be awfully good. Generally speaking, owners seem to be more likely to discuss difficulties of dosing their pets with nurses. A practice may want to consider having a nurse responsible for contacting owners after a few days to have a chat about how they are getting on with medicating their pets and offer advice on any problems they may be encountering. It is prudent to avoid sounding as if the practice is checking up on the owner as this may be taken the wrong way – ideally it should come across as further practice support.

The general principles of chronic pain management are similar to acute pain management – the multimodal approach should be used, i.e. add in more types of analgesic drug with increasing pain intensity to get synergistic analgesia, and tailor protocols according to individual patient requirements and responses. Regular reassessment is needed to monitor the success of treatments; owner input is essential for this. Traditional analgesics can be used alongside adjunctive methods of analgesia (see Chapter 10), which are particularly useful for chronic pain. Some of the options available are as follows and further details are given under individual disease conditions later in the chapter.

Opioids

Opioids tend be to given by injection, often by the i.m. route, and only have a few hours duration of action. This makes them suitable for hospitalised patients, but not those being treated at home. Oral preparations of morphine are available for humans, but the risks of dispensing controlled drugs that are off licence need to be carefully considered. The owner also needs to be aware of concurrent sedation that opioids can cause. Fentanyl skin patches are very useful for providing good quality opioid analgesia over days rather than hours, but the problem of dispensing a controlled drug remains – it is very easy for a patch to be eaten by the pet or handled by children with potentially fatal consequences. Their disposal is also a problem, so again they are really best restricted to inpatients. An oral form of butorphanol is available (off licence for animals) and this may be an option for chronic pain relief in outpatients as it is not a controlled drug. Although it is a controlled drug, oral buprenorphine is also worth considering in cats (this is actually absorbed through the oral mucous membrane; see Chapter 9). As mentioned before, a transdermal skin patch delivering buprenorphine is now available for humans, but its use in cats has not yet been closely studied.

NSAIDs

Currently, NSAIDs are the mainstay of long-term pain relief in animals. There are several oral formulations designed specifically for easy once-daily dosing that may help with owner compliance and that are licensed for long-term use in dogs. They provide good quality analgesia but the main drawback of these drugs is the potential for side effects and the lack of safety data and licensed products for long-term use in cats. NSAIDs tend to have a long and variable half-life in cats, so the worry about repeat dosing relates to the potential for an accumulation of drug leading to toxic effects. It is advisable to contact the manufacturers of individual drugs to ask for the most recent anecdotal off licence dose rates for use in cats where necessary. However, as is always the case, all drugs have the potential for side effects and although the benefits of analgesia almost always out-weigh the risks associated with medication, potential problems should be carefully considered in discussion with the owner who should be informed of the signs of side effects.

The main side effects to monitor with NSAIDs are gastrointestinal ulceration, and renal and hepatic dysfunction. Blood sampling of all patients prior to medication is one option but not always necessary, and depends on individual practice policy. The clinical picture and history should give an indication as to whether further tests are necessary and are only worth doing if the results are actually acted upon. Withholding analgesia is not an option, but dose adjustment, concurrent administration of gastrointestinal protectants (see Chapter 7), adjunctive analgesic therapies or alternative classes of analgesic may be indicated. In higher risk patients it is pertinent to do a baseline PCV (to check for internal bleeding), renal and hepatic tests, e.g. ALT, ALP, BUN, creatinine. These can be repeated 7–14 days after NSAID therapy is initiated to monitor the patient's progress, and then repeated as clinically indicated longer term.

Other analgesics

Local anaesthetics, NMDA antagonists and alpha 2 agonists are not suitable for use in outpatients long-term, however repeat doses and infusions may be indicated for inpatients hospitalised over a few days. One technique to continue epidural analgesia over several days is to place an epidural catheter. Corticosteroids may have a role in the management of chronic pain and discomfort (such as pruritus, see below) but are not considered a first-line analgesic and their array of side effects warrants particular consideration of the risks and benefits to the patient of their use.

Adjunctive analgesic therapies (see Chapter 10 for further details)

Antidepressants, anticonvulsants, benzodiazepines and nutraceuticals are all alternative therapies with a role in chronic pain relief. Physical therapies such as acupuncture, massage and environmental enrichment can also be used alongside analgesics in chronic pain management and to improve quality of life (see below).[5] Fig 11.1 is an example

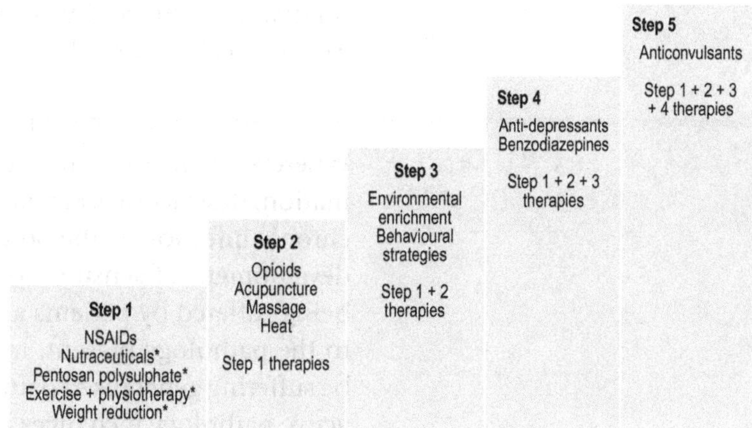

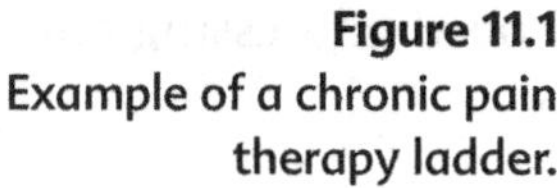
Figure 11.1 Example of a chronic pain therapy ladder.

of a pain therapy ladder and suggests different types of adjunctive analgesic therapies that can be considered for cases of chronic pain such as osteoarthritis. Further levels of therapy can be added in depending on patient response and complexity of the causes of pain.

SURGERY FOR CHRONIC PAIN RELIEF

Sensory neurectomy

In horses with navicular disease, sensory neurectomy may be performed; this involves cutting the nerve supplying the area causing intractable and incurable pain. It can be achieved by surgery or local injection of a toxic chemical to ablate the nerve. However, this is a pretty drastic technique and there are a couple of problems; firstly a painful neuroma can develop at the site of nerve section, and the target body part will be desensitised and therefore can be subject to severe injury unbeknown to the animal.

Therapeutic surgery

Sometimes a surgical procedure will remove the physical source of pain, e.g. spinal surgery to remove disc material causing spinal cord compression, resection of a tumour that's squashing surrounding tissue and releasing inflammatory mediators. Removing the source of pain appears to be the ultimate pain management technique, but in the case of limb amputation may lead to its own problems such as phantom limb pain. Other curative techniques may adversely impact on quality of life and this will need addressing after surgery, e.g. enucleation, maniblectomy.

CAUSES OF CHRONIC PAIN

Wherever there is chronic disease – e.g. chronic tissue inflammation, destruction or irritation, space-occupying lesions and chronic infections – the potential for chronic pain exists. The development of sensitisation can lead to the degree of pain being suffered by patients apparently being disproportionate to the pathology present, in fact it is possible for patients to be suffering generalised pain syndromes in the absence of any active pathology if changes in pain processing have been irreversible and severe enough. Clinically the commonest causes of chronic pain in dogs and cats include osteoarthritis and cancer but there are many other conditions warranting the use of analgesia as well as treatment of the underlying problem that are not always obvious, e.g. chronic eye pain from corneal ulcers, glaucoma, chronic ear pain from otitis externa, chronic dental pain, interstitial cystitis in cats, and neuropathic pain to name just a few. It is also possible that animals may suffer from chronic pain conditions that are only currently recognised in humans such as myofascial pain (see below) and these patients may be presenting as 'behaviour' cases.

There are many less obvious causes of pain and suffering that may warrant the use of analgesics and measures to improve quality of life. Chronic pruritus associated with skin disease such as atopic dermatitis, some medical conditions (e.g. uraemia) and liver failure can result in long-term unpleasant feelings of nausea and 'grogginess' from the presence of toxins in the blood. Congestive heart failure is a common cause of discomfort that affects quality of life by producing feelings of breathlessness and exhaustion. Endocrine disease and associated polydipsia with a constant feeling of thirst is also likely to be significantly unpleasant for patients. Some of these conditions are discussed in more detail below.

Osteoarthritis

Osteoarthritis is the commonest cause of chronic pain in dogs – it is estimated that at least 20% of the UK adult dog population has osteoarthritis. The prevalence of osteoarthritis is unknown in cats and could be more common than previously thought because it may be widely under-diagnosed. A recent retrospective study in the USA examined radiographs of 100 cats over the age of 12 years that had been referred for non-related diagnostic work-ups. Radiographic signs of osteoarthritis were found in 90% of the cats (joints of the spine and sternum were also included, as well as the limbs).[6] Even though radiographic joint changes do not correlate well to clinical signs or severity of arthritis, the study findings suggest osteoarthritis may potentially be an important cause of chronic pain in cats. Osteoarthritis is also amongst one of the oldest diseases; apparently signs of it can be found in dinosaur fossils.

Definition

Osteoarthritis can be defined as joint pain and dysfunction. It is a degenerative disease of moveable joints, characterised by abnormal changes and eventual loss of cartilage, inflammation and thickening of the synovial membrane, the formation of osteophytes (new bone) at joint margins and subchondral bone remodelling. The condition is progressive and irreversible and can affect one or more different joints. Osteoarthritis can be classified as primary, secondary or erosive. The secondary form is by far the commonest type in dogs and follows an initial joint disease, injury or instability, such as a ruptured cruciate ligament, elbow osteochondrosis or traumatic injury. The primary form is seen in humans and affects joints in the absence of an obvious primary problem. Erosive osteoarthritis includes the autoimmune diseases and involves destructive changes in the bone and cartilage. The structural joint changes that are characteristic of secondary osteoarthritis are thought to represent the joint's response to any type of injury, i.e. they represent a disease process that is the final common end-point of joint injury.

Risk factors

Several factors are thought to influence the site, severity and risk of developing osteoarthritis in dogs: genetic factors, breed, age, gender, body weight and concurrent disease. For example, for a given degree of hip laxity the risk of developing hip osteoarthritis has been found to be 5 × higher in German Shepherds than the risk for Rottweilers, Labrador retrievers and Golden retrievers combined.[7] Other studies have shown that limiting food intake over the lifetime of dogs to keep them slim and trim can actually reduce the development of osteoarthritis in the first place.[8,10] The hips of a group of 24 Labrador retrievers fed a calorie-restricted diet from the age of 8 weeks to 8 years and kept at an ideal body weight were compared to another 'plump' group fed 25% more calories over the same period. The prevalence of radiographic signs of hip osteoarthritis was 68% in the group of plump dogs compared to only 14% in the slim group. Not only that but the heavier dogs had a significantly higher incidence of multiple joints being affected with osteoarthritis – 77% had at least two different joints affected compared to only 10% of the lighter dogs.[10]

Clinical signs and diagnosis

The clinical signs of osteoarthritis can be due to both changes in joint structure that affect joint function and joint pain, which results in the animal being unwilling to use the joint normally and causes less specific behaviour changes. Chronic pain due to sensitisation and wind-up of the pain pathway associated with affected joints is an integral part of the disease itself, and one of the main targets of therapy. The common clinical signs found on examination in dogs are:[9]

- lameness
- stiffness
- joint thickening or swelling
- reduced range of joint movement
- pain on joint manipulation
- joint crepitus on movement
- muscle atrophy.

The owner often notices the behavioural signs associated with joint pain (similar to the general signs of chronic pain listed earlier in the chapter) such as:

- avoidance and reluctance to exercise
- difficulty climbing stairs and jumping into car or onto the sofa
- general inactivity
- anxiety, depression, apparent disobedience
- restlessness such as prolonged circling before lying down
- changes in sleep patterns and location
- reduced social interaction with humans and other dogs

- difficulty getting up, stiffness or doddery gait after rest and exercise, especially in the mornings
- increased aggressiveness and irritability
- reduced play activities
- changes in eating patterns
- breaking of house training.

Overt lameness may not always be present, and unfortunately the owner often associates these behavioural signs with acceptable signs of old age rather than unacceptable and treatable pain. Diagnosis of osteoarthritis is usually based on the history, clinical examination and sometimes the use of radiographs and arthrocentesis to rule out other causes of joint pain and complications. Radiographs will only show the bony changes associated with arthritis, the presence of osteophytes rather than any cartilage pathology, and radiographic changes correlate poorly with clinical severity. It is not unusual to see a truly horrible pair of arthritic hips on x-ray with severely remodelled femoral heads attached to a clinically normal dog (Fig 11.2).

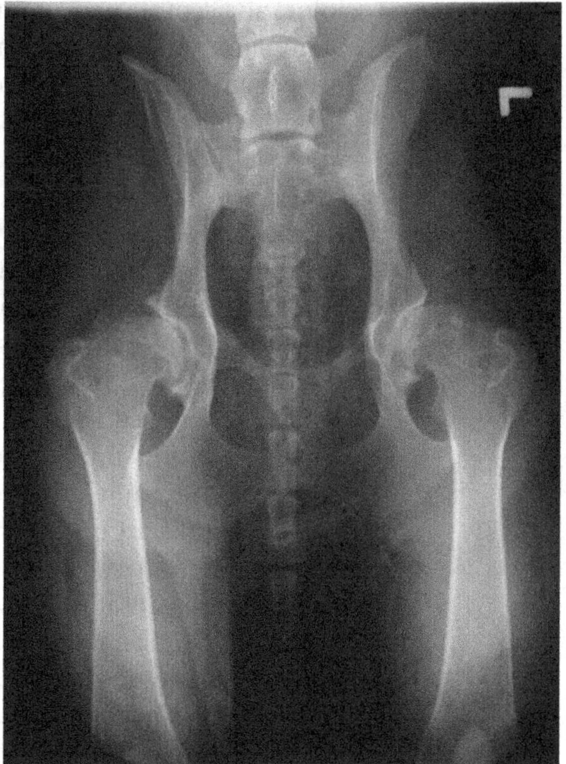

Figure 11.2
Joint osteophytes and bone remodelling are characteristic changes associated with osteoarthritis seen in the radiograph of these canine hips.

Pain in osteoarthritis

In humans the pain associated with osteoarthritis is said to be generally insidious in onset and quite well localised, it is described as a persistent ache interspersed with episodes of stabbing pain provoked by movement of the affected joint(s).[11] Words used by patients often include throbbing, aching and sharp pain. People often report that the pain gets worse when using the joint, e.g. going up and down stairs; it is worse in the evenings but is then eased by rest. The pain is said to vary day to day and can be worse at night. Although commonly located at the affected joint, referred pain is not unusual – people with hip arthritis can feel referred pain in the knee, and spinal pain may be felt in the hip.

There are two main sources of pain in osteoarthritis – synovial inflammation and sensitisation of the pain pathway of the joint (cartilage itself is not innervated). As cartilage is broken down in osteoarthritis the breakdown products are released into the joint and cause inflammation of the synovial membrane. The synovial cells in turn release lots of pro-inflammatory mediators including prostaglandins, cytokines, interleukins and various enzymes that will stimulate further cartilage degradation by chondrocytes and directly stimulate joint nociceptors generating pain. Chronic low-grade inflammation of the synovial membrane seems to exist in osteoarthritic joints, and episodes of more acute severe inflammation may occur over time associated with worsening of clinical signs.

Most of the afferent nerves in joints are C and Aδ nociceptor fibres, silent nociceptors that are normally unresponsive, and Aβ mechanoreceptors. They all richly innervate the synovium, ligaments, tendons, periosteum and fibrous joint capsule. Continual cartilage damage and degradation in osteoarthritis provides a constant supply of inflammatory mediators released into the joint that not only directly stimulate nociceptors but also sensitise them so their thresholds drop. At the same time silent nociceptors will become activated and start generating pain signals in response to innocuous stimuli such as stretch and weight bearing. This peripheral sensitisation plays a key part in the clinical manifestations of osteoarthritis – the patient initially starts to experience pain when joints are actively used and as the neuronal changes in the pain pathway continue, pain is experienced even with normal weight bearing, and eventually at rest. The pain will also continue when there is minimal inflammation ongoing in the joint.

Central sensitisation is bound to be involved as well, but the peripheral changes in neurone activity are probably more important in osteoarthritis in the generation of chronic pain.[11] It is possible that the formation of osteophytes may be painful if they result in elevation and stretching of the periosteum which is heavily innervated with nociceptors. There is also evidence that intraosseous pressure is raised in osteoarthritis, which again could result in pain even at rest. Osteotomy and simple drilling into the bone of affected joints can reduce this pressure and both techniques have been shown to provide rapid pain relief in humans.[11] Stretching of soft tissue structures of the joint due to joint swelling – i.e. the synovial membrane, fibrous joint capsule and ligament and tendon insertions – is another potential source of pain.

There is another unproven hypothesis that some of the pain in osteoarthritic joints emanates from the presence of micro-thrombi in the venules of subchondral bone and synovial tissues. If this occurs the venous occlusion could produce painful oedema and anoxia of the bone and soft tissue. This may be one mechanism by which pentosan polysulphate may be beneficial; it may help break down micro-clots. Patients with osteoarthritis usually develop an altered gait in an attempt to minimise use of affected joints, leading to abnormal body posture, muscle spasm and pain. Massage can therefore be beneficial to relieve this secondary pain.

Pain management in osteoarthritis

Medical management of osteoarthritis falls into two types of drugs – symptom-modifying drugs that aim to relieve pain and thereby improve joint function, and structure-modifying drugs that aim to restore normal cartilage structure. It is still debateable as to whether any truly structure-modifying drugs are yet available but the nutraceuticals are often classed as potentially structure-modifying, as well as being adjuncts to analgesia and therefore symptom modifying. The aim of pain control in arthritic patients is to allow the patient to be able to use their affected joints and allow a controlled exercise protocol to be instigated. By providing analgesia the patient can increase joint mobility and this will prevent or minimise mechanical stiffness and disuse atrophy of muscles supporting the joint. This is very important, as stiffness and muscle atrophy are difficult to revise once established; both worsen the clinical picture and may well hasten deterioration of the clinical picture. Controlled exercise guidelines, physiotherapy (and hydrotherapy), reduction in bodyweight, and the treatment of other concurrent problems and complications are also essential features of a comprehensive osteoarthritis management plan and will depend on the stage and severity of disease.

The mainstays of long-term pain relief for osteoarthritis are NSAIDs. Several are licensed for long-term use, e.g. carprofen and meloxicam, a reflection of a good safety profile. A common approach is to use a first line NSAID for 1–2 weeks, reassess the patient and then reduce the NSAID to a maintenance dose if possible. If there is a poor response after several weeks, it may be worth trying a different NSAID as efficacy can vary between individuals. Maintenance programmes can be adjusted to establish a minimum effective dose. The clinician may decide to reduce dosing to every other day, or titrating the dose right down to the minimum licensed one, or even using intermittent dosing on an as-needed basis. It is common practice now to add in a nutraceutical, e.g. glucosamine, with the aim of enhancing analgesia or for potential long-term benefits to cartilage structure (see Chapter 10). The dose of NSAID may need to be periodically increased as acute flare-ups can occur when the patient suffers breakthrough pain. The exact causes of acute flare-ups is not definitely established but seem to arise after excessive exercise, trauma, or in cold damp weather, or in association with concurrent disease.

The potential for side effects of NSAIDs are one of the main limitations to their use, particularly as a lot of osteoarthritis patients are geriatric and often have other health problems. Measures can be taken to minimise side effects in high-risk patients by dose reduction and the use of gastro-protectants (see Chapter 7) but a risk–benefit assessment should be made in each case and the owner informed of the signs of potential side effects. All cases should be carefully monitored for signs of problems such as gastric irritation, ulceration, melaena (black faeces due to the presence of blood), and renal and hepatic problems. Some cases will warrant pre-

Box 11.4 **Adjunctive analgesics useful in osteoarthritis**

(In addition to NSAIDs ± opioids)

- Nutraceuticals
- Corticosteroids (low dose intra-articular or oral doses)
- Pentosan polysulphate (should not be used concurrently with NSAIDs, it can be used first line)
- NMDA antagonists (oral)
- Tricyclic antidepressants
- Anticonvulsants
- Acupuncture
- Massage

treatment blood tests (see above) that are repeated at regular intervals long-term as a monitoring tool. In the occasional patient where NSAIDs cannot be given, opioid analgesia should be considered alongside all the adjunctive methods of analgesia available to see if adequate pain relief and quality of life can be achieved. All cases should be regularly reassessed to ensure the best and most appropriate long-term care continues to be provided.

The adjunctive analgesics listed in Box 11.4 have been reported as being useful in the control of chronic osteoarthritis pain as part of a multimodal approach, mainly in addition to NSAIDs.[12] Evidence for the benefits of some of those listed may be anecdotal and not conclusive but they are still worth considering.

Management of osteoarthritis also involves maintaining an ideal bodyweight. There is evidence that weight reduction alone can substantially reduce lameness and presumably a degree of pain associated with the condition. One study on nine client-owned dogs with hip osteoarthritis fed a calorie controlled diet found that an 11–18% reduction of their initial body weight resulted in a significant decrease in hindlimb lameness.[13] Unfortunately 'obesity blindness' (along with 'flea denial'), is one of the commonest diseases of owners and it can take a lot of tactful discussion to persuade owners and their families to embark on a weight reduction plan for their pets. The expertise of veterinary nurses and well-run weight clinics are invaluable in the overall management of osteoarthritis cases.

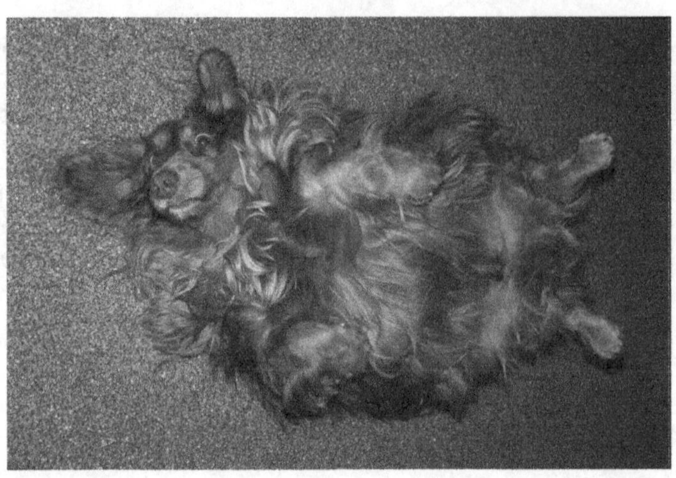

Figure 11.3 Contrary to owner belief this dachshund is not 'big boned' but very overweight, and weight loss alone will significantly reduce lameness associated with osteoarthritis.

Box 11.5	Physical adjunctive measures useful in osteoarthritis
	■ Weight loss ■ Controlled exercise ■ Physiotherapy ■ Hydrotherapy ■ Passive joint movement to warm animal up before exercise ■ Provision of ramps to avoid steps and jumping ■ The use of slings to aid mobility and access around the home ■ Soft supportive bedding ■ Bed positioned for easy access (away from draughts) ■ Raised food and water bowls for easy access ■ Environmental enrichment and behavioural strategies ■ Avoid slippery surfaces (e.g. put rugs on laminate flooring)

Other physical measures, in addition to the essential controlled exercise plan, that help improve patient comfort are shown in Box 11.5.[9]

It is noteworthy on the human side that the prevalence of depression has been found to be higher amongst arthritis sufferers than the general population and depression can worsen or amplify the severity of pain experienced by the patient. It is considered likely that a vicious cycle develops whereby chronic joint pain results in psychological distress (primarily anxiety and depression), which in turn results in pain amplification. It is not unreasonable to suspect this may occur in

a

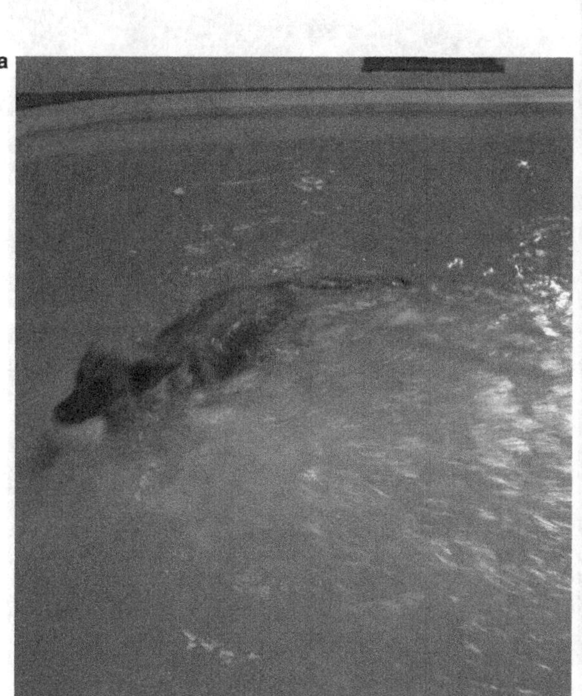

b

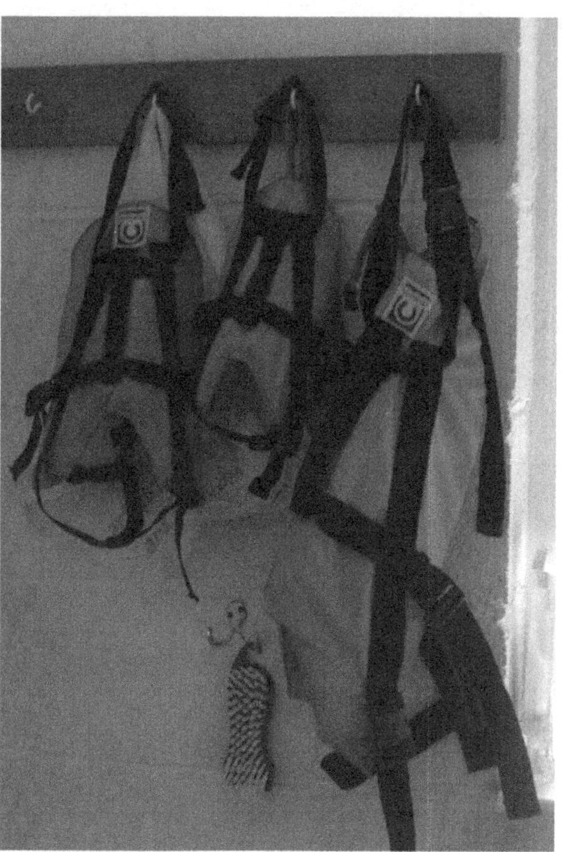

Figure 11.4
(a) Hydrotherapy is a useful tool in the management of osteoarthritis. The water supports the joints allowing exercise that will improve muscle tone, cardiovascular fitness and reduce joint stiffness. (b) Some patients may benefit from the use of a flotation aid during hydrotherapy.

animals and therefore the adjunctive methods of chronic pain management such as behavioural strategies and environmental enrichment may play a crucial role in improving the quality of life of these patients (see later).

Cancer

Cancer is a major cause of chronic pain in older companion animals. The dog population of the USA is estimated to be 50 million and the incidence of cancer is about 20–25%, which means approximately 12 million dogs are suffering from cancer at any one time.[12] It is important that appropriate pain management for cancer patients is provided as well as treatment of the underlying disease. It is also important to

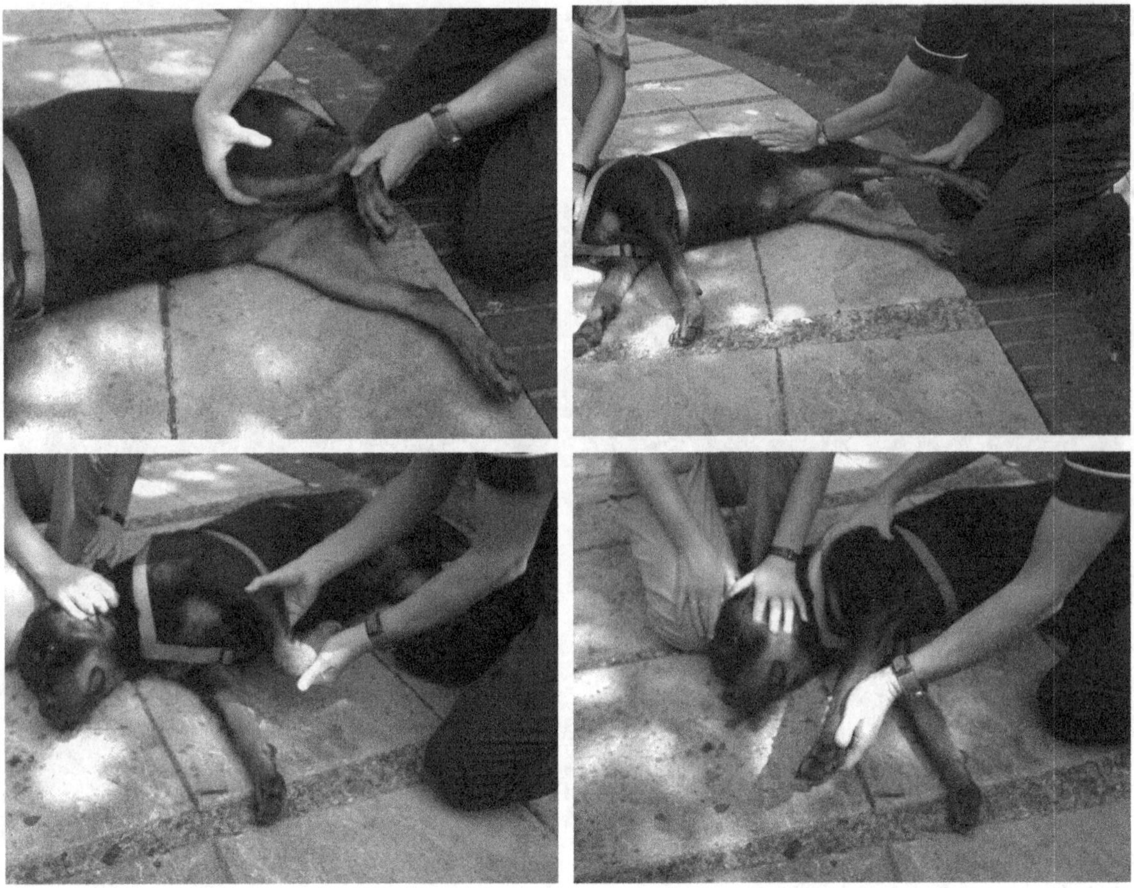

Figure 11.5
Passive joint movements can be performed before exercise in osteoarthritic patients to warm up the joints and reduce stiffness.

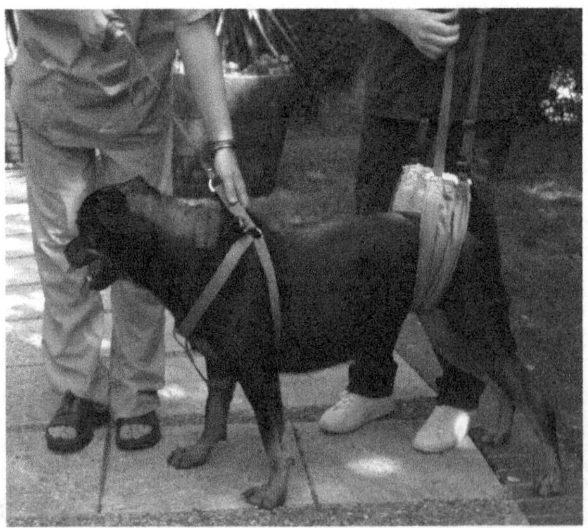

Figure 11.6
Slings may be useful for owners to help their arthritic pets with mobility around the home.

involve owners in their pet's therapy by giving explanations and education to try to avoid feelings of guilt or anger that can arise if they feel their pet is suffering unnecessarily. The detrimental consequences of leaving animals in clinically unrelieved pain are discussed in Chapter 2 and include impairment of the immune system, delayed wound healing, increased catabolism and weight loss, and increased blood pressure. These negative effects in cancer patients can adversely affect their prognosis and response to treatment.

Unrelieved surgical pain has also been shown to increase the risk of metastatic spread of tumours in cancer patients (see Chapter 2). A detailed assessment of pain and analgesic requirements (acutely and long-term) should be an inherent part of any approach to the cancer patient. A detailed history and examination is essential to evaluate the location, nature and severity of pain – owner input is essential to assess behaviour changes indicative of pain. Once treatment is in place, owners need to be closely involved in assessing and monitoring the pet's progress, pain relief and quality of life.

Cancer pain

Cancer pain arises from direct primary and secondary tumour involvement of soft tissue, bone, nerves and viscera, causing tissue destruction, inflammation, pressure, ischaemia and stretch. Pain and discomfort also arises from cancer therapies and procedures such as surgery, chemotherapy, and radiotherapy. Chronic tumour pain often increases as the tumour grows in size, but can conversely reduce if the tumour shrinks in response to treatment. Acute pain breakthrough can occur, in addition to chronic pain, as malignant tumours invade surrounding tissues. Cancer patients can suffer from multiple types of pain depending on the location and type of tumour:

- Somatic pain originates from damage to soft tissues and bones, joints and skin. Humans describe it as constant, throbbing, sharp, aching and well-localised. Bone pain from tumour invasion or metastases is the commonest form of cancer pain in humans; it is notoriously severe and can have both somatic and neuropathic origins. It tends to respond to NSAIDs and the use of biphosphonates should also be considered.

- Visceral pain can arise from the stretch, distension, injury and inflammation of viscera and is described as being deep, cramping, gnawing and poorly localised. Visceral pain is often accompanied by feelings of nausea and would indicate the use of anti-emetics as well as analgesics.

Both visceral and somatic chronic pains usually respond well to NSAIDs (and opioids and local anaesthetics in the more acute situation).

- Neuropathic pain can be a component of cancer pain if the tumour infiltrates peripheral or central nerves, or causes compression of axons. Neuropathic pain is described as burning and shooting, involves sensory or motor deficits and is particularly difficult to treat (see Chapter 5). It is often poorly responsive to both NSAIDs and opioids, whereas anticonvulsants and antidepressants can provide better long-term analgesia.

Management of chronic cancer pain

An individualised pain management approach needs to be taken with each patient depending on the nature and location and stage of the tumour, in addition to the treatment protocol for the cancer itself. Acute pain management around the time of surgery is discussed in detail in Chapter 9. Chronic pain management of cancer patients tends to rely on NSAIDs combined with opioids for more severe pain, and the use of pharmacological and non-pharmacological adjunctive therapies. NSAIDs have a ceiling effect for analgesia; pain relief cannot be increased above a certain dose, whereas pure agonist opioids, e.g. morphine and fentanyl, have no ceiling effect so their dose can be increased with increasing levels of pain. Adjuvant analgesics such as the tricyclic antidepressants and anticonvulsants can be used alongside opioids to further enhance pain relief.

Systemic lidocaine could also be considered, and corticosteroids may have a role in the management of tumours that are compressing the brain and spinal cord. Corticosteroids can reduce both nerve tissue oedema and abnormally high intracranial pressure. The lowest possible dose of corticosteroid should be used, ideally every other day, dosing to minimise side effects, and they should not be used concurrently with NSAIDs because of the higher risk of gastrointestinal ulceration. The World Health Organization (WHO)

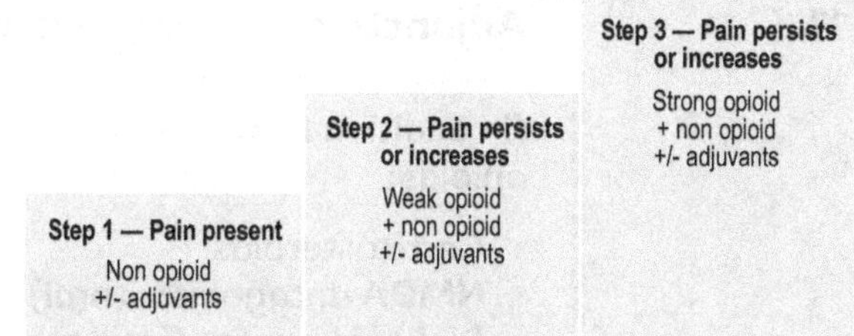

Figure 11.7
WHO pain therapy ladder for human cancer patients. (From Twycross RG. Opioids. In: Wall PD, Melzack R, eds. Textbook of pain, 4th edn. Edinburgh: Churchill Livingstone; 1999:1187–1214, reproduced with permission.)

has devised a pain therapy ladder for human cancer patients (Fig 11.7),[14] which is really taking a multimodal approach adding in more types of analgesia as pain intensity increases alongside more potent opioids.

The first step in the treatment of mild to moderate cancer pain in the WHO ladder is NSAIDs, usually used at the maximum licensed dose, with or without an adjuvant analgesic. If pain persists or increases, then a weak opioid is added, such as codeine or a partial agonist-antagonist, which will have synergy with the NSAID. These partial agonists have a ceiling effect so if the pain becomes uncontrolled then the next step is to use a pure opioid agonist with the NSAID and adjuvants. The dose of pure opioid agonist, most commonly morphine, can be titrated to effect. If the patient develops a tolerance to the opioid it is worth changing to a different pure agonist. Ideally oral preparations should be used in outpatients to minimise patient stress. In veterinary patients, oral sustained-release formulations of morphine have been used successfully as have fentanyl patches for longer-term pain relief.[15] The use of opioid/alpha 2 agonist infusions, epidurals and local anaesthetic techniques may be required for more acute episodes of pain associated with surgery or diagnostic procedures (see Chapter 9).

Some of the adjunctive analgesics and therapies that may contribute to pain relief in cancer patients (in addition to conventional analgesic drugs) and improve quality of life are shown in Box 11.6.

Starvation and anorexia is a serious complication in cancer patients, either from an inability to eat because of the primary lesion or secondary to chemotherapy and radiotherapy. It is

Box 11.6 **Adjunctive analgesics useful in cancer pain**

(In addition to conventional analgesics, e.g. NSAIDs + opioids)

- Corticosteroids
- NMDA antagonists (oral)
- Biphosphonates (for bone pain)
- Tricyclic antidepressants
- Anticonvulsants
- Acupuncture
- Massage
- Environmental enrichment and behaviour strategies

crucial to implement feeding strategies at the start of treatment, and there may be times when placement of feeding tubes is indicated to ensure nutritional support and as a route of drug administration.

Palliative radiation therapy can be used in terminal cancer cases to try and improve quality of life by reducing the tumour size, improve function and relieve pain and extend life. Unfortunately inflammation of the mouth lining (oral mucositis) and throat can develop as a complication after radiation therapy for neck, oral or head-based tumours. This can be painful and severely impair eating and drinking and will require analgesia – NSAIDs, lidocaine preparations and sucralfate can be used. Palliative radiation therapy is commonly used in humans to relieve pain from bone metastases and it has been used in dogs for osteosarcomas,[16] where amputation is not indicated (e.g. dogs with 'wobbler' syndrome). Radiation therapy can achieve pain relief in about two-thirds of dogs with osteosarcoma, and the average survival time is 5 months compared to 10 months for amputation plus chemotherapy. Analgesia can be seen after only one dose of radiation, although the exact mechanism for the effect is unknown.

In humans, neurectomies are occasionally performed as a last resort to relieve localised cancer pain. The nerves innervating the painful area are surgically cut or ablated with alcohol or phenol. This produces permanent anaesthesia of the body part but also motor and sympathetic blockade. There is very limited information on the use of this technique in animals.

Neuropathic pain

Neuropathic pain arises from injury to peripheral or central nervous tissue and is characterised by abnormal pain sensations combined with sensory and motor deficits from the area innervated by the affected nerves (see Chapter 5 for more details). It is very difficult to treat and is often unresponsive to traditional analgesic drugs. Human sufferers describe it as spontaneous, continuous, shooting, scalding, paroxysmal with referred pain and abnormal radiation and duration. It comprises hyperalgesia, severe allodynia and hyperaesthesia (increased sensitivity to stimulation) and even dysaesthesia (an unpleasant abnormal sensation that is spontaneous or evoked). It is difficult to diagnose in animals but experimental models have found animals with nerve damage show hyperalgesia to thermal and mechanical stimuli over the site of injury. Self-mutilation is also thought to be indicative of neuropathic pain in animals.

Management of neuropathic pain

It seems opioids alone may not be particularly effective for neuropathic pain whilst NMDA antagonists in combination with opioids and alpha 2 agonists give a better response.[17] Ketamine has been made into a paste and applied topically for longer-term treatment in humans (epidural ketamine is useful for acute analgesia). Gabapentin, originally used as an anticonvulsant, is now widely used as a treatment in humans for neuropathic pain and anecdotal reports of its use in animals are starting to appear. Antidepressants and topical capsaicin with or without local anaesthetic cream applied to the affected area have also been used successfully in people. The drugs found to be effective for neuropathic pain in people are shown in Box 11.7.

Box 11.7 **Analgesics useful for neuropathic pain**

- Opioids + ketamine
- Anticonvulsants (gabapentin)
- Antidepressants
- Topical capsaicin ± local anaesthetic

Phantom limb and stump pain

These pain states essentially incorporate a degree of neuropathic pain and are discussed further in Chapter 5. Their long-term treatment in people includes the use of conventional analgesics, antidepressants, anticonvulsants, ketamine, TENS, acupuncture, massage and even hypnotherapy. Epidurals and nerve blocks may also be incorporated into the treatment along with physiotherapy.

Chronic idiopathic cystitis in cats

Chronic idiopathic cystitis or interstitial cystitis in cats is not an uncommon diagnosis and refers to cats that have recurrent or persistent signs of haematuria (blood in the urine), pain, straining and increased frequency of urine voiding with no apparent underlying cause. It is thought to have multifactorial risk factors and pain is likely to play an important role in the perpetuation of the condition. NSAIDs could help relieve bladder pain and inflammation in the short-term in cats. Amitriptyline, a tricyclic antidepressant, and glucosamine have recently been suggested as useful additions to traditional treatment protocols, both of which may provide a degree of analgesia.[18] Oral administration of the injectable form of buprenorphine has also been used anecdotally.[18]

Pruritus

Pruritus, like pain, involves stimulation and transmission of nerve impulses by nociceptors. Afferent pruritus messages are closely linked to motor efferent messages that lead to reflex scratching, which can be controlled by higher centres of the brain. Tickling induces a similar motor response but does not actually induce scratching; it is associated with pleasure rather than discomfort and will diminish with repeated stimulation, unlike pruritus. Pruritus only develops in the skin, whilst pain can arise in internal tissues as well. Apart from histamine, the mediators involved in eliciting pruritus are still unclear but probably include several inflammatory mediators such as kinins, prostaglandins and neuropeptides. Chronic pruritus, e.g. atopic dermatitis, is an important and common cause of chronic pain and discomfort in both people and animals. Corticosteroids are widely used to help control pruritus whilst the underlying cause is treated. There are also adjunctive therapies available such as antihistamines, fatty acid supplements, topical shampoos, etc. to name just a few that can be incorporated into management protocols to help alleviate discomfort, depending on the primary disease process. Further information can be found in dermatology texts.

Myofascial pain

Myofascial pain syndromes are a large group of painful muscle disorders seen in people characterised by the presence of hypersensitive painful points within one or more muscles, called trigger points. The clinical signs include pain, muscle spasm, tenderness, stiffness, reduced range of movement and weakness. Trigger points can sometimes be palpable as taut tender bands within muscles. The formation of trigger points seems to be multifactorial and can involve tissue trauma, peripheral neuropathy, intense cold or heat, repetitive movements, mechanical overloading, poor posture, prolonged immobility, and possibly genetic, psychological and systemic factors.[19] Pain impulses originate from these trigger points and bombard the CNS to produce local or referred pain. Myofascial pain can be most effectively treated by placing needles in the trigger points, trigger point therapy (a form of acupuncture), or by injecting low doses of local anaesthetic, steroids or saline into the trigger point. Massage and ultrasound therapy are additional adjunctive therapies that may be helpful to alleviate myofascial pain. NSAIDs and muscle relaxants may need to be used whilst physical therapies take effect. It would be difficult to prove but it is possible veterinary patients may suffer chronic pain from similar pathology.

Complex regional pain syndromes (CRPSs)

This is another set of chronic pain syndromes seen in humans that has a less than clear aetiology and pathology. It could be classed as a subtype of neuropathic pain. Currently there are two types of CRPS; type 1 follows a soft tissue injury, whereas type 2 follows a well-defined nerve injury. Both types are characterised by continuing pain, with disproportionate hyperalgesia and allodynia for the initial injury. The site of pain usually shows oedema, changes in skin colour and temperature. Eventually in the final stages there can be extensive tissue atrophy and fixing of joints due to flexor contracture. Most patients have CRPS involving a single limb, following trauma such as fracture or surgery. Risk factors are not clearly established but could include prolonged immobilisation, genetics and psychological factors.[20] The exact mechanism underlying CRPS is still controversial – there maybe involvement of aberrant healing and inflammation, sympathetic nerve dysfunction, myofascial dysfunction and psychological factors. Treatment requires an individualised multidisciplinary approach, using conventional and adjunctive pharmacological treatments, physiotherapy, psychological approaches (e.g. stress management), TENS and acupuncture, and may necessitate nerve blocks. Similarly to myofascial pain, it is possible CRPS is a cause of chronic pain in animals.

Non-physical pain

Traditionally in veterinary medicine the word pain is used to refer to the pain associated with stimulation of the nociceptive pathway by a physical cause such as tissue damage. However, this physical pain is only one cause of suffering, another cause is emotional pain whereby discomfort arises from unpleasant feelings. Unpleasant feelings can have a physical or psychological cause.

Physical causes of unpleasant feelings

- pain
- hypoxia
- thirst
- hunger
- toxicosis
- nausea
- urinary bladder distension
- pruritus
- temperature extremes.

Emotional or psychological causes of unpleasant feelings

- fear
- anxiety
- social isolation
- frustration
- boredom
- grief
- anger.

There is scientific evidence that unpleasant feelings or emotional states are a form of pain and are related to perceptions of pain in the brain. Anatomically the areas of the brain associated with the emotional systems of separation anxiety, social isolation and loneliness are located next to those areas generating physical pain responses. Endogenous opioids involved in the regulation of physical pain intensity also regulate the emotional states of separation anxiety and loneliness. Evolutionary studies strongly suggest that the biochemical and neurological systems involved in physical pain have been adapted to handle unpleasant feelings as well.[2]

There is also evidence that emotional pain may induce greater suffering than physical pain.[2] Studies have shown that emotional factors can have more influence on an animal's choice of actions than physical pain. One paper reported that puppies crossed an electric grid to reach a person to whom they had formed a bond, despite receiving small electric shocks en route. In another study, mother rats able to hear the cries of their offspring crossed an electric grid to get to their litters, picked them up and carried them back across the grid to return them to the nests. The mother rats were subject to small electric shocks during their journeys in both directions. Work like this demonstrates that emotional distress can outweigh the suffering from physical pain, i.e. non-physical pain can induce a greater degree of suffering than physical pain.[2] Clinicians need to address both physical and non-physical causes of pain when treating patients – this becomes particularly relevant when managing outpatients with chronic diseases.

Like physical pain, emotional pain will determine an animal's overall quality of life – as referred to earlier on in this chapter, a good quality of life is the ultimate aim of medical care, not just quantity of life.

Box 11.8

Non-physical or emotional pain

- **This is pain arising from unpleasant feelings**
- **It is regulated by neuronal and biochemical systems in the brain related to physical pain**
- **It can induce more suffering than physical pain**
- **Both physical and emotional pain need to be alleviated in patients**

Quality of life

Quality of life is basically a general enjoyment of life – it is how an individual feels about his or her own life. Where the individual concerned is a less than chatty veterinary patient, quality of life needs to be estimated by another person, namely the owner – under guidance of the clinician. Quality of life could also be viewed as psychological wellbeing, or overall happiness or contentment with life. Each individual has their own unique definition of what constitutes a good quality of life and this is based on genetic make-up, personality and learned experiences, which result in different values and priorities being assigned by the individual to different aspects of their life. For example the value of human companionship can vary greatly between two dogs. A well-socialised family pet would be quite distressed if it was deprived of human interaction, whilst a working foxhound living outside would be unaffected. Quality of life for an individual depends upon what matters to that individual, and this varies enormously among individual people and animals. It is important to know what matters to the patient when embarking on chronic pain management programmes so the aims and priorities of treatment and measures of success are relevant to the patient, not just the owner and clinician.

Feelings or emotional states are the main constituents of the quality of life of an individual. The vast and continuous array of internal and external stimuli which a conscious animal receives are given a basic value by the brain as to whether they are important for survival and reproduction.

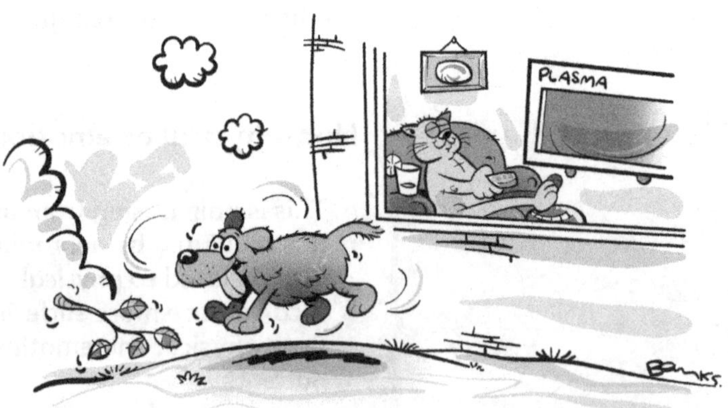

Figure 11.8 Factors that determine quality of life differ between individuals.

This value is the 'feeling' that the stimulus generates in the animal. An unpleasant feeling is elicited by stimuli that have a negative effect on survival whilst a pleasant feeling is elicited by stimuli that have a positive effect on survival. The intensity of the feeling reflects the importance of the stimuli. All feelings have either a pleasant or unpleasant quality and may have a physical or emotional origin. Therefore feelings are a good representation of what matters to an individual and how much something matters to them, i.e. feelings are what comprises quality of life. Something that does not affect an animal's feelings, such as the colour of its collar, will not elicit any feelings and will not affect the animal's quality of life.

Unpleasant feelings, as discussed above under non-physical pain, can be elicited by both physical and non-physical stimuli and have a range of intensity – they serve to alert the animal to threats to their wellbeing and motivate the animal to take actions to reduce this threat. The intensity of an unpleasant feeling will correlate to how life threatening or detrimental the stimulus is to wellbeing and often the intensity will increase over time. For example, the most intensely unpleasant feelings can arise from hypoxia secondary to pleural effusion or pulmonary oedema, whilst distress caused by loneliness or boredom will increase more over time. The presence of unpleasant feelings will reduce overall quality of life.

Pleasant feelings are highly desirable and serve to benefit an animal's life and wellbeing. Pleasure results from the feelings arising from play, social interaction, companionship, mental stimulation, tasty food, nurturing youngsters (female mammals) and sexual activity.[3] Pleasant feelings raise an individual's overall quality of life. Unfortunately unpleasant feelings contribute disproportionately to overall quality of life compared to pleasant ones. This is because they have a higher priority and urgency to an individual than pleasant feelings, to ensure they command an animal's attention so the threat or problem is rectified before harm occurs. In addition, as the threat grows, such as an increasingly full bladder, or increasingly painful joints, the feeling of discomfort and unpleasantness increases in intensity until the animal's attention is almost entirely focussed on the problem and diverted away from all other less urgent matters. This diversion of attention will continue as long as the unpleasant feelings persist, which will severely impair the animal's ability to enjoy any pleasant experiences such as playing with a toy. As a consequence, unpleasant feelings not only directly reduce quality of life, but they indirectly reduce the contribution made by any pleasant feelings.

Maximising quality of life

When assessing an individual patient and putting together a chronic pain management programme, it is essential to look at the likely priorities of the animal in terms of their unpleasant and pleasant feelings, i.e. what is likely to contribute most to their quality of life, and how is the underlying disease and pain producing unpleasant feelings and limiting behaviour and activities that generate the pleasant feelings? Realistically, can therapies be incorporated to manage the pain (and associated disease process) sufficiently to allow pleasant feelings to outweigh unpleasant ones? If the answer to these questions is no, either at the outset or with time, then euthanasia ought to be considered as an option. Fig 11.9 shows the balance model for an animal's quality of life and lists the various pleasant and unpleasant feelings thought to contribute to quality of life. Ideally the aim of treatment is to tip the scales as far as possible in the direction of pleasant feelings to provide the best quality of life, i.e. minimise unpleasant feelings and maximise pleasant feelings.[3] After all, the foremost goal or whole point of veterinary medicine is to minimise the discomfort of patients.

To improve a patient's quality of life, the clinician needs to establish what factors will most effectively tip the scales in the right direction. Factors that require the most urgent attention are those that are the greatest threat to survival and therefore cause the most distress, e.g. pain, difficulty breathing, fear, etc. This usually equates to treating the underlying disease and associated pain as the priority. The next set of

Box 11.9	Maximising quality of life
	Minimise factors contributing to unpleasant feelings AND Maximise factors contributing to pleasant feelings

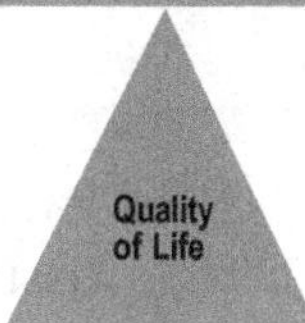

Figure 11.9 Balance model for quality of life. (From McMillan FD. Maximizing quality of life in ill animals. JAAHA 2003; 39:227–235, reproduced with permission.)

feelings to attend to are those that may have grown important depending on their duration, such as loneliness and boredom. Finally the feelings that are more variable in importance between individuals because they are dependent on personality need to be identified. Owner input is essential to elucidate priorities, e.g. is social interaction with humans of more importance than lots of food, or does the pet enjoy playing with toys more than anything, etc. Once a chronic pain management programme has been put in place, regular reassessments are necessary to see whether quality of life is being sufficiently improved, and to provide the information necessary to decide on any changes to the treatment.

Chronic pain and disease will disproportionately reduce quality of life because of the strength of unpleasant feelings they generate but the scales analogy demonstrates how the identification and optimisation of the factors that elicit pleasant feelings in patients will increase their quality of life beyond the level provided by analgesic drugs alone. The provision of more pleasant feelings can be very beneficial in addition to reducing the unpleasant ones. This is one of the roles of some adjunctive methods of pain relief and environmental enrichment detailed in Chapter 10. 'Pampering' is really just the provision of as many pleasurable feelings as possible, including petting, stroking, play, novel toys and outings, etc. It is important to allow the patient to have control or choices so it has the ability to enhance its own life (as long as neither of these strategies adversely affect the animal's health). Sometimes a balance needs to be reached, for example an arthritic dog may enjoy walks tremendously, but too much exercise will exacerbate joint pain, which outweighs the benefit and reduces quality of life. Table 11.2 lists the factors that can contribute to quality of life, how they affect it, and specific strategies for improving quality of life in patients.

FUTURE CONSIDERATIONS

Radical procedures involving resection of large amounts of tissue, cancer therapies, transplantation, etc. are now feasible in small animal veterinary medicine. However, just because a treatment can be carried out, does it automatically mean it should be? Is it in the best interests of the patient, and not just a means of furthering science or meeting unreasonable owner expectations to maximise life longevity at the expense of quality? It is not just the ability or means to carry out a procedure that should be of importance but the availability of appropriate postop care and impact on the patient's quality of life. These issues ought to be addressed with owners before embarking on treatment.

For example, a dog with an invasive squamous cell carcinoma of the maxilla can have radical surgery to excise the

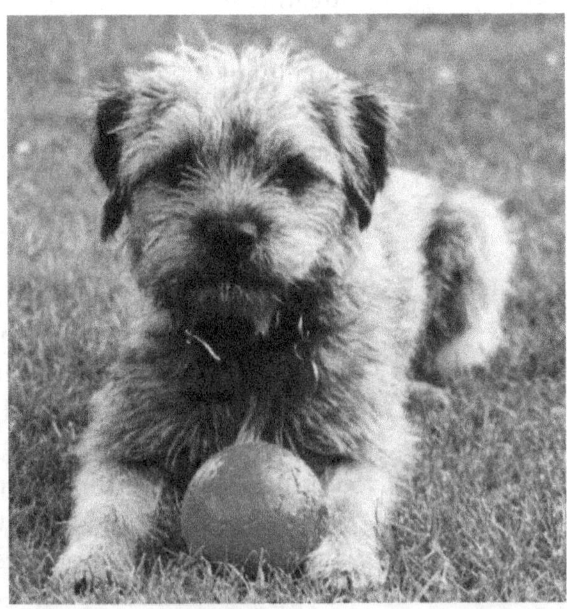

Figure 11.10 Novel toys and playing can significantly enhance quality of life of some veterinary patients and can be used to enhance the management of chronic pain.

Table 11.2

Factors contributing to quality of life (QoL) and strategies for maximising them

Factor contributing to QoL	How QoL can be affected	How QoL can be increased
Social relationships	Separation and isolation can cause unpleasant feelings	Provide plenty of human and other animal social interaction and companionship
Mental stimulation	Too little causes boredom and this can cause severe distress	Provide stimulation to elicit pleasant feelings Novelty, variety, activities, play, fun, recreation, challenges, exploration, etc., e.g. working for food or hiding food in toys and environment, interactive toys, supply novel objects to investigate and explore, outings to parks, new walks, new games
Health	Severe discomfort can arise directly from hypoxia, pain, pruritus, nausea, etc. Unpleasant feelings can arise indirectly from urinary incontinence, skin odour, and the resulting social rejection from human family such as being banished outside resulting in loneliness Physical impairment from disease can limit experience of pleasant feelings, such as joint pain or congestive heart failure preventing running and play	Treat the underlying disease and provide analgesia Aim to restore function and physical comfort to increase ability to have pleasurable experiences Consider adjunctive pharmacological and physical methods of pain relief and behavioural therapy to reduce the intensity of unpleasant feelings
Food	Inadequate food creates hunger, which is very unpleasant Excessive food leads to obesity, which can reduce function and impair ability to experience pleasurable activities	Feed high-quality palatable food to maintain a correct body weight Offer treats in moderation

Table 11.2
Factors contributing to quality of life (QoL) and strategies for maximising them—*cont'd*

Factor contributing to QoL	How QoL can be affected	How QoL can be increased
Stress (ability to cope with environmental demands and changes)	Generates unpleasant feelings of fear, anxiety, pain, loneliness, boredom, anger and frustration	Alleviate the specific unpleasant feeling Reduce stressful stimuli Provide coping strategies for the patient, e.g. more control (see below), predictability of events, social support
Control (control over the ability to escape from, or lessen the threat of an adverse stimulus and control over the ability to enjoy pleasurable stimuli)	A lack of control over stressful stimuli intensifies their negative impact A lack of control generates a severely unpleasant feeling of helplessness and distress	Offer meaningful choices as this imparts control, e.g. allow pet to choose to stay inside or go outside; provide a choice of food and toys Recognise and act on requests made by pet, e.g. respond to a dog's signals that it wants a walk, or would like to play Provide pet with means for alleviating unpleasant feelings, e.g. provide toys to avoid boredom, provide hiding places, act on any signs of pain such as applying heat/massage to painful joints whenever an arthritic dog starts to limp

(After McMillan FD. Maximizing quality of life in ill animals. JAAHA 2003; 39:227–235, reproduced with permission.)

tumour with good margins, effectively providing a cure and removing any pain caused by the tumour eroding into tissues. However, even with a comprehensive peri- and postop analgesic protocol in place the potential for long-term suffering and poor quality of life is still possible. The dog may suffer from hunger and thirst as it struggles to learn to eat post-surgery, and it will be painful when eating or trying to play for some time as all the tissues take time to heal. The change in mouth structure may compromise the dog's ability to play with toys, or have chews, which may have been a source of great stimulation and pleasure prior to treatment. Humans may not be so willing to interact with and pet such a 'funny looking dog' and this can have a dramatic effect on a well-socialised dog. Analgesia and long-term quality of life must not be forgotten or compromised by increasingly sophisticated efforts to prolong life.

Key summary points for chronic pain management

1. **Chronic pain, discomfort and suffering can arise with any chronic disease.**
2. **Analgesia plus measures to alleviate discomfort and maximise quality of life should be an integral part of any treatment plan, in addition to addressing the underlying disease.**
3. **A thorough owner history is essential to establish the severity and nature of chronic pain and its impact on quality of life.**
4. **The aim of chronic pain management is to relieve suffering and maximise quality of life, the latter is a useful and important measure of treatment success.**
5. **Patients require regular monitoring for potential drug side effects and to ensure treatment is effective and appropriate as patient needs may change over time.**
6. **The multimodal approach, using conventional analgesics and adjunctive pharmacological and physical therapies, is particularly useful in the management of chronic pain.**
7. **Clinicians must be aware of and treat the less obvious causes of pain and suffering, e.g. chronic dental pain, pruritus and non-physical pain.**
8. **Patients should be referred to the appropriate veterinary experts for more specialised treatments, e.g. acupuncture, physiotherapy, behavioural strategies, etc.**
9. **Euthanasia is fortunately a humane option for veterinary patients and must be carefully discussed with owners in cases where pain cannot be adequately relieved and quality of life is poor.**

REFERENCES

1. Wiseman-Orr ML, Nolan AM, Reid J, et al. Development of a questionnaire to measure the effects of chronic pain on health-related quality of life in dogs. Am J Vet Res 2004; 65(8):1077–1084
2. McMillan FD. A world of hurts – is pain special? J Am Vet Med Assoc 2003; 223(2): 183–186
3. McMillan FD. Maximizing quality of life in ill animals. JAAHA 2003; 39:227–235
4. Grave K, Tanem H. Compliance with short-term oral antibacterial drug treatment in dogs. JSAP 1999; 40:158–162
5. Lindley S. Thoughts for extending management plans. Proceedings of Rimadyl Extended Care Programme Seminar, Pfizer Animal Health. Hanbury Manor, Hertfordshire, UK 16th July 2004
6. Hardie EM, Roe SC, Martin FR. Radiographic evidence of degenerative joint disease in geriatric cats: 100 cats (1994–1997). J Am Vet Med Assoc 2002; 220(5):628–632
7. Smith GK, Mayhew PD, Kapatkin AS, et al. Evaluation of the risk factors for degenerative joint disease associated with hip dysplasia in German Shepherd dogs, Golden retrievers, Labrador Retrievers and rottweilers. J Am Vet Med Assoc 2001; 219(12): 1719–1724
8. Kealy RD, Lawler DF, Ballam JM, et al. Five year longitudinal study on limited food consumption and development of osteoarthritis in coxofemoral joints of dogs. J Am Vet Med Assoc 1997; 210(2): 222–225

9. Carmichael S. Chronic pain management – osteoarthritis. Proceedings of Rimadyl Extended Care Programme Seminar, Pfizer Animal Health. Hanbury Manor, Hertfordshire, UK. 16th July 2004
10. Kealy RD, Lawler DF, Ballam JM, et al. Evaluation of the effect of limited food consumption on radiographic evidence of osteoarthritis in dogs. J Am Vet Med Assoc 2000; 217(11):1678–1680
11. Creamer P. Ostearthritis. In: Wall PD, Melzack R, eds. Textbook of pain, 4th edn. Edinburgh: Churchill Livingstone; 1999:493–504
12. Lascelles BDX, Main DJ. Surgical trauma and chronically painful conditions – within our comfort levels but beyond theirs? J Am Vet Med Assoc 2002; 221(2):215–222
13. Impellizeri JA, Tetrick MA, Muir P. Effect of weight reduction on clinical signs of lameness in dogs with hip osteoarthritis. J Am Vet Med Assoc 2000; 216(7): 1089–1091
14. Twycross RG. Opioids. In: Wall PD, Melzack R, eds. Textbook of pain, 4th edn. Edinburgh: Churchill Livingstone; 1999:1187–1214
15. Lester PL, Gaynor JS. Management of cancer pain. Vet Clin N Am Small Animal Practice 2000; 30(4):951–966
16. Brearley JC, Brearley MJ. Chronic pain in animals. In: Flecknell P, Waterman-Pearson A, eds. Pain management in animals. London: Saunders; 2000:147–160
17. Pascoe PJ. Problems of pain management. In: Flecknell P, Waterman-Pearson A, eds. Pain management in animals. London: Saunders; 2000:161–177
18. Chew DJ. Upper and lower urinary tract diseases, a complete perspective. Proceedings of a BSAVA Surrey and Sussex regional meeting 12th November 2004, Walton-on the Hill, Surrey, UK
19. Sola AE, Bonica JJ. Myofascial pain syndromes. In: Loeser JD, ed. Bonica's management of pain, 3rd edn. Philadelphia USA: Lippincott Williams & Wilkins; 2000: 530–556
20. Galer BS, Schwartz L, Allen RJ. Complex regional pain syndromes. In: Loeser JD, ed. Bonica's management of pain, 3rd edn. Philadelphia USA: Lippincott Williams & Wilkins; 2000:387–411

Index

A

B

C

D

E

F

G

M

N

O

P

Q

R

U

V

W

X